Allergic and non-allergic Rhinitis
Clinical Aspects

Allergic and non-allergic Rhinitis
Clinical Aspects

EDITED BY

NIELS MYGIND
ROBERT M NACLERIO

MUNKSGAARD · COPENHAGEN

North and South America
W. B. SAUNDERS COMPANY
Philadelphia, London, Toronto

Allergic and non-allergic Rhinitis
Clinical aspects
1st edition, 1st printing

Copyright © 1993 Munksgaard, Copenhagen
All rights reserved

No part of this publication may be reproduced, stored in a
retrieval system, or transmitted in any form or by any means,
electronic, mechanical photocopying, recording or otherwise
without prior permission by the copyright owner.

Cover, layout: Munksgaards Tegnestue/Peter Lind
Cover, illustration: Art Factory / Lena Untidt and
Henning Dahlhof
Drawings and diagrams: Lars Thorsen
Graphic designer: Lars Thorsen
Typesetting: P.J.Schmidt A/S, Vojens
Printer: TL Offset I/S, Copenhagen
Paper: Arctic 115 g.

ISBN 87-16-10911-2

Preface

Seven years ago, the 1st edition of 'Allergic and Vasomotor Rhinitis: Clinical Aspects' was published by Munksgaard. Since then there has been considerable progress in both the diagnosis and treatment of allergic and non-allergic rhinitis, and it is now time for an updated version which we have entitled 'Allergic and Non-allergic Rhinitis: Clinical Aspects'. In this book, we have combined European and North American approaches to the management of allergy and rhinitis. In fact, there is an equal number of authors from the Old and the New Worlds, all of whom are leading clinicians and researchers in the field of allergy and otorhinolaryngology.

Before writing their chapters, all the authors discussed their topics at a workshop in Copenhagen. The workshop was sponsored by the University of Copenhagen, and by the Johns Hopkins University in Baltimore, and was made possible by a generous grant-in-aid from Astra-Draco AB, Lund, Sweden.

We asked the authors to write primarily for the practicing clinician, which they have done. However, some of them could not resist the temptation to include recent research data, which will hopefully prove stimulating.

Niels Mygind   Robert M Naclerio

Contents

Contributors 8

1. Definition, classification, terminology 11
   Niels Mygind, Robert M Naclerio

2. Epidemiology 15
   Jeanne Montgomery Smith

3. Allergens 23
   Robert A Wood

4. Air pollution 32
   Rebecca Bascom

5. Food allergy and intolerance 46
   Carsten Bindslev-Jensen

6. Rhinoscopy 51
   Heinz Stammberger

7. X-ray, CT-scan, MR-imaging 58
   P Clement, P Van der Veken, P Iwens, Th Buisseret

8. Cytology 66
   Eli O Meltzer, H Alice Orgel, Alfredo A Jalowaiski

9. Allergy diagnosis 82
   Sten Dreborg

10. Vasoconstrictors 95
    Lars Malm, Anders Änggård

11. Cromoglycate 101
    Peter Howarth

12. Anticholinergic medication 105
    Jerry Dolovich, Niels Mygind

13. Systemic steroids 111
    Elliott Middleton Jr

14. Intranasal steroids 114
    Robert M Naclerio, Niels Mygind

15. Antihistamines 123
    F Estelle R Simons

16. Immunotherapy 137
    Jean Bousquet, Francois-B Michel

17. Surgical treatment 149
    Ian S Mackay

18. Allergic rhinitis 153
    Michael A Kaliner

19. Non-allergic rhinitis 159
    Alkis G Togias

20. Nasal polyps 167
    Adrian B Drake-Lee

21. Rhinitis in children 174
    Sheldon C Siegel

22. Rhinitis and asthma 184
    Ronald Dahl

23. Rhinitis and otitis 189
    Paul Van Cauwenberge, K Ingels

Index 195

Contributors

ANDERS ÄNGGÅRD
Associate Professor, Department of Otorhinolaryngology, Karolinska Hospital, Stockholm, Sweden

REBECCA BASCOM
Associate Professor, Division of Pulmonary and Critical Care, Department of Medicine, University of Maryland Hospital, Baltimore, Maryland, USA

CARSTEN BINDSLEV-JENSEN
Assistant Professor, Allergy Unit, Department of Internal Medicine, Rigshospitalet, Copenhagen, Denmark

JEAN BOUSQUET
Professor, Clinique des Maladies Respiratoires, Centre Hospitalier Universitaire, Montpellier, France

PAUL VAN CAUWENBERGE
Professor, Department of Otorhinolaryngology, State University Hospital, Ghent, Belgium

PETER CLEMENT
Professor, Department of Otorhinolaryngology, Akademisch Ziekenhuis V.U.B., Brussels, Belgium

RONALD DAHL
Associate Professor, Department of Respiratory Diseases, University Hospital, Aarhus, Denmark

JERRY DOLOVICH
Professor of Pediatrics, McMaster University, Hamilton, Ontario, Canada

ADRIAN B DRAKE-LEE
Consultant ENT Surgeon, The Queen Elisabeth Hospital, Birmingham, UK

STEN DREBORG
Associate Professor, Department of Pediatrics, University Hospital, Linköping, Sweden

PETER HOWARTH
Senior Lecturer in Medicine, Department of Medicine, Southampton General Hospital, Southampton, UK

MICHAEL A KALINER
Chief, Allergic Disease Section, National Institutes of Health, Bethesda, Maryland, USA

IAN S MACKAY
Consultant ENT Surgeon, Brompton and Charing Cross Hospitals, London, UK

ELI O MELTZER
Clinical Professor of Pediatrics, Division of Allergy and Immunology, University of California, San Diego, California, USA

ELLIOTT MIDDLETON JR
Professor of Medicine, Director, Division of Allergy and Clinical Immunology, State University of New York at Buffalo, Buffalo, New York, USA

NIELS MYGIND
Senior Lecturer, Otopathological Laboratory, Department of Otorhinolaryngology, and Allergy Unit, Department of Medicine, Rigshospitalet, Copenhagen, Denmark

ROBERT M NACLERIO
Associate Professor of Medicine and Otolaryngology, The Johns Hopkins Asthma and Allergy Center, Baltimore, Maryland, USA

SHELDON C SIEGEL
Professor of Pediatrics, University of California at Los Angeles School of Medicine, Los Angeles, California, USA

F ESTELLE R SIMONS
Professor and Head, Section of Allergy and Clinical Immunology, Department of Pediatrics, University of Manitoba, Winnipeg, Manitoba, Canada

JEANNE MONTGOMERY SMITH
Associate Professor of Allergy and Immunology, Department of Internal Medicine, University of Iowa, Iowa City, Iowa, USA

HEINZ STAMMBERGER
Professor, Department of Otorhinolaryngology, University Hospital, Graz, Austria

ALKIS G TOGIAS
The Johns Hopkins Asthma and Allergy Center, Baltimore, Maryland, USA

ROBERT A WOOD
Assistant Professor of Pediatrics, Department of Pediatrics, The Johns Hopkins University School of Medicine, Baltimore, Maryland, USA

Chapter 1

Definition, classification, terminology

NIELS MYGIND
ROBERT M NACLERIO

The problem of classification ...
"It is very seldom that diseases are found pure and unmixed, as they are commonly described by authors; and there is almost an endless variety of constitutions. The treatment must be adapted to this mixture and variety in order to be as successful as circumstances will permit".
Mathew Baille

Introduction

The definition of bronchial asthma has plagued chest physicians and allergists for years, so it is not surprising that the definition and classification of rhinitis, involving etiologic criteria (infectious, allergic), has caused even more confusion. There is no universally accepted system for the definition, classification or the terminology of rhinitis. Use of different terms for the same disease and of the same term for different diseases has, in the past, made reports on rhinitis confusing to read and difficult to compare.

In daily work, the diagnosis is of importance for proper counselling, as a guide to therapy, and is necessary for unambiguous communication between clinicians. In the presentation below, we have made the classification simple in order to ensure that a patient will be given the same diagnosis when examined by different doctors (Table 1.1).

Rhinitis or rhinopathy?

The term 'rhinitis' implies an inflammatory disease of the nasal mucous membrane. Demonstration of local inflammation is, however, not practical. Clinical diagnoses are based on the presence of symptoms: itching, sneezing, discharge and blockage. As these symptoms may occur without inflammation, 'rhinopathy' is, strictly speaking, a more correct term – but it is rarely used.

Normal state or disease?

In addition, it is difficult to make a clear distinction between a normal state and a disease. Everyone occasionally has nasal symptoms, but this does not necessarily imply that she/he suffers from rhinitis.

For the above reason, quantitative criteria and objective parameters are necessary for making a clear distinction between a normal state and a disease. But there are at present no epidemiological investigations using stringent criteria that allow us to define the borderline between normal and abnormal. The clinician can be guided by asking the patient how many hours a day he has symptoms, how many times he sneezes and blows his nose. Most reliable is daily recording on a symptom card, for example over a 2-week period.

Anatomic abnormalities

All patients with chronic nasal symptoms need an ENT examination in order to exclude anatomic abnormalities (see Chapters 6 and 7). The com-

Table 1.1. *Simple classification of rhinitis.*

1. Infectious (purulent) rhinitis
2. Seasonal allergic rhinitis = hay fever = pollinosis
3. Perennial allergic rhinitis
4. Perennial non-allergic rhinitis (eosinophilic or non-eosinophilic)

bined use of an endoscopic examination and a CT-scan imaging (when necessary and when possible) gives a much better presentation of anatomic and mucosal abnormalities than do simple rhinoscopy and plain x-ray examination.

Infectious or non-infectious?

Often, a diagnosis of infectious rhinitis is supported by associated symptoms from the throat and the lower airways, but it may occasionally be confused with non-infectious rhinitis. As a matter of clinical routine, a diagnosis of viral or bacterial disease is not based on identification of the specific microorganism. The distinction made is between purulent and non-purulent rhinitis based on the macroscopic character of the nasal discharge (cloudy and milky/colored, or clear and watery/mucoid), preferably supported by microscopy ($\pm$ neutrophilia). The reliability of this sign, however, is not absolute. Neutrophilia can be caused not only by viral and bacterial infection but also by exposure to air pollution (see Chapter 4).

Allergic or non-allergic?

The diagnosis of inhalant allergy can usually be agreed on when history, physical examination, and skin test/RAST results are combined. This is not the case with food allergy, which is a controversial topic. Food allergy as a cause of isolated rhinitis is debatable; but, as a part of documented IgE-mediated allergy to foods, nasal symptoms may occur, especially in children.

The term 'vasomotor rhinitis' is often used for non-infectious, non-allergic rhinitis. However, there is no evidence for the existence of a 'vasomotor pathogenesis'. In addition, it is confusing that the term is presently used with different meanings in Europe (non-allergic rhinitis) and in North America (non-allergic non-eosinophilic rhinitis). For these reasons, it may be wise to drop the term 'vasomotor rhinitis', as it confuses more than it clarifies, and it gives a false impression of a well-defined pathogenesis.

Seasonal or perennial?

Seasonal allergic rhinitis is a generally accepted term for pollinosis or hay fever. But pollen allergy is often perennial in the tropics, and a seasonal increase of symptoms can be caused by allergy to mites and molds in temperate zones. Seasonal refers to short exposures lasting for a few months, while perennial implies continuous or intermittent exposure with chronic or periodic symptoms. The symptomatology of seasonal rhinitis is characterized by sneezing, whereas in perennial rhinitis congestion often dominates.

Eosinophilic or non-eosinophilic?

Non-allergic rhinitis is a heterogenous syndrome consisting of two main groups. One is characterized by nasal secretion eosinophilia, frequent occurrence of nasal polyps, hyperplastic sinusitis, non-allergic or intrinsic asthma, intolerance to acetylsalicylic acid and other NSAID preparations.

Most clinicians do not examine nasal smears and are not familiar with microscopic evaluation. In addition, the specificity, sensitivity and reproducibility of this test has not been properly analyzed. Serial examinations seem to be necessary for a reliable characterization of the disease. The classification of patients with non-allergic rhinitis into an eosinophilic and a non-eosinophilic group is, therefore, not entirely suitable for clinical diagnosis. The presence of eosinophils usually portends a response to glucocorticosteroids.

Other causes of chronic nasal symptoms

Rhinitis medicamentosa develops after prolonged use of vasoconstrictor sprays. Nasal congestion can be caused by medication with antihypertensives and psychosedatives, which act as alpha-adrenoceptor antagonists. Pregnancy is, in a number of cases, associated with persistent nasal blockage and sinusitis symptoms, which disappear after delivery (Table 1.2).

Congenital choanal atresia can be a cause of nasal obstruction, with discharge, in infants. A foreign

Table 1.2. *Other causes of nasal symptoms.*

Mechanical factors

Septal deviation
Nasal polyps
Foreign body
Tumors of nose and paranasal sinuses
Tumors of the nasopharynx
Congenital choanal atresia
Meningocele/Encephalocele
Adenoidal hypertrophy

Infections

Viral infection (common cold)
Bacterial infection
Sinusitis
Leprosy
Immunodeficiency
Primary ciliary dyskinesia

Miscellaneous

Rhinitis medicamentosa
Pregnancy
Antihypertensives
Wegener's granulomatosis
Cystic fibrosis
Leak of cerebrospinal fluid

body is much more common at that age. Enlarged adenoids are a frequent cause of mouth breathing. Septal deviation is another well-known cause of nasal obstruction, often bilateral (S-shaped deviation). A nasal blockage, developing in an adult, cannot be ascribed exclusively to septal deviation, unless the patient has had a traumatic fracture. However, the swollen mucous membrane of rhinitis can make a septal deviation clinically significant, so this type of patient has a combined problem.

Malignant tumors in the nose, paranasal sinuses and nasopharynx, and Wegener's granulomatosis usually start with uncharacteristic symptoms. A first diagnosis of 'perennial non-allergic rhinitis' is not uncommon is these cases, and nasal endoscopy and imaging of paranasal sinuses are obligatory in patients with unilateral symptoms, hemorrhagic secretions or pain.

A practical approach to the diagnosis of rhinitis

First, exclude other diseases and structural abnormalities. Then make a distinction between infectious and non-infectious disease (history, character of discharge), and separate allergic from non-allergic patients on the basis of history and allergy testing as indicated in Chapter 9. Subclassification of the non-allergic patients into an eosinophilic and a non-eosinophilic group is helpful, as it relates to the responsiveness to pharmacotherapy. When repeated sampling and microscopy of a nasal smear are not feasible, the alternative is a therapeutic trial with, e.g., a steroid spray.

The case history, preferably supported by daily symptom recording for 2 weeks in perennial cases, allows a characterization of the patient according to the most prominent symptom. 'Sneezers' (sneezing and discharge), 'nose-blowers' (watery discharge), and 'blockers' (nasal blockage) show varying response to drugs, e.g. antihistamines, and require different therapies.

Conclusion

The different types of rhinitis are at present poorly defined, and the limits between 'normal' and 'disease' are fluid. Rhinitis can be infectious (purulent), allergic or non-allergic. The latter is a heterogenous syndrome consisting of at least two main groups, an eosinophilic and a non-eosinophilic: a distinction which is not entirely suitable for clinical practice.

References

1. Connell JT. Nasal disease: mechanisms and classification. *Ann Allergy* 1983; *50*: 227-35.
2. Flowers BK, Naclerio RM. The nose. In: Naspitz CK, Tinkelman DG, eds. *Childhood rhinitis and sinusitis: pathophysiology and treatment*. New York: Marcel Dekker, 1990: 147-92.
3. Jacobs RL, Freedman PM, Boswell RN. Nonallergic rhinitis with eosinophilia (NARES Syndrome). *J Allergy Clin Immunol* 1981; *67*: 253-62.
4. Mackay IS. Introduction. In: Mackay IS, ed. *Rhinitis: mechanisms and management*. London: Royal Society of Medicine, 1989: 1-10.

5 Meltzer EO, Schatz M, Zeiger RS. Allergic and nonallergic rhinitis. In: Middleton Jr E, Reed CE, Ellic EF, Adkinson NF, Yunginger JW, eds. *Allergy: principles and practice*, 3rd edn. Saint Louis: CV Mosby Company, 1988: 1253-89.
6 Mullarkey MF. The classification of nasal disease: an opinion. *J Allergy Clin Immunol* 1981; 67: 251-2.
7 Mullarkey MF, Hill JS, Webb R. Allergic and nonallergic rhinitis: their characterization with attention to the meaning of eosinophilia. *J Allergy Clin Immunol* 1980: 65: 122-6.
8 Mygind N. *Nasal allergy*, 2nd edn. Oxford: Blackwell Scientific Publications, 1979.
9 Mygind N, Weeke B. Allergic and nonallergic rhinitis. In: Middleton Jr E, Reed CE, Ellic EF, eds. *Allergy: principles and practice*, 2nd edn. Saint Louis: CV Mosby Company, 1983: 1101-17.
10 NIAID Task Force Report. U.S. Department of Health, Education and Welfare. Asthma and the other allergic diseases. Bethesda: NIH Publications 1979; no 79: 387.
11 Settipane GA. Rhinitis: Introduction. In: Settipane GA, ed. *Rhinitis*, 2nd edn. Rhode Island: The New England Regional Allergy Proceedings, 1991: 1-11.

CHAPTER 2

Epidemiology

JEANNE MONTGOMERY SMITH

Prevalence of rhinitis

For most diseases epidemiological studies are the first basis on which we form our ideas about likely causes. For conditions of unknown etiology like those involving atopy this should remain a primary function. This chapter will focus on observations about the occurrence and natural history of allergic rhinitis and its related conditions, hoping that the reader will recognize that many of our basic assumptions can be questioned and that many basic questions about atopy and other possibly related conditions await answers.

The large numbers of people affected by atopic diseases world-wide and big differences from one community to another present a picture of a very important group of conditions where potentially alterable environmental factors certainly must play a major role.

Data from studies done differently are difficult to compare but it seems almost certain that there has been an increase in the occurrence of both allergic rhinitis and asthma in many if not all the industrialized nations. The increase may have begun as early as the 1930s but seems to have accelerated over the last two decades, at least in some populations.[1-5] Asthma and probably atopic disease have also become more common in a variety of previously little-affected groups in the Third World.[6-10] Unfortunately, a great many of the more recent studies are primarily concerned with asthma and give data on allergic rhinitis only secondarily. Figures given in Table 2.1 for asthma and rhinitis in Swedish conscripts is a good example of what seems to be changing prevalence in a developed country.[3]

One group of studies of asthma in a Third World country needs to be mentioned even though language difficulties were blamed for an inability to study allergic rhinitis. These studies are the work of several Australian authors who have been following the development of asthma in the Fore group of New Guinea islanders.[10-13] About 20 years ago the first 7 cases of asthma were recognized. Six of these were in adults who had returned to the villages after working in the European-influenced community. The villages were surveyed in 1972 and 2 cases in adults were found in a 1500-strong population. In 1976, another survey found 20 asthmatic adults and 2 children among 900 adults and 14,000 children. The affected children were found in households with affected adults. Since then, there have been increasing numbers of cases. At last report, 7.3% of the adult population had asthma but as yet only 0.6% of the children. House dust mites seem to be the major allergens related to this epidemic of asthma but it is difficult to understand why the children should be spared. Some other New Guinea groups still have little asthma. This phenomenon presents an unparalleled opportunity to study environmental factors in the development of atopy in a newly-affected population and, if at all possible, an effort should be made to study nasal symptoms and seasonal allergens as well as dust mites.

A 1978 Danish study of 2,000 randomly selected people over the age of 15 found an incidence rate for allergic rhinitis of 1% (new cases in the past year per 100 population) and cumulative

Table 2.1. *Prevalence of asthma and rhinitis in 55,000 Swedish conscripts.*

	1971	1981
Asthma	1.9	2.8
Rhinitis	4.4	8.4

prevalence of 7% (ever having had symptoms).[14] A sample of about 70 people selected from the group reporting allergic rhinitis were skin tested and completed a questionnaire with medical help. Allergic rhinitis was confirmed in 2/3, thus it was estimated that the 1-year prevalence rate was really 5%. Cumulative prevalence figures depend on age and effort to remember, so it is not surprising that in a Swedish twin study in the 1960s 15% of men and 14% of women over the age of 42 reported having had allergic rhinitis.[15]

American cumulative prevalence figures range from 9 to 21% for allergic rhinitis in most studies and from 4 to 8% for asthma.[16-19] In American figures, subjects with hay fever who also have asthma are usually counted as asthma and left out of the hay fever numbers. European rates have generally been a little below the American numbers.[14, 15, 20-22] Australia and New Zealand report the highest rates for childhood asthma, with about 20% of children affected. Australian rates for rhinitis in children are also high, with 27.6% reported to have hay fever.[23] This figure for hay fever in Australian children includes those who also have asthma. (Often figures for hay fever do not include those who have asthma.)

Inter-relationships make it necessary to decide which conditions should really be considered in studying the epidemiology of allergic rhinitis. Allergic rhinitis and extrinsic asthma are clearly members of a group of conditions associated with atopy. Atopy was the name coined by allergists early in this century who recognized "a hereditary group of spontaneously appearing allergies". Robert Cooke, a pioneer in American allergy studies, felt that the term should be used to denote "spontaneously occurring long-lasting wheal reacting allergy" regardless of family history.[24] That is how most allergists use the term today. It is important to recognize that IgE is produced normally and that some antigens, for example many parasites and some viruses, call forth an IgE response more readily than others. Thus not all raised IgE levels or all positive skin tests are signs of atopy. For clinical and for epidemiologic purposes it is important to know that positive tests can reflect IgE responses to currently met antigens and not the abnormal, long-lasting, sometimes (but not always) very high levels of atopic disease.

In the 1950s Michael Schwartz of Denmark undertook a classic study that identified the conditions that were and were not epidemiologically interconnected in the families of patients with asthma.[25] These were allergic rhinitis, infantile eczema, asthma both with and without atopy and rhinitis with nasal polyps. Schwartz's findings seemed to settle the question of inter-relatedness for these conditions, but it is important to realize that his findings will be affected by the fact that his study started with an asthmatic patient population.

Most people dealing with these diseases still feel that we may be dealing with several overlapping tendencies or diseases and make efforts to define and separate them. This is particularly true when infantile eczema, rhinitis, and asthma occur without demonstrable atopy. Good modern examples of these efforts in asthma are studies by Sibald et al[26] in Britain. Of 1166 possible subjects with asthma they decided to compare the 89 with negative skin tests, late onset and no exacerbations related to allergens with 327 allergic asthma patients who had developed symptoms at an early age. This choice of patients from the two extremes of what seems to be a spectrum left another 750 patients somewhere in between and illustrates the difficulty we have in defining groups because of clinical and epidemiologic overlap. If we arranged the equivalent group of skin test-negative older-onset nasal disease at one end of a spectrum and the larger group of young-onset atopic disease at the other we would probably also find that there is a big middle group with mixed characteristics.

Nasal disease with polyp formation is clearly associated with a particularly chronic form of asthma. Both nasal polyps and asthma have a family-related epidemiology which sometimes overlaps with family atopy.[27] Settipane et al,[28] in an allergy practice population, found that 2.2% of patients with allergic rhinitis or extrinsic asthma had nasal polyps, compared with 12.5% of asthmatics without demonstrable allergy. The 2.2% is probably greater than the general population occurrence of nasal polyps, but for comparison we have only the 0.3% of the population who reported nasal polyps in the American General Health Survey of 1980.[29]

One must be careful as to where the figures from clinical practices, or even one's own experience, come from. For example Settipane et al[28] in an allergy practice found that 71% of their patients with polyps had asthma, while two separate groups of otolaryngologists, Malony[30] and Drake-Lee et al,[31] found only 21% and 29% asthmatic. In the otolaryngologist experience, 2 to 3 times as many men had nasal polyps compared with women, but women with polyps were twice as likely to have asthma. In the 445 nasal polyp patients studied by Drake-Lee et al[31] positive skin tests to pollens were found in 10.5% and another 15% reacted to dust mite. At a time when the head of our Otolaryngology Clinic sent all patients with polyps to us, we found that 17% of 140 had positive skin tests to seasonal allergens or animal danders or marked reactions to house dust. Less strongly positive skin tests to dusts or dust mites are very common in asymptomatic populations and therefore hard to interpret. We think of nasal polyps and intrinsic asthma as relatively late-onset conditions but of our 140 cases with nasal polyps 46% had their first nasal symptoms, though not necessarily polyps, before the age of 20. The inflammatory cells in nasal polyps are usually like those of allergic inflammation and since polyps are often associated with asthma, it is tempting to suppose that they are part of the atopic disease spectrum. Currently available epidemiologic information does not clearly separate the two kinds of asthma or their nasal equivalents.

It is difficult to study nasal allergy in young children because of their many viral colds. When nasal polyps are found in childhood the child should be tested for cystic fibrosis in which about 20% of children have nasal polyps. This is another similarity between the epidemiology of nasal polyps and atopy since atopy is also more common in patients with cystic fibrosis than in the general population.[32, 33]

There are some families who have more eczema with their atopy than others, some families who have more hay fever than asthma, and some families where almost everyone with allergic rhinitis has asthma. Still other families have nasal polyps with or without asthma and with or without atopy. Table 2.2 from a study of patients joining a prepaid medical plan is a good example of this family tendency to develop similar manifestations.[3, 4]

Where the aim of epidemiology is to look for interconnections that may give clues about the cause of these diseases it is important to study the whole group, defining each subset carefully.

For epidemiologic purposes, it is also important to recognize that the form taken by atopic disease can be modified by intercurrent viral infections, age at onset, excessive allergen exposure and by the nature of the allergen.

Risk factors for the development of atopic conditions, nasal polyps, and asthma

The family

There can be no doubt that the family is the single most important risk factor for the development of all these conditions in childhood. However, the influence of family diminishes sharply in adulthood; over the age of 25 in our experience.

In a study of an Iowa rural population looking at those under the age of 20 at the time of interview, 16% of the girls and 27% of the boys born into households with allergic members had developed allergic rhinitis or asthma while 0.8% of the girls and 1.5% of the boys born into households without allergy were affected.[16]

There is a strong tendency for the form of the disease to be characteristic of a particular family[34] (Table 2.2). On the other hand, this can be overcome by environmental factors such as excessive allergen exposure or lower respiratory tract infection. Family allergic disease also is a determining factor for an early onset and, in turn, an early age at onset is a risk factor for the development of asthma in the atopic child. Seasonal sensitivities developing in adults are more often manifested as allergic rhinitis except where exposure is heavy, as in occupational asthma.[35] Figures from an Iowa rural survey are given in Table 2.3 to show most common ages at onset for rhinitis and asthma. These are fairly typical of the experience of other workers. The Iowa farming population, but not the city subjects, studied by us had somewhat more asthmatic relatives for the allergic rhinitis group, possibly because of an excess of occupational asthma in adult men (Tables 2.2 and 2.4).[16]

Table 2.2. *Allergic rhinitis and asthma in relatives of patients with allergic rhinitis with and without asthma.*

Subjects' disease	Relatives' disease	
	Iowa rural area, general population under age 20	Population of all ages, initial examination for a health insurance plan
Rhinitis	42% rhinitis	41% rhinitis
	28% rhinitis and asthma	9% rhinitis and asthma
	30% negative family	50% negative family
Rhinitis and asthma	24% rhinitis	25% rhinitis
	52% rhinitis and asthma	44% rhinitis and asthma
	24% negative family	31% negative family

The role of genetic factors in atopic disease

Since it is clear that the family is a very important risk factor, it has been assumed that this was entirely on a genetic basis. One theory is that the genetic tendency relates to specific purified allergens. There is good evidence for this but it is also true that in the same families there are often other affected individuals allergic to other things.[36-38]

Identical twins both develop respiratory allergy more often than dizygous twins but it is clear that environmental factors also contribute significantly even in monozygous twins.[15, 39, 40]

Whatever the role of genetic factors in specific sensitivities, it seems very likely that genetic permissiveness is required for the development of atopic disease. Yet from the maximum rates encountered in various countries one can assume that at least 25% of the population are susceptible.

Allergen

Allergen exposure and possibly the nature of the allergen seem to have more to do with the form of taken by atopic disease than with the total number of cases. A recent study in Australia comparing two populations with different allergen prevalence demonstrates this phenomenon quite well.[23] A good example of the effect of allergen exposure in the development of a specific allergy is seen in a French study comparing a mountainous area having little mite allergen with Marseille. Ten percent of the mountain dwellers had positive mite skin tests compared with 27% in Marseille.[4] In spite of differences in allergen exposure, the prevalence of atopic diseases is also very similar in most parts of the United States except where families with allergic disease have sought refuge in desert areas like Arizona. In the most recent report from the Arizona studies, 55% of the general population being followed by Barbee et al complain of allergic rhinitis.[42] (This appears to be an interview report without clinical confirmation.)

An early age at onset is associated with strong and multiple allergies but not all patients with an early onset of symptoms have positive skin tests or probable allergy. There are several studies showing an increased risk for the development of pollen allergy for those born a month or so before the season.[43, 44] On the other hand, hay fever with positive skin tests can develop for the first time in old

Table 2.3. *Age of onset of seasonal allergy.*

Age	Male (n = 135)	Female (n = 123)
0-9	60%	39%
10-19	17%	32%
20-29	21%	24%
30-39	23%	12%
40-49	10%	8%
50-59	2%	6%
60+	2%	2%

Table 2.4. *Age of onset of asthma in subjects drawn from general populations.*

Age	Urban (n = 193)		Rural (n = 277)	
	Male	Female	Male	Female
0-9	80 (75%)	51 (59%)	117 (65%)	68 (70%)
10-19	13 (12%)	18 (21%)	16 (9%)	9 (9%)
20+	14 (13%)	17 (20%)	47 (26%)	20 (21%)

age, even to allergens to which there has been life-long exposure.

Certain allergens such as the enzymes used in laundry detergents seem to be particularly prone to cause occupational asthma rather than just nasal symptoms. With this particular allergen most cases represent new symptoms in already atopic individuals and the development of altogether new cases occurs at about the same rate as new cases in a general population of adults.[17, 45] There has been little study of occupational allergic rhinitis though it is sometimes mentioned in studies such as those of laboratory animal allergy.

In the New Guinea studies more mites were found in the blankets of households with asthmatic members and it is likely that the nature of the allergen and heaviness of exposure affect the presentation of atopic disease. This may explain the prevalence of asthma in the New Guinea population but does not explain the sparing of children.[46]

Infection

Respiratory infection clearly affects the occurrence of asthma in the very young child, both the initial development and recurrences are often related to virus infections.[47] There is also evidence that viral infections can promote IgE responses to other allergens.[48a] Falliers[48b] made a study of two pairs of monozygous twins, one of each set having severe asthma and the other only hay fever. Both were apparently equally atopic and the only difference was a history of lower respiratory tract infection at the onset in the asthmatic twin. A relationship between allergic rhinitis and respiratory infection may not be discernible because of the ubiquity of upper respiratory infections.

In the New Guinea studies one cannot postulate a primary role in asthma for the usual epidemic respiratory viruses because there is no reason why children and adults would not be equally affected by such viruses.[10-13, 45]

Race

Race as a factor in atopy has been difficult to separate from environmental factors. For example a much quoted study in Singapore has found more atopic disease in Malaysians than in Chinese and Indians.[49] However, the 16% of Chinese immigrant students who developed ragweed hay fever at the University of Michigan years ago suggests that the Chinese are by no means non-susceptible to atopic disease in another setting.[50] Without knowing the social relationships and customs of the two groups in Singapore one cannot say that, because they live in the same geographic area, their environment is the same.

There are many examples of very different prevalences of atopic disease comparing racial groups but also enough examples of different rates in the same ethnic group in different environments to make it impossible to know whether there is any real racial difference in susceptibility.

The natural course of atopic disease

Population studies that follow atopic patients over many years are scarce. It has been known for a long time that people can develop atopic sensitivity in the sense of markedly positive skin tests several years before respiratory symptoms begin. It is also true that, occasionally, symptoms develop before skin tests become positive. An example is found in a study of German baker's apprentices who were followed from the beginning of their employment in order to study the development of baker's asthma. Most developed skin reactivity first, but the reverse order also occurred.[51]

Hagy and Settipane followed students with positive skin tests but no symptoms from the beginning of their college years until their 4th year and then to 7 years. They found that the most strongly positive skin tests were predictive of symptoms (71%) but lesser reactions were less certain to predict symptoms.[52] Sixty-four percent of the 1836 students originally tested 23 years ago have recently been followed up once more. Seventeen new cases of asthma have developed in the 162 subjects who previously only had hay fever (10.5%). Nineteen new cases of asthma have developed in the 528 without previous symptoms (3.2%). Subjects without symptoms but with previous positive skin tests were also somewhat more likely to have developed asthma than people with negative tests, 10.6% compared with 3.2%.[53]

In clinical practice we require correlation of skin tests with symptoms for diagnosis and the same requirement should apply in epidemiologic studies because some of the positive skin tests may represent normal IgE from recent exposure to some allergens.[54] For example, years ago Schwartz found 50% of subjects in a study of Danish bakers to be skin test-positive, but only about 20% were symptomatic.[25] It is probable that some of the skin test positivity represented normal IgE in response to recent allergen exposure and not the abnormal, atopic IgE response that persists long after the stimulus is gone.

A most important characteristic of atopy is this long-lasting, self-perpetuating, abnormally high level of specific sensitivity without the need for further allergen exposure.

The natural course of atopic sensitization has not received much attention. Several workers have demonstrated that abnormal IgE levels can develop *in utero* and have some value as predictors of atopic disease.[55, 56] We know from clinical experience that very strong and multiple positive skin tests are mainly developed in youth. On the other hand, both asthma and hay fever with strongly positive skin tests (usually to only one or a very few allergens) can develop at any age, even in people who have been exposed to the same allergen all their lives.

Forty years ago it was a fairly common practice to skin test every year to see if new allergies had developed. This was given up long ago because usually the pattern of allergies remains the same over many years. This is an important observation in need of much more study. The long-term localization of the abnormal immune response that, unlike normal IgE responses, has become self-perpetuating, suggests resistance to further involvement.

We wrote to the people who had been skin tested or treated with allergens during their years at university.[57] Two-hundred-and-forty-five (88%) of these subjects responded. There were only 10 who thought that they had developed a new allergy. The 10 had developed new springtime symptoms, but 5 of these had had positive skin tests to spring pollens in our tests years before. There were 29 subjects who thought that their problems had increased over the years and 14 of these reported nasal polyps. If these observations are correct, sensitization usually occurs over a limited period of time under unknown circumstances that are only rarely repeated. There is great need for more data on the occurrence of new allergies. When we go to meetings, we ask fellow allergists how our patients do when they move to another part of the country. We forget that they will not have seen those whose condition had resolved. They will also usually not have knowledge of previous skin tests.

Discussion

Probably most allergists think of the atopy-eczema-allergic rhinitis and asthma group of conditions as a collection of overlapping, genetically-determined susceptibilities. For example, it has been postulated that atopy is a genetically-determined tendency to mount excessive IgE responses and that excessively reactive bronchial membranes are a second inherited trait that is prone to cause asthma, to which the atopic population is particularly susceptible. There is a great deal of evidence to suggest that environmental factors must play a part in both atopic sensitization and the development of asthma.

It is also possible to explain the epidemiologic interconnections if we think of atopy-eczema-allergic rhinitis and extrinsic asthma as manifestations of a single disease in which several self-perpetuating abnormalities develop over a period of time, influenced by both host factors and environmental factors. First, there is the localized long-term specific IgE-mediated allergy that may be evident on skin test for several weeks or several years before the development of symptoms. Then there is possible involvement of the skin, nose and lower respiratory tract with a chronic inflammation response in which the eosinophil is an important player. Development of lesions in these various areas may occur simultaneously, or there may be intervals of years between the development of disease in one area and its spread to involve another. At least for asthma, the beginning of chest symptoms is often related to intercurrent viral infection, trauma to the respiratory membranes or excessive allergen exposure. The very similar inflammation of infantile eczema, rhinitis with nasal polyps and asthma without atopy could also be manifestations of a similar disease that may or may not be related to the atopic group.

It is important to develop and test a variety of working hypotheses clearly recognizing that the cause of atopy and related diseases is unknown. Nasal conditions, and not asthma alone, should be carefully scrutinized in epidemiologic studies.

Conclusion

Over the past 20 years, and especially the last 10 years, there has almost certainly been a substantial increase in the occurrence of allergic nasal disease and asthma in the industrialized countries. Asthma with allergy has also been developing in some previously unaffected Third World populations. Unfortunately, nasal conditions have not been studied in these groups because of language problems. In the Nordic countries the cumulative prevalence for allergic rhinitis in the general population is about 7%. It is probably somewhat higher in North America with prevalence figures ranging from 9 to 21%. Australia reports a very high figure of 27.6% for hay fever in children and also very high rates for asthma. It is quite clear that, although the family occurrence of these diseases points to a possible role for genetic susceptibility, the short-term increase within a generation must involve environmental factors. Since environmental factors are often alterable it is of the utmost importance to determine the nature of such factors. Neither indoor nor outdoor pollution, or new allergens, explain the increasing numbers of cases and it will be important to ask new questions if we are to get new answers.

References

1 Smith JM. Studies of the prevalence of asthma in childhood. *Allergol Immunopathol* 1975; *3:* 127.
2 Varonier HS, De Haller J, Schopfer C. Prevalence de L'allergie chez les enfants et les adolescents. *Helv Paediat Acta* 1984; *39:* 129.
3 Åberg N. Asthma and allergic rhinitis in Swedish conscripts. *Clin Exp Allergy* 1989; *19:* 59.
4 Wüthrich B, Schnyder VW, Honauer SA, Heller A. Thirteenth Congress of the European Academy of Allergology and Clinical Immunology. Budapest, 1986: 656.
5 Denis J, Perdrizet S, Levallois M. Increased frequency of allergic diseases in Parisian students from 1968 to 1982 (abstract 93), presented at the International Symposium on Prevention of Allergic Diseases, Florence, Italy, 1984.
6 Godfrey RC. Asthma and IgE levels in rural and urban communities of the Gambia. *Clin Allergy* 1975; *5:* 201.
7 Van Niekerk CH, Weinberg EG, Shore SC, et al. Prevalence of asthma: a comparative study of urban and rural Xhosa children. *Clin Allergy* 1979; *3:* 319.
8 Wolstenholme RJ. Bronchial asthma in the southern Maldives. *Clin Allergy* 1979; *9:* 325.
9 Waite DA, Eyles EF, Tonkin SL, O'Donnell TV. Asthma prevalence in Tokelauan children in two environments. *Clin Allergy* 1980: *10:* 71.
10 Woolcock AJ, Green W, Alpers MP. Asthma in a rural highland area of Papua New Guinea. *Am Rev Respir Dis* 1981; *123:* 565.
11 Dowse GK, Smith D, Turner KJ, Alpers MP. Prevalence and features of asthma in a sample survey of urban Goroka, Papua New Guinea. *Clin Allergy* 1985; *15:* 429.
12 Dowse GK, Turner KJ, Woolcock AJ, Alpers MP. Emerging asthma in the Okapa District of the Eastern Highlands Province of Papua New Guinea: the problem and its implications. *Papua New Guinea Med J* 1983; *26:* 33.
13 Turner KJ, Dowse GK, Stewart GA, Alpers MP, Woolcock AJ. Prevalence of asthma in the South Fore People of the Okapa District of Papua New Guinea. *Int Archs Allergy Appl Immunol* 1985; *77:* 158.
14 Weeke ER, Pedersen PA, Backman A, Siegel SC. Epidemiology. In: Mygind N, Weeke B, eds. *Allergic and vasomotor rhinitis: clinical aspects.* Copenhagen: Munksgaard, 1985: 21-30.
15 Edfors-Lubs MI. Allergy in 7000 twin pairs. *Acta Allergol (Kbh)* 1971; *26:* 249.
16 Smith J Montgomery, Knowler LA. Epidemiology of asthma and allergic rhinitis. I. In a rural area. II. In a university-centered community. *Am Rev Respir Dis* 1965; *92:* 16.
17 Broder I, Higgins MW, Mathews KP, Keller JB. Epidemiology of asthma and allergic rhinitis in a total community, Tecumseh, Michigan. *J Allergy Clin Immunol* 1974; *54:* 100.
18 Hagy GW, Settipane GA. Risk factors for the development of asthma and allergic rhinitis: a 7-year follow-up of college students. *J Allergy Clin Immunol* 1976; *58:* 330.
19 Freman GL, Johnson S. Allergic diseases in adolescents. I. Description of survey: prevalence of allergy. *Am J Dis Child* 1964; *107:* 549.
20 Burr ML, Butland BK, King S, Vaughan-Williams E. Changes in asthma prevalence: two surveys 15 years apart. *Arch Dis Childh* 1989; *64:* 1452.
21 Skarpaas IJK, Gulsvik A. Prevalence of bronchial asthma and respiratory symptoms in schoolchildren in Oslo. *Allergy* 1985; *40:* 295.
22. Haahtela T, Jokela H. Asthma and allergy in Finnish conscripts. *Allergy* 1978; *34:* 413.
23 Peat JK, Britton WJ, Salome CM, Woolcock AJ. Bronchial hyperresponsiveness in two populations of Australian schoolchildren. III. Effect of exposure to environmental allergens. *Clin Allergy* 1987; *17:* 291.
24 Cooke RA. *Allergy in theory and practice.* London: W. B. Saunders Company, 1947.
25 Schwartz M. *Heredity in bronchial asthma.* Copenhagen: Munksgaard, 1952.
26 Sibbald B, Turner-Warwick M. Factors influencing the prevalence of asthma among first degree relatives of extrinsic and intrinsic asthmatics. *Thorax* 1979; *34:* 332.
27 Lockey RF, Rucknagel DL, Vanselow NA. Familial occurrence of asthma, nasal polyps and aspirin intolerance. *Ann Intern Med* 1973; *78:* 57.
28 Settipane GA, Chafee FH. Nasal polyps in asthma and rhinitis: a review of 6,037 patients. *J Allergy Clin Immunol* 1977; *59:* 17.
29 Vital and health statistics. Prevalence of selected chronic conditions, USA. Series 10, No. 155, p. 25.
30 Maloney JR. Nasal polyps, nasal polypectomy, asthma and aspirin sensitivity. *J Laryngol Otol* 1977; *91:* 837.

31. Drake-Lee AB, Lowe D, Swanston A, Grace A. Clinical profile and recurrence of nasal polyps. *J Laryngol Otol* 1984; *98:* 783.
32. Rachelefsky GS, Osher A, Dooley RE, et al. Coexistent respiratory allergy and cystic fibrosis. *Am J Dis Child* 1974; *128:* 335.
33. Wönne R, Hofmann D, Posselt H-G, et al. Brochial allergy in cystic fibrosis. *Clin Allergy* 1985; *15:* 455.
34. McKee WD. The incidence and familial occurrence of allergy. *J Allergy* 1966; *38:* 226.
35. Ramirez DA. The natural history of mountain cedar pollinosis. *J Allergy Clin Immunol* 1984; *73:* 88.
36. Marsh D, Hsu SH, Roebber M, et al. HLA-Dw2: A genetic marker for human immune response to short ragweed allergen RAS: I. Response resulting primarily from natural antigenic exposure. *J Exp Med* 1982; *155:* 1439.
37. Freidhoff LR, Ehrlich-Kautzky E, Meyers DA, Ansari AA, Bias WB, Marsh DG. Association of HLA-DR3 with human immune response to Lol p I and Lol p II antigens in allergic subjects. *Tissue Antigens* 1988; *31:* 211.
38. Blumenthal MN, Yunis E, Mendell N, Elston RC. Preventive allergy: genetics of IgE-mediated diseases. *J Allergy Clin Immunol* 1986; *78 (Part 2):* 962.
39. Wüthrich B, Baumann E, Fries RA, Schnyder UW. Total and specific IgE (RAST) in atopic twins. *Clin Allergy* 1981; *11:* 147.
40. Ericsson CH, Svartengren M, Mossberg B, Pedersen N, Camner P. Bronchial reactivity and allergy-promoting factors in monozygotic twins discordant for allergic rhinitis. *Ann Allergy* 1991; *67:* 53.
41. Charpin D, Kleisbauer J-P, Lanteaume A, et al. Asthma and allergy to house-dust mites in populations living in high altitudes. *Chest* 1988; *93:* 758.
42. Barbee RA, Halonen M, Kaltenborn WT, Burrows B. A longitudinal study of respiratory symptoms in a community population sample: correlations with smoking, allergen skin-test reactivity, and serum IgE. *Chest* 1991; *99:* 20.
43. Korsgaard J, Dahl R. Sensitivity to house dust mite and grass pollen in adults. Influence of month of birth. *Clin Allergy* 1983; *13:* 529.
44. Björksten F, Suoniemi I, Koski V. Neonatal birch pollen contact and subsequent allergy to birch pollen. *Clin Allergy* 1980; *10:* 585.
45. Slavin RG, Lewis CR. Sensitivity to enzyme additives in laundry detergent workers. *J Allergy Clin Immunol* 1971; *48:* 262.
46. Turner KJ, Stewart FA, Woolcock AJ, Green A, Alpers MP. Relationship between mite densities and the prevalence of asthma: comparative studies in two populations in the Eastern Highlands of Papua New Guinea. *Clin Allergy* 1988; *18:* 331.
47. Busse WW. The relationship between viral infections and onset of allergic diseases and asthma. *Clin Exp Allergy* 1989; *19:* 1.
48a. Frick OL, German DF, Mills J. Development of allergy in children. I. Association with virus infections. *J Allergy Clin Immunol* 1979; *63:* 228.
48b. Falliers CJ, Cardoso A, Bane MS, et al. Discordant allergic manifestations in monozygotic twins. *J Allergy* 1971; *47:* 207.
49. Ross I. Bronchial asthma in Malaysia. *Br J Dis Chest* 1984; *78:* 369.
50. Maternowski CJ, Mathews KP. The prevalence of ragweed pollinosis in foreign and native students at a midwestern university and its implications concerning methods for determining the inheritance of atopy. *J Allergy* 1962; *33:* 130.
51. Borchert J. Beobachtungen über die Entwicklung des allergischen Asthmas und der allergischen Rhinitis bei Backern. *Acta Allergol (Kbh)* 1972; *27:* 195.
52. Hagy GW, Settipane GA. Risk factors for developing asthma and allergic rhinitis. *J Allergy Clin Immunol* 1976; *58:* 330.
53. Settipane RJ, Hagy GW, Settipane GA. Development of new asthma and allergic rhinitis in a 23-year follow-up of college students. *J Allergy Clin Immunol* 1991; *87:* 232.
54. Cserhati E, Kiss AG, Mezei G, et al. Positive skin prick tests of immediate type of non-allergic children. *Acta Paediatr Hung* 1983: *24:* 189.
55. Michel FB, Bousquet J, Greillier P, et al. Comparison of cord blood immunoglobulin E concentrations and maternal allergy for prediction of atopic diseases in infancy. *J Allergy Clin Immunol* 1980; *65:* 422.
56. Kjellman N-IM. Development and prediction of atopic allergy in childhood. Theoretical and Clinical Aspects of Allergic Diseases. In: Skandia international Symposia 1982. Stockholm: Almqvist and Wiksell, 1983: 52-73.
57. Smith, JM. The long-term effect of moving on patients with asthma and hay fever. *J Allergy* 1971; *48:* 191.

CHAPTER 3

Allergens

ROBERT A WOOD

Introduction

IgE-mediated reactions to aeroallergens are common causes of rhinitis in both children and adults. This chapter focuses on the allergens themselves and on strategies that can be utilized to reduce or even prevent such reactions through allergen avoidance.

Allergens can be grouped in a variety of ways but we will use two general categories, those found in outdoor environments and those found in indoor environments. Outdoor allergens are comprised primarily of pollens of various trees, grasses, and weeds, as well as some mold species. They are generally present on a seasonal basis and produce the typical symptoms of seasonal allergic rhinitis, occurring at very predictable intervals each year in a given geographical region. Indoor allergens are usually present on a perennial basis; most important among these are dust mites and animal danders, with cockroaches and certain mold species also being important in some areas. These allergens tend to produce chronic symptoms that are more persistent but usually less dramatic, and hence less clinically obvious, than those of seasonal allergic rhinitis.

Allergens: General characteristics, identification, and quantification

Aeroallergens share several important characteristics.[1-5] For each allergen, one or more component(s) serve as the antigen against which IgE is generated and are referred to as major allergens (see Tables 3.4, 3.7 and 3.9). They are all proteins or glycoproteins with molecular weights that generally range from 10,000 to 40,000 Daltons. They are carried on particles that range in size from less than 5 µm to greater than 60 µm. In general, the clinical importance of any allergen is determined by the interplay of two major factors: its concentration in the environment, which relates to both source production and aerodynamic characteristics, and its allergenicity, or ability to stimulate specific IgE production in susceptible individuals. Thus, the "ideal" allergen would be present in high concentrations, would remain airborne for extended periods, and would stimulate a brisk IgE response.

The aerodynamic characteristics of an allergen are critically important for several reasons. First, the particle size of an allergen is a major determinant of its buoyancy (Table 3.1).[5] Allergens carried on small particles will tend to remain airborne for longer periods of time, disseminate more widely, and have a generally greater chance of coming in contact with the human airway. Thus, some pollens are so large that they fall rapidly after release and are virtually incapable of causing disease, even though they may be released in high numbers. Second, once an allergen reaches the human airway, its particle size largely determines its site of deposition (Table 3.2) and therefore has major impli-

Table 3.1. *Allergen particle size and buoyancy.*

Particle source	Size range (µm)	Persistence (still air)
Cat	0.05–20+	6 min–75 days
Dust mite	6+	<36 min
Pollens	10–100	9 sec–13 min
Tobacco smoke	0.01–1.0	19 h–400 days

Table 3.2. *Allergen particle size and airway deposition.*

Particle size	Percent reaching lower airways
> 10 μm	0%
5 μm	20%
1–2 μm	100%

cations with regard to the location of the allergic response.[6]

Allergens can be identified and quantitated by several different means. For outdoor allergens, pollen and mold spore counts have been used for decades and are still the primary means used to both identify and quantitate these allergens. The counts are accomplished by exposing a collecting unit, usually a greased slide, to outdoor air using one of several different sampling devices (Table 3.3).[2,7] These slides are then viewed under a microscope such that pollens and spores can be identified and counted. Although they are semi-quantitative at best, they do serve as an excellent means of following trends in outdoor allergen levels and are highly correlated with symptoms in sensitized individuals.

The other major means of identifying and quantitating allergens is the use of immunochemical assays. These techniques, which include ELISAs, radioimmunoassays, and RAST inhibition, allow for the specific quantitation of a variety of allergens. They have been particularly useful for the assessment of indoor allergen exposure, with assays now available for the measurement of dust mite, cat, dog, and cockroach allergens.[8-13] These assays are highly accurate and reproducible and have added greatly to the study of indoor allergens. Similar techniques have been applied to the study of outdoor allergens but they are not routinely available.[14] Although there is relatively little data with regard to allergic rhinitis, it has been shown that exposure to high levels of dust mite allergen as measured immunochemically is a risk factor for asthma exacerbations.[15,16]

Diagnostic considerations

Although the laboratory diagnosis of allergic rhinitis will be covered in detail in a subsequent chapter, a few points are particularly relevant here with regard to the interpretation of historical data regarding allergen exposure. For seasonal rhinitis, the history is often very clear and extremely helpful. An experienced clinician can often predict a patient's allergy test results by utilizing a careful history and a detailed knowledge of local aeroallergen patterns. For indoor allergens, however, the history may be far more difficult to interpret and a high index of suspicion must be maintained. This is because both the exposures and the symptoms tend to be more chronic and low grade. In addition, emotional factors may be very important when household pets are involved, commonly invoking a strong sense of denial. These situations can be approached either by challenge studies, which are not routinely available, or by trials of avoidance, which rely on careful observation of symptoms during an extended vacation or trial period of pet removal. It is critical to note, however, that the pet must be out of the home for at least 4 to 6 months before allergen levels will be sufficiently reduced in most instances to make any valid conclusions.[17]

Table 3.3. *Common air sampling devices.*

Type	Advantages	Disadvantages
Gravity sampler	Simplicity	Non-volumetric, misses small particles, influenced by wind speed
Rotating arm impactors	Volumetric, not influenced by wind speed	Poor sampling of small particles
Suction filters	Good sampling of all particle sizes	Requires proper wind orientation and air speed
Suction impinger	Can assess counts over time or by size	Also requires proper wind orientation and air speed

Allergen distribution and environmental control

Pollens

The major allergens for many pollens, particularly the grasses and ragweed, have been identified and characterized (Table 3.4).[3-4] For example, for rye grass about 90% of sensitive patients react to the major allergen *Lol p* I, while 60 to 70% react to the minor allergens *Lol P* II and *Lol p* III. Substantial cross reactivity, which generally follows botanical relationships, has been demonstrated between many of these allergens. In the United States, most grass pollens fall into two general cross-reacting groups, those associated with timothy grass and those associated with Bermuda grass. Such data are very useful in the interpretation of allergy test results and in the development of effective immunotherapy strategies.

Although pollens are located predominantly in the outdoor environment, they may also be present in house dust samples at substantial concentrations in a seasonal fashion.[18, 19] Knowledge regarding the specific pollen seasons in your area can make patient care more effective and should be sought by anyone caring for allergic patients.

Although it is usually not possible to dramatically reduce pollen exposure through environmental control, certain steps can be taken that may help to provide some relief for patients with seasonal allergic rhinitis (Table 3.5). Although difficult, source control should be undertaken whenever possible. Windows should be closed to reduce allergen exposure in both the home and automobile. Air conditioners may provide added benefit. Certain activities, particularly in the hours when pollen counts tend to be highest, may have to be avoided altogether. It has been shown that ragweed pollen counts peak in the late morning and grass in the early to mid-afternoon. Finally, masks may help to filter some pollen and may be helpful for particularly sensitive individuals.

Mold allergens

Although there is a huge variety of fungi in both indoor and outdoor environments, relatively few are of clinical importance.[20-21] Most important among these are *Alternaria* and *Cladosporium*, which are most prevalent in outdoor environments, and *Aspergillus* and *Penicillium*, which are most prevalent in indoor environments. Both spore and mycelial antigens have been described but the exact site of the major allergens for most molds remains unclear. Similarly, with the exception of *Alternaria* (*Alt a* I) and *Cladosporium* (*Cla h* I and *Cla h* II), major allergens have not been identified for most fungal species. These facts have made the preparation of reliable mold extracts for diagnostic and therapeutic use difficult, with mold sensitivity remaining one of the more confusing areas in clinical allergy.

Molds grow best in warm areas with high humidity and are therefore most prevalent in the summer and fall. Outdoors, they commonly grow in

Table 3.4. *Examples of well-characterized pollen allergens and their molecular weight.*

Rye grass	*Lol p* I	27,000
(*Lolium perenne*)	*Lol p* II	11,000
	Lol p III	11,000
	Lol p IV	56,800
	Lol P X	12,000
Timothy grass	*Phl p* V	15,000
(*Phleum pratense*)	*Phl p* VI	15,000
	Phl p VII	34,000
	Phl p VIII	8,000
Orchard grass	*Dac g* I	33,000
(*Dactylis glomerata*)		
Short ragweed	*Amb a* I	37,800
(*Ambrosia artemisii folia*)	*Amb a* II	38,200
	Amb a III	12,300
	Amb a IV	22,800
	Amb a V	4,990
	Amb a VI	11,500
Giant ragweed	*Amb t* V	4,390
(*Ambrosia trifida*)		
Silver birch	*Bet v* I	22,500
(*Betula verrucosa*)		

Table 3.5. *Environmental control: pollens.*

1. Remove sources if possible
2. Close windows (home and auto)
3. Use air conditioners
4. Avoid certain activities, certain times of day
5. Wear masks if necessary

leaves, soil, thatch, moist debris, and on moist surfaces. They may become airborne in extraordinary numbers with lawn mowing, raking of leaves, farming, and other similar activities. Mold spore counts have been reported to peak in the afternoon. Their numbers are often markedly reduced by the first frosts in the late fall or early winter.

The approach to the patient with sensitivity to outdoor molds is similar to that described above for pollen allergy. In addition, however, it may be more feasible to eliminate local sources of mold growth than it is for pollens. Proper drainage around the home should be ensured and leaves and other debris should be removed promptly. Similarly, activities such as lawn mowing and raking or playing in leaves may have to be avoided.

Indoors, fungi grow well wherever sufficient surface moisture and adequate temperature are present. There may be significant seasonal variation related to temperature and humidity but they commonly persist on a year-round basis to some degree, particularly in warmer climates. Basement walls, window moldings, and bathroom walls and fixtures are common sites of mold growth. In addition, food storage areas, garbage containers, decaying upholstery and foam rubber, household plants, and poorly maintained humidifiers or vaporizers can all contribute to indoor mold exposure. The most important measures to control growth are aggressive dehumidification, proper ventilation, and the use of fungicides to control mold growth (Table 3.6). A good deal of detective work may be required to identify areas of mold growth so that these measures can be maximized.

Dust mites

Dust mites of the genus *Dermatophagoides* are overall the most important indoor allergens and sensitivity to mites comprises a significant proportion of what has for decades been called "house dust" allergy.[22-23] Dust mites are eight-legged animals that are close relatives of ticks and spiders. They grow best in warm areas with high humidity (60-70% relative humidity) and feed on human skin scales. They have been found in high numbers in house dust samples from Europe, the United States, Central and South America, the Far East, and Australia.[9,24-30] The only areas that appear to be relatively spared of mite contamination are those with very dry climates or those at high altitudes (>3,000 meters elevation).[31-33] In addition, it has been postulated that the design of homes in the last 20 years, particularly the manufacture of more "tight", energy-efficient homes, has led to significant increases in mite levels by reducing ventilation and increasing indoor temperatures and humidity.

Two major mite species, *Dermatophagoides farinae* and *D. pteronyssinus*, are the most important causes of dust mite allergy.[25] Other species, such as *D. microceras* and *Euroglyphus maynei*, may also be important in more limited geographical regions. It has been shown that *D. farinae* is capable of surviving periods of low humidity and therefore tends to predominate in climates that are less consistently humid. *D. pteronyssinus* is more likely to be the dominant mite in areas, such as London, where humidity is consistently high. Seasonal variation in mite numbers may occur in some areas, with peaks occurring in the summer and fall.[18] Mite antigen levels may then remain elevated through the fall and early winter, a time when mite-induced symptoms tend to be most prominent.

Major dust mite allergens are listed in Table 3.7.[9-11, 25, 34-36] Mite allergens are found in both feces and body parts. They are carried on particles that are relatively large (10-30 μm) that tend to settle rapidly after disturbance.[37] Mite antigen levels have been extensively measured in many areas and some

Table 3.6. *Environmental control: molds.*

1	Remove sources of mold growth (inside and outside)
2	Dehumidify
3	Maximize ventilation
4	Ensure proper drainage around home
5	Use fungicides on contaminated areas (be a detective)
6	Limit vaporizer and humidifier use and clean frequently when in use

Table 3.7. *Dust mite allergens.*

Species	Allergen(s)	Molecular weight
Dermatophagoides farinae	Der f I	24,000
	Der f II	15,000
D. pteronyssinus	Der p I	24,000
	Der p II	15,000
D. microceras	Der m I	24,000

general agreement now exists regarding the levels that should be considered clinically significant for patients with asthma. A level of 10 μg/g of dust is considered a risk factor for the development of acute asthma symptoms and a level greater than 2 μg/g a risk factor for sensitization.[15, 24] No solid data exist to date regarding the correlation of specific mite levels with symptoms of rhinitis.

Mites are not common components of surface dust but instead grow best in fabrics such as mattresses, pillows, bedding, carpets, upholstered furniture, and stuffed animals.[18] Environmental control for mites must therefore focus on these prime areas of mite growth. Mite control strategies follow two general approaches: either the sources of mite growth are removed from the immediate environment or impermeable barriers are placed between the mites and the patient. New methods that may kill mites or denature mite allergens have also recently been introduced and will be discussed.

Although there is relatively little data on the value of environmental control measures for mite-induced rhinitis, substantial data exist to support their role in the management of patients with asthma.[38-42] A comprehensive program for mite reduction in the home is outlined in Table 3.8. The bedroom should be tackled most aggressively both because of the particular predilection of mites for mattresses and bedding and the prolonged contact with mites that may occur while sleeping. Mattresses, box springs, and pillows should be encased with plastic covers. Stuffed animals and other soft toys should be removed. All bedding should be washed in a hot (>130 degrees F=55°C) cycle at least every 2 weeks. Carpets, upholstered furniture, and curtains should be removed and humidifiers should be avoided.

For very sensitive individuals, similar measures should be considered for other areas of the home. Carpets should never be installed over a cement slab in the basement as this may promote extraordinary mite growth. In addition, carpets and upholstered furniture might be removed from the family room or other areas where large amounts of time are spent. If carpets do remain, they should be vacuumed at least once a week. Unfortunately, however, vacuuming removes relatively little mite allergen from carpets and should not be considered a substitute for carpet removal. Finally, any measures that might help to increase home ventilation and decrease indoor relative humidity should be undertaken.

The final step that should be considered for patients with significant mite sensitivity is the use of chemical substances that may help to decrease mite allergen levels.[25, 43-45] These are of two general varieties, those that work by denaturing mite allergens and those that actually kill mites (acaricides). Tannic acid, which is said to denature mite allergens, has now been marketed for several years. Although it does appear capable of reducing mite levels in carpets, clinical trials have not yet been reported to document any clinical efficacy. The only acaricide currently marketed in the United States is benzyl benzoate; natamycin is another agent that is marketed in Europe. Other agents, such as lindane and primiphos methyl, are also under study but may be too toxic for routine use. These products have been shown to reduce both mite counts and mite allergen levels but, as with

Table 3.8. *Environmental control: dust mites.*

1. Encase mattress, box spring, and pillows with plastic covers
2. Remove carpets (especially in bedroom and basement)
3. Remove upholstered furniture
4. Vacuum any remaining carpets and upholstered furniture weekly
5. Hot wash bed linens every 1-2 weeks (>130 degrees F=55°C)
6. Control humidity (relative humidity <50%)
   - Limit humidifier use
   - Use dehumidifiers if necessary
   - Increase ventilation (if indoor humidity > outdoor humidity)
7. Remove stuffed animals, soft toys, curtains
8. Consider acaricides and tannic acid

tannic acid, their clinical efficacy has not been documented. The most reasonable conclusion at this time is to say that they may have some value but that they should by no means be considered substitutes for the other measures listed above, particularly mattress covers and carpet removal.

Animal danders

Animal allergens are another extremely important cause of allergic rhinitis. This is both because many are highly immunogenic and because humans insist on close contact with them. Currently, over half of all the homes in the United States have at least one cat or dog, with a total pet population of over 100 million. In addition, cat and dog allergens have been found in household dust from almost every home sampled[26] and most commercially available house dust extracts contain measurable concentrations of cat allergen.[46] Rodents, including guinea pigs, hamsters, rabbits, rats, and mice, are also commonly kept as pets in the home, as well as in schools and even pediatric hospitals. Animal danders are also potential occupational sensitizers for veterinarians and laboratory animal workers.[47]

Several major animal allergens have now been defined (Table 3.9).[48-53] In most cases, these allergens are found in secretions. For example, *Fel d* I, the major allergen of the domestic cat, is produced predominantly in cat saliva and to a lesser extent in sebaceous glands of cat skin.[48-49, 54] In dogs, major allergens have been identified in saliva, dander, and possibly urine.[49-50] It is presumed that these secretions dry on fur, bedding, carpeting, and other objects and then become airborne when these reservoirs are disturbed. Airborne cat and rat allergens have been best studied and have been demonstrated to be associated with particles that range in size from less than 1 μm to larger than 20 μm, with a significant proportion on particles less than 5 μm.[37, 55-56] Particles of this size tend to remain airborne for hours after they are produced. Cat allergen also appears to be "sticky" and to adhere to walls, clothing, and other surfaces.[57] As a consequence, the allergens are virtually ubiquitous and are widely distributed even in homes that have never had pets.[26]

Whenever possible, avoidance is the treatment of choice for all animal allergy (Table 3.10). Unfortunately, however, many problems may be encountered with this approach in both the home and the work place. In particular, the patient or the family may refuse to give up the offending pet. If symptoms are mild, this may be a reasonable decision when considering the importance of the pet to the family. When symptoms are more severe, however, compromises may no longer be appropriate and the physician's recommendations should clearly reflect that sentiment. The refusal to remove a pet from the home of a child with severe asthma and documented sensitivity to that pet should be considered tantamount to child abuse.

If a pet is removed from a home, aggressive cleaning measures should be instituted to reduce the residual allergen content as rapidly as possible. In most homes, it will take 4 to 6 months to reduce allergen levels in settled dust to a level found in homes that never housed a pet (Figure 3.1).[17] The process can be accelerated, however, by removing the major reservoirs for the allergen, particularly carpets and upholstered furniture, and by increasing ventilation. It does not appear that steam cleaning or frequent vacuuming accelerates the rate of cat allergen removal. Further, several homes have been identified with persistently elevated levels of cat allergen in spite of cat removal and routine cleaning.[17]

Some degree of avoidance may also be possible without actually removing the pet from the home. It may be possible to reduce the allergen content

Table 3.9. *Representative major animal allergens.*

Animal	Allergen	Source
Cat	*Fel d* I	Saliva, pelt
Dog	Multiple Ag's	Saliva, pelt
Rat	*Rat n* I + II	Urine
Mouse	*Mus m* I	Urine
Horse	*Equ c* I, II + III	Pelt

Table 3.10. *Environmental control: animal allergens.*

1 Remove source!

2 If source cannot be removed:
   – Limit mobility
   – Remove carpets
   – Remove upholstered furniture
   – Wash cat weekly (? for other animals)
   – ? Air filters

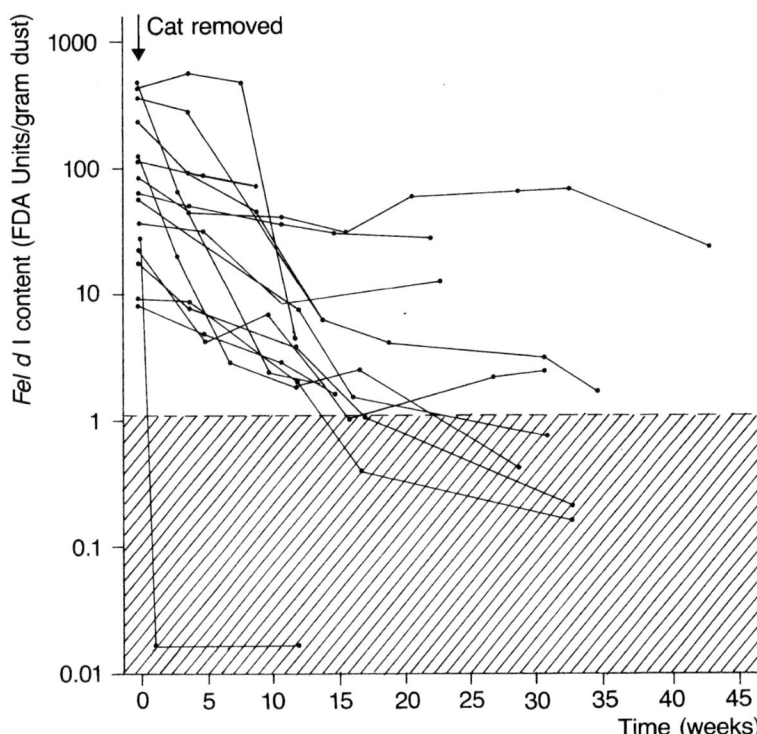

Fig. 3.1. Rate of decline of *Fel d* I in household dust samples after cat removal. From Wood RA, Chapman MD, Adkinson NF, Eggleston PA. The effect of cat removal on allergen content in household dust samples. *J Allergy Clin Immunol* 1989; *83:* 730-5.

in a particular room or area of a home by limiting the pet's access to that area, removing carpets and upholstered furniture, and increasing ventilation.[58] For cats, it has also been shown that allergen levels may be reduced by bathing the animal frequently.[58-59] Room air cleaners, particularly those using HEPA or electrostatic filters, may also be helpful. This may be particularly true for cat allergen (and any other allergen carried on relatively small particles) because the allergen will tend to remain airborne for longer periods of time and thus be more available for air filtration. The true impact of any of these measures on patient symptoms awaits further study.

Cockroach

Cockroaches have now also been shown to be sources of important indoor allergens in many areas, particularly inner city dwellings.[60-61] Major allergens from both the German (*Bla g* I and *Bla g* II) and American (*Per a* I) cockroach have now been identified and characterized.[61-62] These allergens may be located to feces, body parts, and even saliva. In homes, they appear to be widely distributed with the highest allergen levels being in kitchens and other food storage areas.

No studies on environmental control for cockroach allergens have as yet been reported. Unfortunately, there is reason to be pessimistic about the probable success of any such programs. Even though pesticides are widely available for the control of cockroaches, reinfestation is expected to be very common, particularly in the multiple unit dwellings that characterize inner city housing. In addition, cockroach body parts and feces may remain for extended periods after extermination. With our current state of knowledge, the following recommendations should be made for cockroach-sensitive patients: aggressive extermination of all units in a dwelling, careful attempts to reduce reinfestation, and good general housekeeping to help reduce sources of food for cockroaches.

Conclusion

A great deal of knowledge has been gained in recent years regarding aeroallergens and their relationships to rhinitis and other allergic diseases. Many major allergens have been identified and characterized and much has been learned regarding their aerobiology. These data are not only of academic interest but also of great practical importance. They have allowed for the production of better extracts for both diagnostic testing and immunotherapy, provided new means to study the distribution of allergens in our environment and have permitted the study and implementation of allergen-specific environmental control measures.

Although there is relatively little data available on the efficacy of allergen avoidance measures for allergic rhinitis, there is every reason to believe that they are at least as effective as those for asthma. Thus, they should be considered the first line of treatment for all patients with allergic disease. This approach has the beauty of being logical, risk-free and, in all likelihood, very effective.

References

1 Aas K. What makes an allergen an allergen. *Allergy* 1978; *33:* 3-14.
2 Solomon WR, Mathews KP. Aerobiology and inhalant allergens. In: Middleton E, Reed CE, Ellis EF, Adkinson NF; Yuninger JW, eds. *Allergy: Principles and Practice.* St. Louis: C. V. Mosby Company, 1988.
3 Marsh DG. Allergens and allergen nomenclature. In: Marsh DG and Blumenthal N, eds. *Genetic and Environmental Factors in Clinical Allergy.* Minneapolis: University of Minnesota Press, 1990.
4 Weber RW, Nelson HS. Pollen allergens and their interrelationships. *Clin Rev Allergy* 1985; *3:* 291-318.
5 Solomon WR. Aerobiology of pollinosis. *J Allergy Clin Immunol* 1984; *74:* 449-61.
6 Corn M. Assessment and control of environmental exposure. *J Allergy Clin Immunol* 1983; *72:* 231-41.
7 Solomon WR. Sampling airborne allergens. *Ann Allergy* 1984; *52:* 140-6.
8 Chapman MD. Allergen specific monoclonal antibodies: New tools for the management of allergic disease. *Allergy* 1988; *43(5):* 7-14.
9 Chapman MD, Heymann PW, Wilkins SR, Brown MB, Platts-Mills TAE. Monoclonal immunoassays for measuring major dust mite (*Dermatophagoides*) allergens, Der P I and Der f I, and quantitative analysis of the allergen content of mite and house dust extracts. *J Allergy Clin Immunol* 1987; *80:* 184-94.
10 Lind P. Enzyme linked immunosorbent assay for determination of major excrement allergens of house dust mite species *D. pteronyssinus, D. farinae,* and *D. microceras.* *Allergy* 1986; *41:* 442-50.
11 Luczynska CM, Arruda LK, Platts-Mills TAE, Miller JD, Lopez M, Chapman MD. A two-site monoclonal antibody ELISA assay for the quantitation of the major *Dermatophagoides* spp. allergens, Der P I and Der f I. *J Immunol Methods* 1989; *118:* 227-35.
12 Chapman MD, Aalberse RC, Brown MB, Platts-Mills TAE. Monoclonal antibodies to the major feline allergen Fel d I. Single step affinity purification of Fel d I and development of a sensitive two site immunoassay to assess Fel d I exposure. *J Immunol* 1988; *140:* 812-8.
13 Pollart SM, Platts-Mills TAE, Chapman MD. Identification, quantification and purification of cockroach allergens using monoclonal antibodies. *J Allergy Clin Immunol* 1989; *83:* 293.
14 Bose R, Rector ES, Fisher J, Taronno R, Delespesse G. Production and characterization of mouse monoclonal antibodies to allergenic epitopes on Lol p I. *Immunology* 1986; *59:* 309-15.
15 Pollart SM, Chapman MD, Fiocco GP, Rose G, Platts-Mills TAE. Epidemiology of acute asthma: IgE antibodies to common inhalant allergens as a risk factor for emergency room visits. *J Allergy Clin Immunol* 1989; *83:* 875-82.
16 Wood RA, Trent PA, Mudd KE, Bowes SE, Eggleston PA. Determinants of upper and lower airway responses to cat allergen. *J Allergy Clin Immunol* 1991; *87:* 169.
17 Wood RA, Chapman MD, Adkinson NF, Eggleston PA. The effect of cat removal on allergen content in household dust samples. *J Allergy Clin Immunol* 1989; *83:* 730-5.
18 Platts-Mills TAE, Hayden ML, Chapman MD, Wilkins SR. Seasonal variation in dust mite and grass pollen allergens in dust from the houses of patients with asthma. *J Allergy Clin Immunol* 1987; *79:* 781-91.
19 Chang WWY. Pollen survey. In: Paterson R, ed. *Allergic Diseases – Diagnosis and Management.* Philadelphia: J. B. Lippincott Co, 1985.
20 Burge HA. Fungus allergen. *Clin Rev Allergy* 1985; *3:* 319-29.
21 Salvaggio J, Aukrust L. Mold induced asthma. *J Allergy Clin Immunol* 1981; *68:* 327-46.
22 Voorhorst R, Spieksma FThM, Varekamp H, Leupen MJ, Lyklema AW. The house dust mite (*Dermatophagoides pteronyssinus*) and the allergen it produces: Identity with the house dust allergen. *J Allergy* 1967; *39:* 325-33.
23 Bullock JD, Frick OL. Mite sensitivity in house dust-allergic children. *Am J Dis Child* 1972; *123:* 115-23.
24 Dust mite allergens and asthma – a worldwide problem. Report of an International Workshop in Bad Kreuznach, FRG, Sept 1987. *J Allergy Clin Immunol* 1989; *83:* 416-27.
25 Platts-Mills TAE, Chapman MD. Dust mites: Immunology, allergic disease and environmental control. *J Allergy Clin Immunol* 1987; *80:* 755-77.
26 Wood RA, Eggleston, Lind BA, et al. Antigenic analysis of household dust samples. *Am Rev Respir Dis* 1988; *137:* 358-63.
27 Smith TF, Kelly LB, Heymann PW, Wilkins SR, Platts-Mills TAE. Natural exposure and serum antibodies to house dust mite of mite allergic children with asthma in Atlanta. *J Allergy Clin Immunol* 1985; *76:* 782-8.
28 Tovey ER, Chapman MD, Wells CW, Platts-Mills TAE. The distribution of dust mite allergen in the houses of patients with asthma. *Am Rev Respir Dis* 1981; *124:* 630-5.
29 Arlian LG, Bernstein IL, Gallagher JS. The prevalence of dust mites, *Dermatophagoides* spp., and associated environmental conditions in homes in Ohio. *J Allergy Clin Immunol* 1982; *69:* 527-32.
30 Korsgard J. Mite asthma and residency. *Am Rev Respir Dis* 1983; *128:* 231-5.
31 Vervolet D, Penaud A, Razzouk H, et al. Altitude and house dust mites. *J Allergy Clin Immunol* 1982; *69:* 290-5.
32 Charpin D, Kleisbauer JP, Lanteaume A. Asthma and allergy to house dust mites in patients living in high altitude. *Chest* 1988; *93:* 758-66.
33 Moyer DB, Nelson HS, Arlian LG. House dust mites in Colorado. *Ann Allergy* 1985; *55:* 680-2.
34 Lind P. Purification and partial characterization of two major allergens from the house dust mite *Dermatophagoides pteronyssinus.* *J Allergy Clin Immunol* 1985; *76:* 753-61.
35 Yasueda H, Mita H, Yui Y, Shida T. Isolation and characterization of two allergens from *Dermatophagoides farinae.* *Int Arch Allergy Appl Immunol* 1986; *81:* 214-23.

36. Arlina LG, Bernstein IL, Geis DP, Vyszenski-Moher DL, Gallagher JS, Martin B. Investigations of culture medium-free house dust mites. III. Antigens and allergens of body and fecal extract of *Dermatophagoides farinae*. *J Allergy Clin Immunol* 1987; *79:* 457-66.
37. Platts-Mills TAE, Heymann PW, Longbottom JL, Wilkins SR. Airborne allergens associated with asthma: particle sizes carrying dust mite and rat allergens measured with a cascade impactor. *J Allergy Clin Immunol* 1986; *77:* 850-7.
38. Sarsfield JK, Gowland G, Toy R, Normal AL. Mite-sensitive asthma of childhood: A trial of avoidance measures. *Arch Dis Child* 1974; *49:* 711-6.
39. Murray AB, Ferguson AC. Dust-free bedrooms in the treatment of asthmatic children with house dust mite allergy: A controlled trial. *Pediatrics* 1983; *71:* 418-24.
40. Korsgard J. Preventative measures in house dust allergy. *Am Rev Respir Dis* 1982; *125:* 80-6.
41. Walshaw MJ, Evans CC. Allergen avoidance in house dust mite-sensitive adult asthma. *Q J Med* 1986; *58:* 199-215.
42. Burr ML, Dean BV, Merrett TG, Neale E, St Leger AS, Verrier-Jones ER. Effects of anti-mite measures on children with mite sensitive asthma: A controlled trial. *Thorax* 1980; *35:* 506-12.
43. Mitchell EB, Wilkins Sr, Deighton JM, Platts-Mills TAE. Reduction of house dust allergen levels in the home: Use of acaricide pirimphos methyl. *Clin Allergy* 1985; *15:* 235-40.
44. de St Georges-Gridelet D. Optimal efficacy of a fungicide preparation, natamycin, in the control of the house dust mite, *Dermatophagoides pteronyssinus*. *Exp Appl Acarol* 1988; *4(1):* 63-72.
45. Lau-Schadendorf S, Rusche AF, Weber AK, Buettner-Goetz P, Wahn U. Short-term effect of solidified benzyl benzoate on mite-allergen concentrations in house dust. *J Allergy Clin Immunol* 1991; *87:* 41-7.
46. Ohman JL, Lorusso JR, Lewis S. Cat allergen content of commercial house dust extracts. *J Allergy Clin Immunol* 1987; *79:* 955-9.
47. Gross NJ. Allergy to laboratory animals: Epidemiologic, clinical, and physiologic aspects. *J Allergy Clin Immunol* 1980; *66:* 158-62.
48. Leiterman K, Ohman JL. Cat allergen I: Biochemical, antigenic, and allergenic properties. *J Allergy Clin Immunol* 1984; *74:* 147-53.
49. Anderson MC, Baer H, Ohman JL. A comparative study of the allergens of cat urine, serum, saliva, and pelt. *J Allergy Clin Immunol* 1985; *76:* 563-70.
50. Larsen JN, Ford A, Gjesing B. The collaborative study of the international standard of dog, *Canis domesticus*, hair/dander extract. *J Allergy Clin Immunol* 1988; *82:* 318-24.
51. Lindgren S, Belin L, Dreborg S, Inarsson RE, Pahlman I. Breed-specific dog-dandruff allergens. *J Allergy Clin Immunol* 1988; *82:* 196-201.
52. Walls AF, Longbottom J. Comparison of rat fur, urine, saliva, and other rat allergen extracts by skin testing, RAST and RAST inhibition. *J Allergy Clin Immunol* 1985; *75:* 242-9.
53. Price JA, Longbottom JL. Allergy to mice: Identification of two major mouse allergens (Ag 1 and Ag 3) and investigations of their possible origin. *Clin Allergy* 1987; *15:* 241-50.
54. Bartholome K, Kisler W, Baer H. Where does cat allergen come from? *J Allergy Clin Immunol* 1985; *76:* 503-8.
55. Luczynska CM, Li Y, Chapman MD, Platts-Mills TAE. Airborne concentrations and particle size distribution of allergen derived from domestic cats. *Am Rev Respir Dis* 1990; *141:* 361-7.
56. Corn M, Koegel A, Hall T. Characterization of airborne particles associated with animal allergy in laboratory workers. *Ann Occup Hyg* 1988; *32:* 435.
57. Wood RA, Mudd KE, Eggleston PA. The distribution of cat and dust mite allergens on wall surfaces. *J Allergy Clin Immunol* (in press).
58. DeBlay R, Chapman MD, Platts-Mills TAE. Airborne cat allergen (*Fel d* I): Environmental control with the cat *in situ*. Am Rev Respir Dis 1991; *143:* 1334-9.
59. Glinert R, Wilson P, Wedner HJ. *Fel d* I is markedly reduced following sequential washings of cats. *J Allergy Clin Immunol* 1990; *85:* 225.
60. Pollart SM, Smith TF, Morris EC, Gelber LE, Platts-Mills TAE, Chapman MD. Environmental exposure to cockroach allergens: Analysis with monoclonal antibody-based enzyme immunoassays. *J Allergy Clin Immunol* 1991; *87:* 505-10.
61. Schou C, Fernandez-Caldas E, Lockey RF, Løwenstein H. Environmental assay for cockroach allergens. *J Allergy Clin Immunol* 1991; *87:* 828-34.
62. Pollart SM, Mullins DE, Vailes LD, et al. Identification, quantitation, and purification of cockroach allergens using monoclonal antibodies. *J Allergy Clin Immunol* 1991; *87:* 511-21.

CHAPTER 4

Air pollution

REBECCA BASCOM

Introduction

Adults breathe 10-20,000 liters of air a day, the majority of which passes through the nose. Air pollution research initially focused on the lungs and dismissed the nose as part of the pulmonary "dead space". However, the nose is ideally suited to filter particles, remove vapors and condition inhaled air. These properties protect the lung from air pollution but make the nose a target. Recent studies demonstrate that some air pollutants cause irritation and drying, alter nasal resistance, reduce mucociliary clearance and induce inflammation. Pollutants may also alter specific immune responses to viruses or antigens. Pre-existing disease or differential sensitivity affect the individual response to pollutants.

It is estimated that 40-50 million Americans have chronic rhinitis. A specific etiologic diagnosis of rhinitis is not clear in approximately ⅔ of all patients, which is a measure of our current ignorance of the pathogenetic mechanisms in many forms of chronic rhinitis.[1] Continued study is therefore needed to determine whether and how pollutant exposure contributes to common nasal diseases in humans.

This chapter will summarize the types and causes of air pollution, sources of information about the health effects of air pollutants, and the direct and indirect effects of air pollution on the nose. Readers interested in occupational upper respiratory disease are referred to a recent chapter.[2]

Air pollution: types and sources

The atmosphere contains 20.94% oxygen, 0.04% carbon dioxide, 78.03% nitrogen and 0.99% inert gases.[3] "Air pollutants" are present in much smaller quantities, yet are so termed because they exert effects at very low concentrations. Ground-level ozone, for example, causes health effects at concentrations between 0.08 and 0.12 parts per million. Table 4.1 summarizes sources and types of air pollution.

Outdoor air pollution

Many chemicals are released into the air each year as by-products of people's activities and the industries that support them. Early air sampling identified a few major pollutants and these have been the focus of most regulations.[4] For these major "criteria pollutants", legal limits to air pollution are established based on scientific evidence of the health effects. In the United States, criteria pollutants are ozone, carbon monoxide, sulfur dioxide, total suspended particulates, nitrogen oxides, and lead. There is also a host of "air toxides" for which legal limits do not exist. The most recent strategy has been to mandate that industries use "maximum achievable control technology" to reduce these emissions.

Ozone. From late spring to early fall, photochemical smog in many regions is dominated by ground-level ozone. It has been stated that ozone "is arguably the most politically and economically intractable environmental problem" facing the United States.[5] Ground-level ozone is generated by a complex photochemical reaction between volatile organic compounds (VOC's), oxides of nitrogen (NO_x) and sunlight. The reaction between ozone precursors and sunlight takes place over several hours so that ozone levels rise, beginning in the late morning, several hours after the morning rush

Table 4.1. *Types and sources of air pollution.*

Name	Sources	Location
Ozone (ground level)	cars, industrial emissions personal products (+sunlight) photocopiers	outdoors in warm populous regions offices
Sulfur dioxide	power plants fossil fuel combustion	near point sources
Environmental tobacco smoke	smokers	home, workplace
Formaldehyde	furnishings, glues	offices, homes
Volatile organic mixtures	furnishings building materials personal products cleaning materials	new or remodeled indoor sites homes or offices
Wood smoke	wood stoves	homes
Oxides of nitrogen	gas stoves, kerosene heaters automobile exhaust	homes
Allergens	cats, rodents, cockroaches dust mites	homes homes
Bioaerosols	moist ventilation systems buildings with leaks/standing water	homes, offices

hour. The highest concentrations of ground-level ozone in the United States occur in southern California. Prevailing winds may transport the air pollution to nearby regions. In the eastern United States, summer winds transport ozone in a northeasterly direction, and ozone air pollution is a regional problem stretching from northern Virginia to Maine. Over 100 million Americans are exposed to concentrations in excess of the current United States ambient air quality standard of 0.12 parts per million.

Ground level ozone (currently present in excess) should be clearly distinguished from stratospheric ozone (currently being depleted). Halogenated hydrocarbons used by people and industries escape up to the stratosphere, react with stratospheric ozone, and result in a depletion of the so-called "ozone layer". Stratospheric ozone, located 31 miles above the earth's surface, serves as a protective filter to block ultraviolet light. Ground-level (tropospheric) ozone is present in the air which people breathe and is also known as "summertime smog". Its sources and health effects are discussed below.

Outdoor ozone air pollution comes from three major source categories: point (stationary) sources, area sources and mobile sources. These designations are useful since remedial strategies may be different for each. Mobile sources are primarily cars. Point sources are large industrial sources, and are often easiest to identify and target for control measures. Area sources are more difficult to control since they include consumer products such as oil-based paints. The relative contribution of these three source categories can vary tremendously. In the eastern United States, mobile sources emit well over half the volatile organic compounds that result in ground level ozone air pollution. In contrast, the nitrogen oxide (NO_x) emissions are predominantly from point sources such as power plants, although mobile sources contribute about one-third of the total. Recent studies suggest that controlling NO_x emissions will be critical to reducing ozone air pollution.

Particles. Particulate air pollution has been associated with increased morbidity and mortality especially in the elderly and those with preexisting respiratory diseases.[6] Sources of particulates include point sources, such as utility plants and quarries, and fugitive sources such as unpaved parking lots. Particles can vary tremendously in their composition, and may serve as an adsorbtive surface for gaseous materials.

Sulfur dioxide. Sulfur dioxide is generated primarily from utility plants and other processing of sulfur-containing fossil fuels. The grade of coal or the type of fuel which is burned will influence the sulfur dioxide concentration of the emissions. This pollutant is ubiquitous, but levels in the air are highest in the vicinity of point sources and in the indoor air of homes heated with kerosene space heaters.[7]

The historic air pollution epidemics in London, in Belgium, and in the United States occurred in the winter and were combinations of particles and sulfur and acidic aerosols which failed to dissipate because of a thermal inversion. These were associated with increased deaths due to respiratory illnesses. In one report, 88% of patients with asthma experienced exacerbation during the pollution episode in Donora, Pennsylvania in 1948.[7]

Indoor air pollution

Pollutants found in the indoor environment may originate in the building's primary structural materials, its heating, ventilation or air conditioning system, or its furnishings. Secondary contamination of the indoor environment can arise from human activities, from outdoor pollutant infiltration, from indoor combustion products, from animal or arthropod infestation, or from accumulation of bioaerosols. Each of these sources will be briefly discussed below.

Air sampling of new buildings shows a host of volatile organic compounds (VOC's) derived from the off-gassing of structural materials and furnishings.[8] The air concentrations of VOC's usually decrease rapidly over the first 1-2 years of a building's existence. The TEAM Study, performed in the 1980's by the United States Environmental Protection Agency, documented the existence of exposure to multiple VOCs in the indoor environment.[9] Unexpectedly, exposures to VOCs were significantly higher indoors than outdoors, even in heavily industrialized regions like Northern New Jersey. Personal activities strongly influenced the exposure profile.

Formaldehyde is still frequently found in indoor environments, not from insulation but from sources such as fabrics. Duct work in some buildings may be lined with fiberglass. Itching related to dermal exposure to the fiberglass has been reported, and fiberglass, if moist, can serve as reservoir for bioaerosols. Other studies have shown that improper maintenance procedures can cause exposure to mucosal irritants. For example, carpets which are not properly rinsed after shampooing may contain a residue of the irritant sodium laurel sulfate.[10]

Approximately 30% of Americans smoke, and 40% of homes have at least one smoker.[11] Environmental tobacco smoke is therefore a dominant indoor air pollutant, despite increasing restrictions in public places and worksites. Tobacco smoke is a complex mixture of over 3,000 compounds. These can be grouped into the particle phase (a semiaerosol dispersion of tar), nicotine and the organic vapor phase which contains potent irritants such as aldehydes.[12] Smoke which is bubbled through media is rich in oxidants.

Outdoor air pollutants enter the indoor environment through ventilation systems or by infiltration. If the intake duct for a building's ventilation system is positioned near a loading dock or parking lot, exhaust fumes including carbon monoxide may be dispersed through the building. The indoor environment usually reduces the concentrations of outdoor pollutants so that ozone and sulfur dioxide are usually 2- to 5-fold lower inside than outside. There are, however, indoor point sources for ozone, including poorly ventilated photocopiers.

The oldest form of indoor air pollution is smoke from fires intended for warmth or food preparation. Combustion products continue to be a source of indoor air pollution. Indoor nitrogen dioxide levels are determined primarily by gas stoves and kerosene heaters. Wood stoves are a source of particulate pollution and aldehydes.

Animal or arthropod infestation is a source of indoor allergen exposure. Proteins derived from rodents and cockroaches are recognized to be important urban allergens and cat allergen is an important suburban allergen. Dust mites proliferate in carpets, beddings and upholstery. These allergens have been shown to play a key role in chronic asthma; their relative importance in chronic rhinitis is less well established, since Turkletaub et al[13] failed to find a relationship between chronic rhinitis and skin test reactivity to house dust extracts.

"Bioaerosols" is broad term describing all materials in the indoor environment which are alive or derive from living materials. These include a diverse array of molds, fungi, and bacteria and their products, such as glucans and lipopolysaccharides. These agents proliferate when water leaks have occurred or standing water is present in ventilation systems. It is currently thought that these agents primarily function as antigens, inducing allergic illness in selected individuals.[10]

Seventy years ago, indoor air ventilation guidelines were established based on the ventilation rates needed to control body odor. In the 1970's, however, the energy crisis resulted in a shift in emphasis to energy conservation and a marked reduction in ventilation rates. There was a simultaneous change in office decor, furniture and equipment. Carpets became common, fabric-covered partitions were often installed, cushioned chairs became common, and the office was automated with computers, printers and copiers. The outbreak of building-related complaints resulted in a reconsideration of ventilation standards. The American Society of Heating, Refrigeration and Air Conditioning Engineers promulgated new standards in 1989 which significantly increased recommended ventilation rates, including a recommended 20 cubic foot/min (0.57 m^3/min) of outside air per person in an office.[14]

Sources of information about the health effects of air pollution

Information about the health effects of pollutants is derived from four sources: epidemiologic studies, animal studies, *in vitro* studies, and short-term human exposure studies. Advantages and disadvantages of each information source are summarized in Table 4.2. Epidemiologic studies of humans in their natural environment are most compelling, but also the most expensive to perform. It is difficult to assess the response to a single pollutant in epidemiologic studies because simultaneous exposure to many pollutants may occur. Few epidemiologic studies of the effect of pollutants on the human nose have been performed. Excellent acute and chronic nasal air pollution studies using animals have been performed;[15] however, significant cross-species differences in anatomic, physiologic and biochemical factors complicate extrapolation to humans.[16] One of the findings from animal studies has been that effects of pollutant inhalation in the nose are non-uniform.[17] Recent *in vitro* studies have begun to explore the cellular response to air pollutants. Cultures of airway epithelium or macrophages can be exposed to pollutants under controlled conditions.[18, 19] Human exposure studies have the advantage of carefully controlled exposures and outcome measures, and the disadvantage of relatively short exposure periods. These studies have traditionally used nasal symptoms, resistance and mucociliary clearance as outcome measures.[20] The technique of nasal lavage has allowed a new look at the acute inflammatory response to common air pollutants in humans.[21, 22, 23]

The overall assessment of the effect of a pollutant on human health requires an integration of information from all available sources. Traditional risk assessment has emphasized relatively rare endpoints such as cancer and virtually ignored far more common conditions such as rhinitis.

The response to an air pollutant: determinants and host defense

Many factors affect the response of the nose to an air pollutant. The dose of the pollutant is critically

Table 4.2. *Sources of information about the health effects of air pollution.*

	Advantages	Disadvantages
Animal studies	Long-term exposure possible Detailed pathology possible Mechanistic studies possible	Must extrapolate to humans
Epidemiologic studies	"Real life" exposures	Many confounding factors Complex, expensive
Human exposure studies	Relevant species Can study biologic variability Careful control of exposures	Limited duration Limited outcome measures

important and is determined by the pollutant concentration, the duration of exposure, the magnitude (rate and depth) of ventilation, and the nasal-oral partitioning of the inhaled airstream. The fraction of an ambient pollutant which is removed by the nose depends on the physical characteristics of the pollutant and the geometry of the individual nose. Nasal deposition increases with particle size, ventilation flow rates and nasal resistance. In a recent study of adults and children inhaling particles from 1-3 μm in diameter, the average deposition percentages were surprisingly similar in children and adults. The lower total ventilation rates in children offset the smaller nose dimensions.[24]

The water solubility of vapor-phase pollutants influences their removal by the nose. Water-soluble gases like sulfur dioxide are almost entirely cleared by the nose during tidal breathing.[25] Less soluble gases such as ozone still undergo significant clearance by the nose.[26] Because of these complexities, methods continue to be developed to directly measure nasal and lung uptake of inhaled vapors.[27]

The nose is an efficient filter for particles. The majority of naturally occurring dusts are deposited in the nose, or exhaled without being deposited.[20] In one study, 45% of smaller particles (<1.8 μm) were removed by the nose while 80% of larger particles (>12 μm) were removed.[28] The deposition characteristics can be determined by the physical size, shape, density and hygroscopicity of a particle. At higher humidity, an increased fraction of an aerosol will deposit in the nose. The mechanisms of particle deposition in the respiratory tract was reviewed extensively by Brain & Valberg.[29] In the anterior nose, particles are captured by the vibrissae or the squamous epithelium, and are expelled through sneezing or wiping. Particles which are deposited on the pseudostratified ciliated columnar epithelium are removed posteriorly by mucociliary transport.

The immune system defends against foreign substances through two types of response: natural immunity and specific (acquired) immunity.[30] Specific immunity is induced through recognition of specific antigens and variability in the host response due to acquired immunity is well-recognized. Air pollutants are not antigenic, so the host response is mediated through the so-called natural immune response. The components of natural immunity which participate in host defense include the mucous membranes (airway epithelium and mucus), complement, phagocytes and their soluble mediators. Variability in the response to air pollutants is increasingly being demonstrated, although the basis for the variability is still poorly understood. In one study, the average flow through the adult nose was 20 l/min, but ranged from 13-25 l/min. Furthermore, nasal mucous flow in normal subjects ranged almost 50-fold, from 2 cm/min to <0.05 cm/min.[28] Intriguing studies show a relationship between low baseline mucous flow rates, and discomfort and ciliostasis induced by SO_2 exposure.[31] It has recently been shown that anti-oxidant is present in nasal lavage fluid, but the role which this plays in the response to oxidant air pollutants is unknown.[32] Irritant neurons also play a role in host defense and interstrain differences in irritant-induced inhibition of respiratory rate have been reported. The nose has a tremendous capacity for xenobiotic metabolism, as was recently extensively reviewed.[33] Genetic differences in one or more of these systems may be important in host variability to air pollutants.

Pre-existing nasal disease might be expected to alter the host response to air pollution, although this has been studied very little. Diseases which result in nasal congestion could alter particle deposition or vapor removal. Ciliary activity may be affected by prior pollutant exposure.[15] Conditions which reduce mucociliary transport could result in prolonged residence time of particles or antigens. Similarly, the effect of non-pathogenic alterations in the quantity or quality of nasal surface fluid could alter the response to pollutants.

Direct effects of pollutants on the nose

Early studies at the University of Aarhus focused on the structure and function of the normal nose under controlled climatic conditions. These are extensively reviewed elsewhere.[20] Changes in the relative humidity of ambient air had no effect on airflow resistance, and mild changes in temperature did not alter nasal resistance. Exercise decreased nasal resistance. Prolonged exposure to very dry air did not alter nasal resistance or mucociliary transport.[34]

Dust

The effects of inert dust on the nose have been studied in controlled chamber studies. Healthy young adults were exposed to inert dust, up to 25 mg/m^3, for 6 hours. Discomfort was reported which was proportional to the concentration of dust, and lagged almost 2 hours behind the changes in dust concentration (Fig. 4.1). The discomfort was rated as "slight", i.e. 20 on a 100-point scale, with exposure to 25 mg/m^3 of dust. However, the maximum discomfort rating was 45/100. The main specific complaints were dryness in the nose and pharynx. Of the 16 subjects, 4 reported dryness after 2 mg/m^3; 10 reported dryness after 10 mg/m^3 and 13 had dryness after 25 mg/m^3. Interestingly, these exposures produced no change in nasal resistance or nasal mucociliary clearance rate.[28] These data suggest that the symptom of dryness may reflect effects other than a decrease in mucociliary clearance. Other investigators have demonstrated ciliostasis in woodworkers exposed to wood dust.[35] The chamber studies suggest that ciliostasis from wood dust is not a dust effect, but occurs in response to another pollutant which may be present in the dust.

Ozone

Ozone is frequently described as a relatively insoluble gas which exerts its main effect in the smaller airways of the lung. Studies by Gerrity recently demonstrated 40% removal of ozone by the extrathoracic airway in the upper respiratory tract of humans, with only modest differences in removal efficiency occurring with different ozone concentrations, modes of breathing and breathing frequencies.[26] In dogs, Yokoyama & Frank showed that changes in nasal congestion and vascularity induced by histamine or phenylephrine did not significantly alter the fractional uptake of ozone.[36]

Human challenge studies show that ozone inhalation (0.4 ppm, 2 hours, intermittent mild exercise) blocks the decongestant effect of exercise in non-allergic subjects.[37] In normal adults, a neutrophil influx occurs with exposure to 0.5 ppm ozone for 4 hours at rest or to 0.4 ppm ozone for 2 hours with exercise.[38, 39] Elevated nasal lavage albumin concentrations were also demonstrated, indicating vascular leakage, or altered albumin flux at the epithelial surface.[39] In subjects with a history of seasonal allergic rhinitis (studied out of season), high-level ozone exposure (0.5 ppm, 4 hours, at rest) induced a mixed inflammatory cell influx including neutrophils, eosinophils and mononuclear cells as well as an increase in nasal lavage albumin concentration (Fig. 4.2).[22]

Twenty-four hours after ozone exposure, several effects have been observed. In non-allergic subjects, a nearly 50% reduction in nasal surface fluid occurs in the anterior nasal septum, while methacholine reactivity increases.[40] Neutrophils in nasal lavage

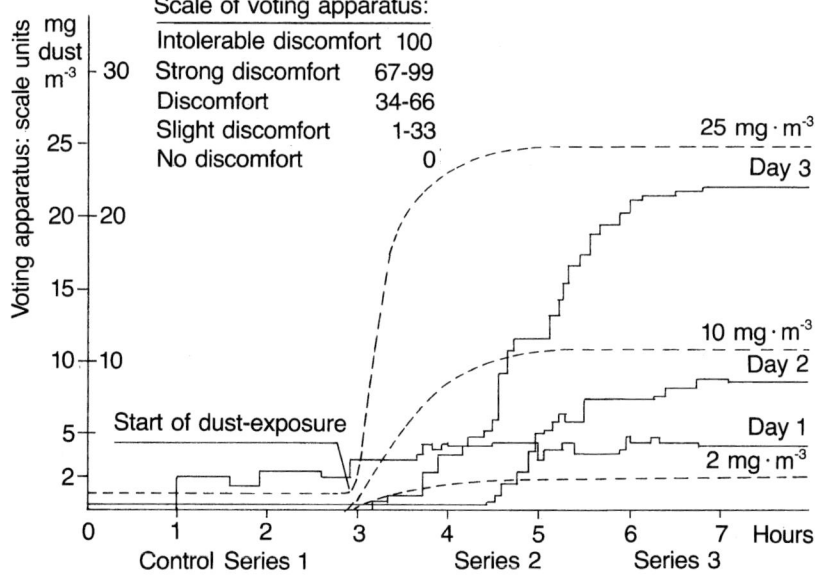

Fig. 4.1. Exposure to inert dust is associated with symptoms of dryness which begin 2 hours after exposure. From Andersen I, Lundqvist GR, Proctor DF, Swift DL. Human response to controlled levels of inert dust. Am Rev Respir Dis 1979; 119: 619-27.

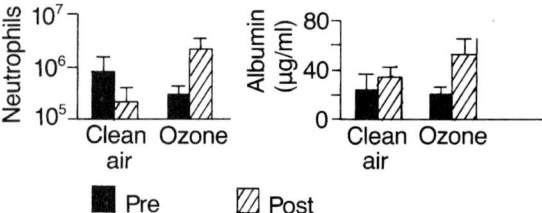

Fig. 4.2. Ozone exposure is associated with an inflammatory cell influx and increased nasal lavage albumin. From Bascom R, Naclerio RM, Fitzgerald TK, Kagey-Sobotka A, Proud D. Effect of ozone inhalation on the response to nasal challenge with antigen of allergic subjects. *Am Rev Respir Dis* 1990; *142:* 594-601.

fluid are 6-fold above clean air values.[39] The concentrations used in these studies occur only in Southern California; exposure to concentrations between 0.08 ppm and 0.16 ppm occurs much more widely in the United States. Recent studies have shown a neutrophil influx and elevations with interleukin 8 in nasal lavage fluid of subjects exposed to these lower ozone concentrations (J. Koenig, personal communication).

Studies of the effects of ambient ozone levels on the nasal mucosa have been performed in macaque monkeys. Monkeys were exposed to 0, 0.15 or 0.3 ppm ozone for 6 or 90 days, 8 hours/day. Light and electron microscopic evaluation showed quantitative changes in the nasal transitional and respiratory epithelium. At 6 or 90 days of exposure to 0.15 or 0.3 ppm, ozone lesions consisted of ciliated cell necrosis, shortened cilia, and secretory cell hyperplasia. Inflammatory cell influx was only present at 6 days of exposure. Ultrastructural changes in goblet cells were evident at 90 days. *In vitro* studies have demonstrated that exposure of tracheal epithelial cells to ozone results in release of arachidonic acid metabolites at concentrations as low as 0.1 parts per million.[19] These data suggest that commonly encountered concentrations of ozone may induce nasal inflammation or alter nasal mucosal biology. Epidemiologic studies have not addressed the effect of ozone on the nose.

Sulfur dioxide

Challenge studies with sulfur dioxide have produced variable results. A 30% increase in the nasal work of breathing occurred with exposure of adolescent asthmatics to sulfur dioxide (0.5 ppm for 30 minutes at rest followed by 10 minuts exposure with exercise) compared to a sham air exposure.[41] The increase in nasal resistance occurred with exposure to SO_2 by facemask as well as by mouthpiece. This raises the interesting possibility that pulmonary exposures can alter the dimensions of the nasal cavity. Exposure to an aerosol of sulfuric acid did not alter the nasal work of breathing. In a separate study, pre-treatment with chlorpheniramine blocked the increased resistance.[42] Tam et al[43] exposed adult subjects with allergic rhinitis for 10 minutes to 4 ppm SO_2 and found no increase in nasal airway resistance. Nasal resistance also did not change in asthmatic subjects who had previously demonstrated bronchoconstriction with SO_2 inhalation.[43] These results suggest that hyperresponsiveness to sulfur dioxide is not uniform throughout the respiratory tract.

Studies in the 1970's determined the effect of longer, higher concentrations of sulfur dioxide on normal volunteers. Sixteen young men were studied for 6-hour exposures to 1, 5, and 25 ppm sulfur dioxide at rest.[31] At the end of the 5 ppm exposure, 5/16 complained about dryness in the nose and pharynx while 10/16 had dryness after 25 ppm SO_2. One week later, 5 subjects still had a feeling of dryness. There was a significant decrease in nasal mucous flow rate. This decrease was greatest in the anterior nose, and was greatest in subjects with an initially slow mucous flow rate (Fig. 4.3). With 3 hours' exposure to 1 ppm SO_2, mucous flow in the middle of the nose was 20% below baseline. After 6 hours' exposure mucous flow was 50% below baseline.[31] Mucous flow was further reduced at higher levels of exposure. Nasal resistance increased at all concentrations, with an 11% drop in estimated nasal cross-sectional area at 1 ppm SO_2. The authors noted that 27% of their subjects reported upper respiratory infection during the week following the study compared with 8% of subjects exposed to dry air in an earlier study. Exposure to a combination of SO_2 and inert dust showed that the effects of these two pollutants were additive, not synergistic.[44]

Formaldehyde

Formaldehyde is a well-recognized upper respiratory irritant, and nasal tumors have been demonstrated in animal studies.[45] Epidemiologic studies have shown an increase in nasal squamous meta-

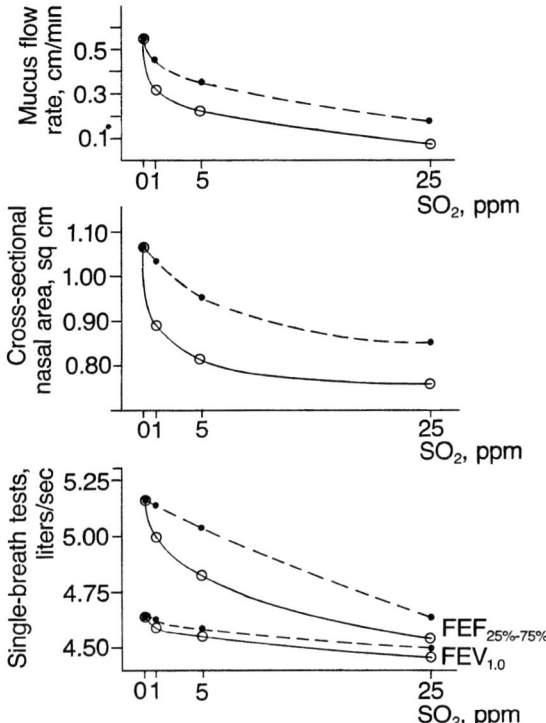

Fig. 4.3 Six-hour exposure to sulfur dioxide decreases mucociliary clearance and increases nasal resistance. From Andersen I, Lundqvist GR, Jensen PL, Proctor F. Human response to controlled levels of sulfur dioxide. *Arch Environ Health* 1974; *28:* 31-9.

plasia in some occupants of homes insulated with formaldehyde.[46] The metaplasia was found in the subset of residents who wanted to move out of their home, and was associated with excess upper respiratory symptoms. Nasal resistance and patch tests to formaldehyde were not different between the two groups.

Volatile organic compounds

Mølhave[8] selected a mixture for challenge studies which was representative of the VOC mixtures found in new buildings in Denmark. His initial studies showed that controlled exposure to a representative mixture of volatile organic compounds caused upper respiratory irritant symptoms in individuals with a history of "sick building syndrome".[47] Subsequent studies have confirmed that upper respiratory irritation occurs in normal Danish individuals as well.[48] While a neutrophil influx was demonstrated in tear fluid following exposure to the VOC mixture, these investigators did not see a nasal neutrophil influx.[48] Koren et al[49] performed challenge studies using the Mølhave mixture at a concentration of 25 mg/m^3 in healthy American subjects. They demonstrated symptoms of mucosal irritation and an increase in nasal lavage neutrophils. The number of neutrophils was 2-fold above clean air controls immediately post-exposure and 9-fold above clean air controls 18 hours post-exposure. Nasal lavage neutrophils have also been demonstrated in a small group of people occupying a newly carpeted office.[51] Studies of the "office eye syndrome" have demonstrated increased tear-film breakup and early corneal ulcerations in some individuals.[50]

Indoor environments: sick building syndrome

The World Health Organization definition of the sick building syndrome included irritation of the eyes, nose and throat, dry mucous membranes and skin.[52] Epidemiologic studies have tried to determine the causes of building-related upper respiratory symptoms. Three major epidemiologic studies in the mid 1980's profiled health complaints of over 9,000 people and building characteristics of over 50 buildings.[10] In one or more studies, symptoms increased in buildings with a higher occupancy rate, with the use of carbonless copy paper, with high estimated office surface areas, and with high fleece factors (perhaps reflecting the presence of a surface onto which irritants or bioaerosols could adsorb). Buildings with natural ventilation had lower symptom rates than those with mechanical systems which used chillers and humidifiers. Women had higher symptom rates than men and clerical/secretarial workers had higher rates than managers. These and other epidemiologic studies have shown a variable prevalence of mucosal symptoms in office buildings. The prevalence of upper respiratory symptoms in building occupants ranges from 5% to 50-60%, and is often around 20%. In one study, 50% of building occupants reported upper respiratory symptoms which "sometimes, often or always begin at work".[53] A smaller group (15-17%) had upper respiratory symptoms which "often or always begin at work".[53]

The occurrence of irritant symptoms in the office setting poses significant practical problems for clinicians. Patients may complain bitterly of their symptoms and report that associated fatigue and difficulty in concentrating are impairing work performance. Psychosocial disruption may well occur. Workers may ask that their workplace be investigated, and supervisors may be evasive, unresponsive or without resources. In these complicated conditions, the physician must judge whether the patient is a reliable reporter of the symptoms. Signs of illness may be absent when the usual screening tests are performed.[10] Most physicians do not have access to the most basic information about their patient's workplace. "Mass hysteria" is probably the cause of only a relatively small number of cases of building-related symptoms.[10] However, specific causal agents are often not identified. The consequences of continued symptomatic exposure in the indoor environment are largely undefined. Work recommendations are therefore difficult to establish. The concern has been raised that some few individuals who remain in buildings despite experiencing mucosal symptoms may develop progressive mucosal irritation, and intolerance of an increasing array of common substances. Objective measures to corroborate these "multiple chemical sensitivity" symptoms are lacking at present, as is a fundamental understanding of the nature of this problem.[54]

Environmental tobacco smoke

Environmental tobacco smoke (ETS) is defined as the combination of the smoke which issues from the burning end of the cigarette (sidestream tobacco smoke, STS) and exhaled mainstream smoke. It is therefore the smoke which nonsmokers inhale. ETS is a well-recognized mucosal irritant, with symptoms occurring at concentrations as low as 1-3 ppm carbon monoxide in controlled challenge studies.[55, 56] Patients often report being "allergic to tobacco smoke", because they have congestion or rhinorrhea with smoke exposure. Speer[57] reported a history of ETS-related nasal symptoms in 67% of a group of 191 allergic patients and 29% of a group of 250 non-allergic patients. More recently, 34% of a group of healthy young adults unselected for allergy reported a history of one or more rhinitis symptoms with tobacco smoke exposure.[23] Subjects were chosen for further study who had a history of ETS-rhinitis (ETS-sensitive) and those with no history of ETS-rhinitis (ETS-nonsensitive). Controlled challenge with a brief, high level of sidestre-

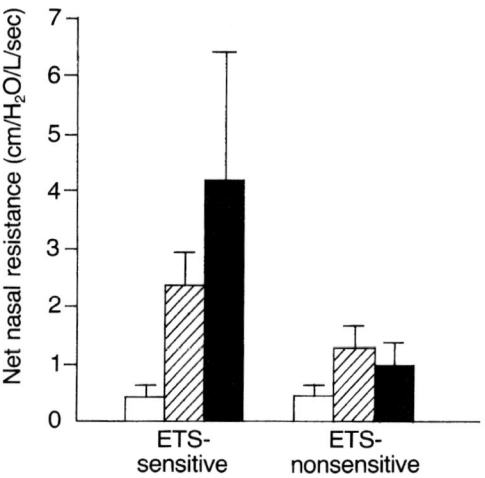

Fig. 4.4. Exposure to environmental tobacco smoke increases nasal resistance in historically sensitive subjects. From Bascom R, Kulle T, Kagey-Sobotka A, Proud D. Upper respiratory tract environmental tobacco smoke sensitivity. *Am Rev Respir Dis* 1991; *143:* 1304-11.

am tobacco smoke (45 ppm carbon monoxide, 15 minutes) caused a significant increase in nasal resistance in the subjects with a history of ETS sensitivity, but not in ETS-nonsensitive individuals (Fig. 4.4).[23] Nasal lavage studies on a separate day showed no increase in the concentration of histamine (indicating a lack of mast cell activation), no increase in kinins or albumin (indicating a lack of vascular extravasation) and no increase in TAME-esterase activity (indicating no significant glandular activation) (Fig. 4.5). These data provide evidence for ETS sensitivity occurring by a mechanism other than IgE allergy, and suggest that vascular congestion is responsible for the increased nasal resistance.

Dose-response studies have subsequently shown that prolonged, 2-hour, exposures to lower doses of sidestream tobacco smoke cause increases in nasal resistance and decreases in nasal volume as determined by acoustic rhinometry.[56] These effects have been observed in both ETS-sensitive and ETS-nonsensitive subjects.

In rats, exposure to tobacco smoke causes an acute increase in vascular permeability of the upper respiratory tract. Exposure to the organic vapor fraction of the tobacco smoke (with the particles and nicotine removed) caused a similar response. In contrast, local anesthesia, neonatal capsaicin and substance P antagonists blocked the response.[58]

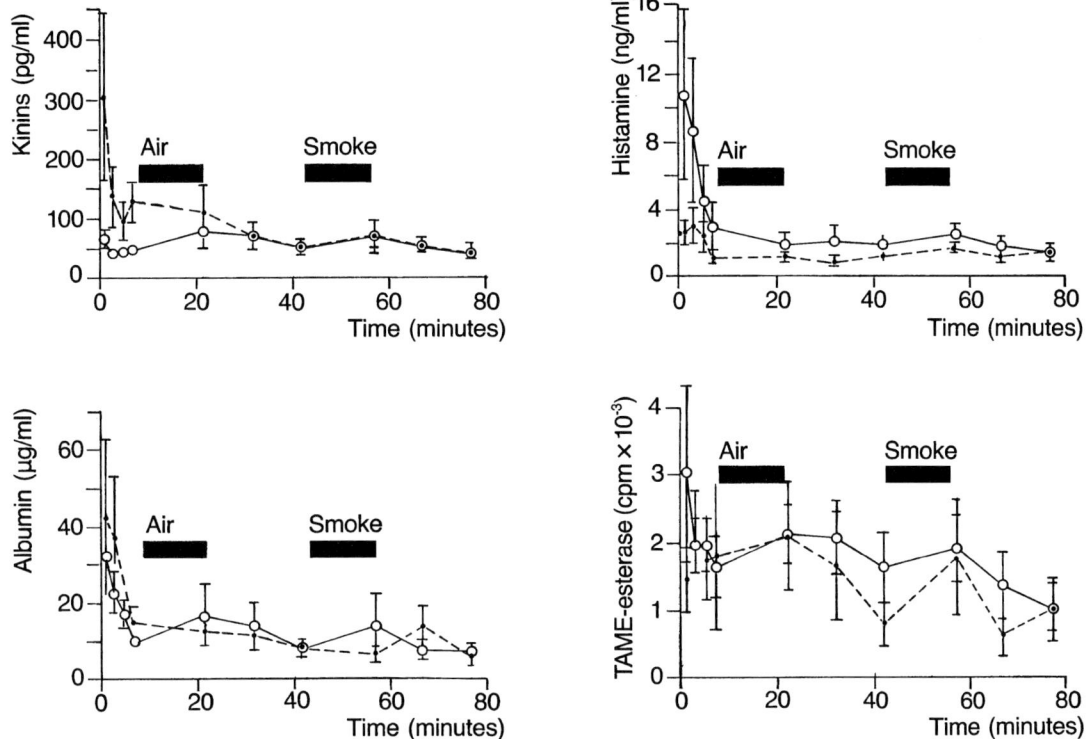

Fig. 4.5. Exposure to brief, high levels of sidestream tobacco smoke does not increase the concentration of histamine, kinins, albumin nor the activity of TAME-esterase in nasal lavage fluid. From Bascom R, Kulle T, Kagey-Sobotka A, Proud D. Upper respiratory tract environmental tobacco smoke sensitivity. *Am Rev Respir Dis* 1991; *143:* 1304-11.

The investigators concluded that tobacco smoke caused a neuroinflammatory response which was mediated by activation of C-fiber neurons.

In humans, increased vascular permeability does not occur with tobacco smoke exposure, as described above. We have hypothesized that differential responsiveness to tobacco smoke occurs through differential function of C-fiber neurons in the human nose. Challenge of ETS-sensitive and ETS-nonsensitive subjects with capsaicin showed increased rhinorrhea symptoms in the ETS-sensitive subjects.[59] Capsaicin challenge was associated with an increase in TAME-esterase activity in nasal lavage fluid in some but not all subjects.[59] The increase in TAME-esterase activity occurred in the absence of an increase in albumin or kinin concentration and was therefore thought to be an index of glandular stimulation. Individuals who were TAME-producers with capsaicin challenge had more sneezes and less nasal burning than TAME-nonproducers (Fig. 4.6). This suggests a relationship between differential irritant symptoms and irritant-induced glandular production.

Indirect effects

Several lines of evidence suggest that air pollution exposure may alter specific immune responses including IgE-mediated anaphylaxis and the immune response to infectious agents. In the 1970's, Matsamura et al[60, 61, 62] showed that intermingling high-dose ozone and antigen inhalation over several days could result in augmented IgE sensitization in guinea pigs. The ozone effect was specific to the respiratory mucosa, since intermingling ozone inhalation and intraperitoneal antigen did not augment sensitization. The investigators further showed that ozone exposure at these concentrations delayed clearance of the antigen in the lung and postulated that an increased residence time of antigen was responsible for the augmented sensitization. Augmented sensitization also occurred with high-dose SO_2 or NO_2 exposure. More recently, Riedel et al[63] demonstrated that low and medium concentrations of SO_2 could facilitate allergic sensitization in the guinea pig (Fig. 4.7). An effect was demonstrated with a 1-week, 8-hour per day SO_2

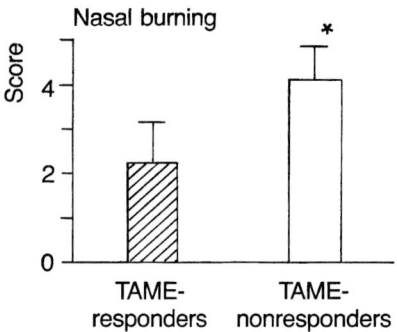

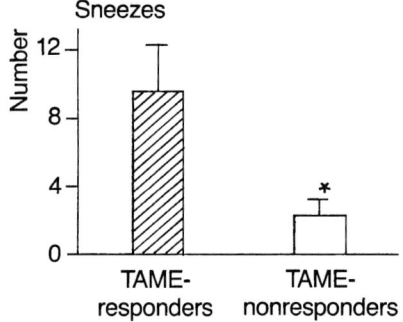

Fig. 4.6. Relationship between production of TAME-esterase activity, and symptoms of sneezes and nasal burning following intranasal capsaicin. TAME-producers had more sneezes and less nasal burning than TAME nonproducers. From Bascom R, Kagey-Sobotka A, Proud D. Effect of intranasal capsaicin on symptoms and mediator release. *J Pharmacol Exp Ther* 1991; *259:* 1323-7.

exposure to 0.1 ppm, which is below the current U.S. standard of 0.14 ppm.

Limited human studies have shown mixed results. Exposure at rest for 4 hours to 0.5 ppm ozone in asymptomatic subjects with allergic rhinitis caused a clear inflammatory cell influx and vascular leak, but did not augment the response to subsequent nasal challenge with antigen.[22] In contrast, a brief, lower dose of ozone (0.12 ppm, 1 hour, at rest), significantly increased the sensitivity of asthmatics to allergen inhalation.[64]

Recommendations for reducing the health effects of air pollution

Ozone exposure can be reduced by avoiding peak exposure periods. Individuals should be advised to stay inside and to avoid exercising in the middle of the day from April through September. Government air quality hot lines can be used to determine air quality on a specific day.

The traditional strategies to reduce the health effects of an environmental or occupational exposure include point source reduction through product substitution, enclosure or ventilation. Personal protection can be achieved through the use of respirators, job reassignment or relocation to low-exposure areas. These principles should be used when seeking a solution in the individual case, particularly with indoor air pollutants.

A practical problem which is often encountered is that overall indoor ventilation may not reflect local ventilation. Some people may have virtually no fresh air because of quirks in the ventilation system or because partitions may create unventilated pockets of air. The best approach is to have an industrial hygienist or other ventilation expert assess local ventilation using smoke tubes. One of the frustrations encountered in building investigations is that a plethora of low-level pollutants may be found, and direct links between reported symptoms and specific triggers are often hard to establish.

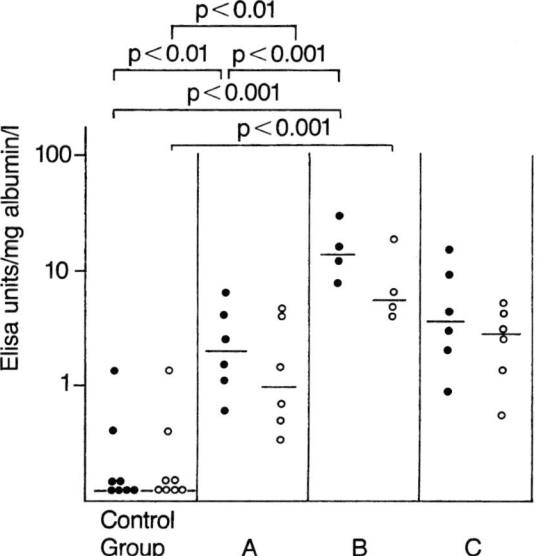

Fig. 4.7. Sulfur dioxide exposure increases allergic sensitization in guinea pigs. Shown is the anti-ovalbumin, total (filled symbols) and IgG_1 (open symbols), in bronchoalveolar lavage fluid in the control and SO_2-exposed groups (A = 0.1 ppm, B = 4.3 ppm, C = 16.6 ppm of SO_2). From Riedel F, Kramer M, Scheibenbogen C, Rieger CHL. Effects of SO_2 exposure on allergic sensitization in the guinea pig. *J Allergy Clin Immunol* 1988; *82:* 527-34.

Nonallergic rhinitis from environmental tobacco smoke (ETS) is recognized and avoidance is recommended in standard textbooks.[65] This may be difficult, however. In 1968, Speer[57] wrote that "relief depends partly on the ingenuity and resources of the patient. Some patients change jobs or even occupations, first making sure that the new position will not involve heavy exposure to smoke."[57] Exposure to ETS is being reduced by vigorous smoking cessation programs and by banning smoking in the workplace. Some anecdotal reports suggest that an air filter next to the desk may be helpful for symptomatic workers who are exposed to smoke at work. Studies are needed to find practical ways to reduce ETS exposure in the home, particularly when people with asthma or allergic rhinitis are present. Smokers should be strongly encouraged to smoke outdoors at home. Pharmacotherapy of ETS-rhinitis and irritation is needed, but is largely unstudied.

Pollutants which cause allergic rhinitis can be treated with topical corticosteroids and antihistamines. Cat allergen exposure can be decreased by removing cats from the home or washing the cat weekly. House dust mite exposure can be limited by enclosure of mattresses in plastic, and by stopping the practice of placing wall-to-wall carpets on cement foundations. The use of agents which denature mite protein is promising.

Bioaerosol exposure can be controlled by prompt repair of leaks and water damage. Ventilation systems should be inspected for the presence of standing water and professional consultation should be sought to determine appropriate maintenance procedures. The advantages of the use of carpets should be weighed against their potential as an antigen reservoir.

Conclusions

The nose is both the first target of, and the first defense against, airborne hazards. An increasing array of indoor and outdoor air pollutants are recognized as affecting the nose. Effects of air pollution range from irritant symptoms, to increased nasal resistance, to reduced mucociliary clearance, to the induction of inflammation. A research need which deserves emphasis is the need to develop methods to evaluate symptoms of nasal drying, which seem to occur with dust or irritant exposure, but not with exposure to dry air. The relationship between acute inflammatory responses to pollutants and chronic nasal diseases is still poorly understood. Differential individual responsiveness to pollutant exposure occurs, but its causes and consequences are largely unexplored. Selected pollutants may modulate the response to viruses and antigens. There is a continuing need to understand pollutant effects, to develop practical strategies to limit pollutant exposure, and to develop practical ways to identify and treat susceptible individuals. It is the responsibility of the personal physician to evaluate complaints triggered by specific environments and to consider remedial action or removal if health is at risk.

References

1. Middleton Jr E. Chronic rhinitis in adults. *J Allergy Clin Immunol* 1988; *81:* 971-5.
2. Bascom R, Raford PR. Disorders of the Upper Airway. In: Cullen MR, Rosenstock L, eds. *Clinical Occupational Medicine*. Philadelphia: WB Saunders Company, 1992 (in press).
3. *Stedman's Medical Dictionary.* Twenty-second edition. Baltimore: The Williams & Wilkins Company, 1972.
4. Summary of the Clean Air Act Amendments of 1990. State and Territorial Air Pollution Program. Administrators and the Association of Local Air Pollution Control Officials (STAPPA/ALAPCO), 1990.
5. Russell M. Ozone pollution: the hard choices. *Science* 1988; *241:* 1275-6.
6. Schwartz J, Dockery DW. Increased mortality in Philadelphia associated with daily air pollution concentrations. *Am Rev Respir Dis* 1991; *143:* A95.
7. Sheppard D. Sulfur dioxide and asthma – A double-edged sword? *J Allergy Clin Immunol* 1988; *82:* 961-4.
8. Mølhave L, Møller J. The atmospheric environment in modern Danish dwellings. Measurements in 39 flats. In: Fænger PO, Valbjørn O, eds. *Indoor Climate*. Hørsholm, Denmark: SB1, 1979: 171-86.
9. Wallace L. The TEAM Study: Personal exposures to toxic substances in air, drinking water, and breath of 400 residents of New Jersey, North Carolina, and North Dakota. *Environ Res* 1987; *43:* 290-307.
10. Kreiss K. The epidemiology of building-related complaints and illness. In: Cone JE, Hodgson MJ, eds. *Problem Buildings: Building-Associated Illness and the Sick Building Syndrome*. Philadelphia: Hanley & Belfus Inc, 1989: 575-92.
11. Reducing the Health Consequences of Smoking: 25 Years of Progress. A Report of the Surgeon General. U.S. Department of Health and Human Services, Public Health Service, Centers for Disease Control, Center for Chronic Disease Prevention and Health Promotion, Office on Smoking and Health, 1989.

12. Corn M. Characteristics of tobacco sidestream smoke and factors influencing its concentration and distribution in occupied spaces. *Scand J Respir Dis* 1974; *Suppl 91:* 21-36.
13. Gergen PJ, Turkeltaub PC. The association of allergen skin test reactivity and respiratory disease among whites in the US population. Data from the second National Health and Nutrition Examination Survey, 1976-1980. *Arch Int Med* 1991; *151:* 487-92.
14. ASHRAE Standard: Ventilation for acceptable indoor air quality. American Society of Heating, Refrigerating and Air-Conditioning Engineers Inc, 1989.
15. Harkema JR, Plopper CG, Hyde DM, St George JA, Wilson DW, Dungworth DL. Response of the macaque nasal epithelium to ambient levels of ozone. *Am J Pathol* 1987; *128:* 29-44.
16. Harkema JR. Comparative pathology of the nasal mucosa in laboratory animals exposed to inhaled irritants. *Environ Health Perspect* 1990; *85:* 231-8.
17. Jiang X-Z, Morgan KT, Beauchamp Jr RO. Histopathology of acute and subacute nasal toxicity. In: Barrow CS, ed. *Toxicology of the Nasal Passages.* Washington: Hemisphere Publishing Corporation, 1986: 51-66.
18. Doupnik CA, Leikauf GD. Acrolein stimulates eicosanoid release from bovine airway epithelial cells. *Am J Physiol* 1990; *259:* L222-9.
19. Leikauf GD, Driscoll KE, Wey HE. Ozone-induced augmentation of eicosanoid metabolism in epithelial cells from bovine trachea. *Am Rev Respir Dis* 1988; *137:* 435-42.
20. Andersen I, Proctor DF. The fate and effects of inhaled materials. In: Proctor DF, Andersen I, eds. *The Nose: Upper Airway Physiology and the Atmospheric Environment.* New York: Elsevier Biomedical Press, 1982: 423-56.
21. Koren H, Hatch GE, Graham DE. Nasal lavage as a tool in assessing acute inflammation in response to inhaled pollutants. *Toxicol* 1990; *60:* 15-25.
22. Bascom R, Naclerio RM, Fitzgerald TK, Kagey-Sobotka A, Proud D. Effect of ozone inhalation on the response to nasal challenge with antigen of allergic subjects. *Am Rev Respir Dis* 1990; *141:* 594-601.
23. Bascom R, Kulle T, Kagey-Sobotka A, Proud D. Upper respiratory tract environmental tobacco smoke sensitivity. *Am Rev Respir Dis* 1991; *143:* 1304-11.
24. Becquemin MH, Swift DL, Bouchikhi A, Roy M, Teillac A. Particle deposition and resistance in the noses of adults and children. *Eur Respir J* 1991; *4:* 694-702.
25. Speizer FE, Frank NR. The uptake and release of SO_2 by the human nose. *Arch Environ Health* 1966; *12:* 725-8.
26. Gerrity TR, Weaver RA, Berntsen J, House DE, O'Neil JJ. Extrathoracic and intrathoracic removal of O_3 in tidal-breathing humans. *J Appl Physiol* 1988; *65:* 393-400.
27. Snipes MB, Spoo JW, Brookins LK, et al. A method for measuring nasal and lung uptake of inhaled vapor. *Fundam Appl Toxicol* 1991; *16:* 81-91.
28. Andersen I, Lundqvist GR, Proctor DF, Swift DL. Human response to controlled levels of inert dust. *Am Rev Respir Dis* 1979; *119:* 619-27.
29. Brain JD, Valberg PA. Deposition of aerosol in the respiratory tract. *Am Rev Respir Dis* 1979; *120:* 1325-73.
30. Abbas A, Lichtman AH, Pober JS. *Cellular and Molecular Immunology.* Philadelphia: WB Saunders Company, 1991.
31. Andersen I, Lundqvist GR, Jensen PL, Proctor F. Human response to controlled levels of sulfur dioxide. *Arch Environ Health* 1974; *28:* 31-9.
32. Peden DB, Brown ME, Berkebile C, Hohman RJ, Kaliner MA. Characterization and partial purification of a nasal mucosal antioxidant. *Am Rev Respir Dis* 1991; *141:* A817.
33. Barrow CS. Toxicology of the nasal passages. *Chemical Industry Institute of Toxicology Series* 1986: 317.
34. Andersen I, Lundqvist GR, Jensen PL, Proctor DF. Human response to 78-hour exposure to dry air. *Arch Environ Health* 1974; *29:* 319-24.
35. Black A, Evans JC, Hadfiled EH, Macbeth RG, Morgan A, Walsh A. Impairment of nasal mucociliary clearance in woodworkers in the furniture industry. *Br J Ind Med* 1974; *31:* 10.
36. Yokoyama E, Frank R. Respiratory uptake of ozone in dogs. *Arch Environ Health* 1972; *25:* 132-8.
37. Willes S, Raford P, Baroody F, Fitzgerald TK, Bascom R. Differential responses to ozone in allergic and non-allergic subjects. *Am Rev Respir Dis* 1991; *143:* A91.
38. Graham D, Henderson F, House D. Neutrophil influx measured in nasal lavages of humans exposed to ozone. *Arch Environ Health* 1988; *43:* 228-33.
39. Graham DE, Koren HS. Biomarkers of inflammation in ozone-exposed humans. Comparison of the nasal and bronchalveolar lavage. *Am Rev Respir Dis* 1990; *142:* 152-6.
40. Baroody F, Fitzgerald T, Raford P, Willes S, Naclerio R, Bascom R. Effect of ozone on nasal methacholine challenge of allergic and nonallergic subjects. *Am Rev Respir Dis* 1991; *143:* A93.
41. Koenig JQ, Morgan MS, Horike M, Pierson WE. The effects of sulfur oxides on nasal and lung function in adolescents with extrinsic asthma. *J Allergy Clin Immunol* 1985; *76:* 813-8.
42. Koenig JQ, McManus MS, Bierman CW. Chlorpheniramine-sulfur dioxide interactions on lung and nasal function in allergic adolescents. *Ped Asthma Allergy Immunol* 1988; *2:* 199-205.
43. Tam EK, Liu J, Bigby BG, Boushey HA. Sulfur dioxide does not acutely increase nasal symptoms or nasal resistance in subjects with rhinitis or in subjects with bronchial responsiveness to sulfur dioxide. *Am Rev Respir Dis* 1988; *138:* 1559-64.
44. Andersen I, Mølhave L, Proctor DF. Human response to controlled levels of combinations of sulfur dioxide and inert dust. *Scand J Work Environ Health* 1981; *7:* 1-7.
45. Acheson ED. Epidemiology of nasal cancer. In: Barrow CS, ed. *Toxicology of the Nasal Passages.* Washington DC: Hemisphere Publishing Corporation, 1986: 135-41.
46. Broder I, Corey P, Cole P, Lipa M. Comparison of the health of occupants and characteristics of houses among control homes and homes insulated with urea formaldehyde foam. II. Initial health and house variables and exposure-response relationships. *Environ Res* 1988; *45:* 156-78.
47. Mølhave L, Bach B, Pedersen OF. Human reactions during controlled exposures to low concentrations of organic gases and vapours known as normal indoor air pollutants. *Indoor Air: Proceedings of the 3rd International Conference on Indoor Air Quality and Climate,* 1984: 431-6.
48. Kjaergaard SK, Mølhave L, Pedersen OF. Human reactions to a mixture of indoor air volatile organic compounds. *Atmospheric Environment* 1991; *25A:* 1417-26.
49. Koren HS, Graham DE, Devlin RB. Exposure of humans to volatile organic compounds (VOC) results in inflammation in the nasal passages. *Arch Environ Health* 1992 (in press).
50. Franck C. Eye symptoms and signs in buildings with indoor climate problems ('office eye syndrome'). *Acta Ophthalmol* 1986; *64:* 306-11.
51. Devlin RB, Koren HS. Inflammatory effect of newly installed carpet on humans. Clinical Research Branch Human Studies Division Health Effects Research Laboratory, Environmental Protection Agency, Research Triangle Park 27711, 1991.
52. Indoor air quality research: report on a WHO meeting. Geneva: World Health Organization, 1986.
53. U.S. Environmental Protection Agency, National Institute for Occupational Safety and Health, Westat, Inc and John B Pierce Foundation Laboratory at Yale University. *Indoor air quality and work environment study.* Volume I. 1989.
54. Cullen MR. Multiple chemical sensitivities: summary and directions for future investigators. In: Cullen MR ed. *Workers with Multiple Chemical Sensitivities.* Philadelphia: Hanley & Belfus, 1987: 801-4.
55. Muramatsu T, Weber A, Muramatsu S, Akermann F. An experimental study on irritation and annoyance due to passive smoking. *Int Arch Occup Environ Health* 1983; *51:* 305-17.

56 Bascom R, Fitzgerald TK, Permutt T, Sauder L, Nadarajah J, Swift DL. Response to environmental tobacco smoke: dose-response studies and the effect of acoustic rhinometry. *Am Rev Respir Dis* 1992; *145A:* 92.
57 Speer F. Tobacco and the non-smoker. A study of subjective symptoms. *Arch Environ Health* 1968; *16:* 443-6.
58 Lundberg JM, Lundblad L, Saria A, Änggård A. Inhibition of cigarette smoke induced oedema in the nasal mucosa by capsaicin pretreatment and a substance P antagonist. *Naunyn-Schmiedeberg's Arch Pharmacol* 1984; *326:* 181-5.
59 Bascom R, Kagey-Sobotka A, Proud D. Effect of intranasal capsaicin on symptoms and mediator release. *J Pharmacol Exp Ther* 1991; *259:* 1323-27.
60 Matsumura Y. The effects of ozone, nitrogen dioxide, and sulfur dioxide on the experimentally induced allergic respiratory disorder in guinea pigs: I. The effect on sensitization with albumin through the airway. *Am Rev Respir Dis* 1970; *102:* 430-7.
61 Matsumura Y. The effects of ozone, nitrogen dioxide, and sulfur dioxide on the experimentally induced allergic respiratory disorder in guinea pigs: III. The effect of the occurrence of dyspneic attacks. *Am Rev Respir Dis* 1970; *102:* 444-7.
62 Matsumura Y. The effects of ozone, nitrogen dioxide, and sulfur dioxide on the experimentally induced allergic respiratory disorder in guinea pigs: II. The effects of ozone on the absorption and the retention of antigen in the lung. *Am Rev Respir Dis* 1970; *102:* 438-43.
63 Riedel F, Kramer M, Scheibenbogen C, Rieger CHL. Effects of SO_2 exposure on allergic sensitization in the guinea pig. *J Allergy Clin Immunol* 1988; *82:* 527-34.
64 Molfino NA, Wright SC, Katz I, et al. Effect of low concentrations of ozone on inhaled allergen responses in asthmatic subjects. *Lancet* 1991; *338:* 199-203.
65 Meltzer EO, Schatz M, Zeiger RS. Allergic and Nonallergic Rhinitis. In: Middleton Jr E, Reed CE, Ellis EF, Adkinson Jr NF, Yunginger JW, eds. *Allergy Principles and Practice.* Washington DC: The CV Mosby Company, 1988: 1253-89.

CHAPTER 5

Food allergy and intolerance

CARSTEN BINDSLEV-JENSEN

Definition of terms

An adverse reaction to a food was defined by the American Academy of Allergy and Immunology Committee on Adverse Reactions to Foods as "a general term that can be applied to a clinically abnormal response attributed to an ingested food or food additive".[1] This definition includes a variety of non-hypersensitivity reactions (food poisoning, pharmacological food reaction, metabolic food reaction) together with food hypersensitivity, often divided into food allergy, characterized by a proven involvement of the immune system and food intolerance, which has not been proven to be immunologic. Food hypersensitivity only occurs in some patients, often immediately after ingestion of small amounts of the substance, and the reaction is unrelated to any physiological effect of the food or food additive. A subgroup of food allergy is the pollen cross-reactivity, where especially birch pollen-sensitized patients experience oral and pharyngeal itching and swelling (OAS, the Oral Allergy Syndrome) following ingestion of, e.g., hazelnut, apple or almond.[2]

The term food hypersensitivity and in particular the term food intolerance have both been widely misused, including all sorts of symptoms and reaction patterns in the definition. This mainly results from uncontrolled reports in the literature claiming a relationship between ingestion of a substance and occurrence of symptoms.[1,3] Food hypersensitivity can only be correctly diagnosed using double-blind, placebo-controlled food challenges (DBPCFC) and by the use of this procedure, only the classic symptoms and signs (e.g. anaphylaxis, OAS, diarrhea, vomitus, urticaria, angioedema, dermatitis herpetiformis, atopic dermatitis, contact eczema, rhinitis, asthma, conjunctivitis, eosinophil duodenitis) have convincingly been demonstrated to be true food hypersensitivity.[4-14]

Sensitization

The route of sensitization is normally via the gastrointestinal tract, where reactions in sensitized patients can be elicited from the mouth (OAS), the stomach or the intestine,[2,15,16] whereas in occupational food hypersensitivity (e.g. Baker's asthma and rhinitis) the patient is sensitized by inhalation.[14] In pollen cross-reactivity, the patient is sensitized to the pollen grain via the respiratory tract, following which symptoms of cross-reaction due to common epitopes on the pollen grain and fruits or vegetables will occur, particularly in the mouth and throat.[2] Whether sensitization is organ-specific is not known, although a dose-relationship seems to exist (Fig. 5.1).

Prevalence

Food hypersensitivity is most prevalent in childhood, and a recent study by Høst & Halken has shown that approximately 2% of newborns will develop hypersensitivity to cow's milk within the 1st year of life.[17] This challenge-controlled study reveals a prevalence markedly lower than questionnaire studies.[14,17] Duration of the clinical disease varies and depends on the allergen type – 90% of the patients in Høst's & Halken's study[17] had developed tolerance before 3 years of age, whereas Sampson[18] reported development of tolerance in 19 to 50% of the patients, depending on the allergen.

Food additives have been claimed to elicit food hypersensitivity reactions in a high proportion of

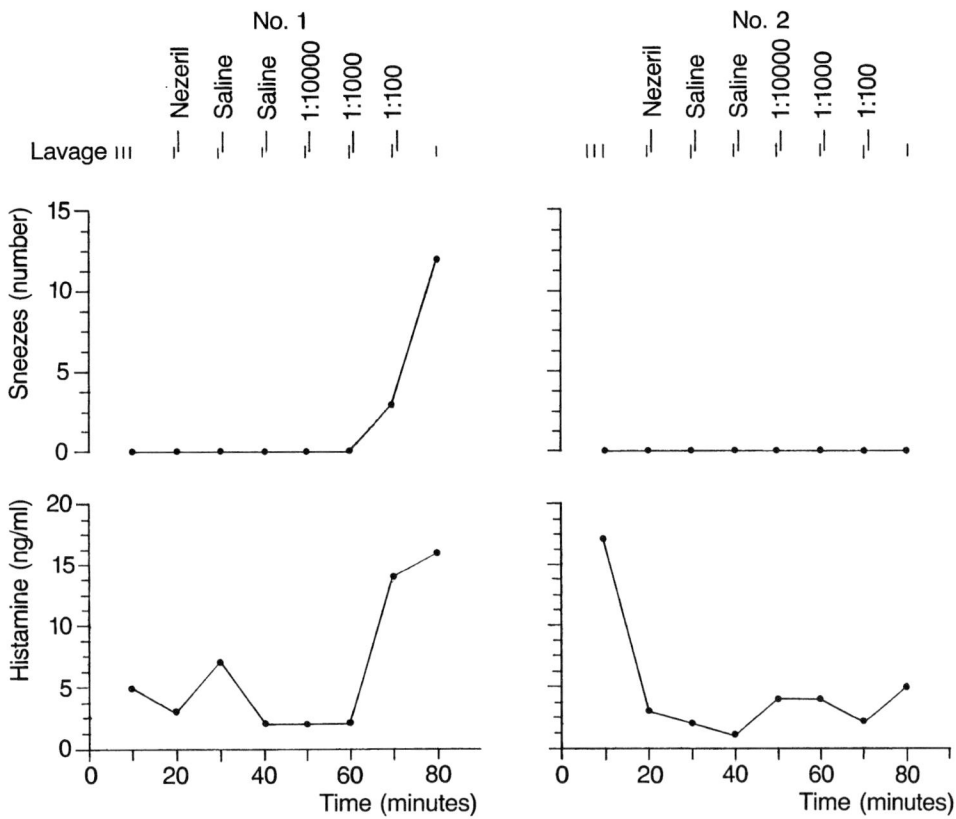

Fig. 5.1. The outcome of nasal provocation with hen's egg in 2 adults with proven food allergy[22] to egg. Patient No. 1 had developed sneezing and watery rhinorrhea (together with vomitus, asthma and diarrhea) when given hen's egg (50 mg) orally in DBPCFC, whereas patient No. 2 did not experience nasal symptoms when reacting with urticaria, vomitus and abdominal cramp to 500 mg of hen's egg. The clinical symptoms to nasal challenge in patient No. 1 were accompanied by increase in nasal lavage histamine content. Data from Pretorius C, Jacobi H, Skov PS, Bindslev-Jensen C.

patients with asthma or rhinitis, but using DBPCFC, Rosenhall[19] found only 2% positive towards preservatives and 3% positive to dyes in a large study of 504 patients with asthma or rhinitis. A link between aspirin intolerance and sensitivity to oral provocation with tartrazine could not be demonstrated by Stevenson in a study of 80 patients with aspirin asthma.[20] The reported number of positive reactions to orally ingested sulfite in asthmatics varies from 0 to 66%,[21] whereas no controlled trials on sulfite sensitivity in rhinitis patients have been published. Twenty per cent of bakers will suffer from baker's asthma and rhinitis after 20 years of exposure.[14]

Diagnosis of food hypersensitivity

A controlled program, beginning with exclusion of other causes for the patient's complaints, is mandatory (Table 5.1). In most of the patients in whom food hypersensitivity can be verified by DBPCFC, multiorgan involvement can be demonstrated.[4-14, 17, 18, 22] Selection of patients for the controlled program should therefore be based on concomitant occurrence of symptoms (among the symptoms listed above) from more than one organ system, where normal standard treatment has proven insufficient.

Patient's case history is mostly of value in obvious cases, where objective signs occur in clear connection to ingestion of a food item. The normal diagnostic tools for diagnosing type 1 allergy (Skin Prick Test (SPT), RAST or histamine release from basophils (HR)) suffer from the lack of standardized extracts, and must always be compared to the outcome of DBPCFC. Some authors report superiority of SPT, whereas others recommend RAST or HR as the primary diagnostic tool. Whether these differences reflect variations in allergen extract quality remains unsettled, but both SPT and HR will yield results which are in significant concordance with the outcome of DBPCFC,

Table 5.1. *Flowchart for a controlled program for diagnosing food hypersensitivity.*

```
┌─────────────────┐     ┌─────────────────┐  Yes  ┌─────────────────┐
│ Case history    │     │ Is there another│──────▶│ Other diagnosis │
│ Objective findings│──▶│ explanation to  │       │ established.    │
│ Indication?     │     │ patient's complaints?│  └─────────────────┘
└─────────────────┘     └─────────────────┘              │
                               │ No                      ▼
                               ▼                  ┌─────────────────┐
                        ┌─────────────────┐       │      Stop       │
                        │   Controlled    │       └─────────────────┘
                        │    program      │
                        │ allergy testing │
                        └─────────────────┘
                               │
                               ▼
┌─────────────┐         ┌─────────────────┐       ┌─────────────┐
│  Symptoms   │◀────────│ Basis registration│────▶│ No symptoms │
└─────────────┘         │   of symptoms   │       └─────────────┘
        │               └─────────────────┘              │
        ▼                                                ▼
┌─────────────┐         ┌─────────────────┐       ┌─────────────┐
│Elimination  │────────▶│    No effect    │──────▶│    Stop     │
│    diet     │         │consider other diet│     └─────────────┘
└─────────────┘         └─────────────────┘
        │                        │
        ▼                        ▼
┌─────────────┐         ┌─────────────────┐
│   Effect    │◀────────│    New diet     │
└─────────────┘         └─────────────────┘
        │
        ▼
┌─────────────┐         ┌─────────────────┐       ┌─────────────┐
│Open provocations│────▶│    Negative     │──────▶│    Stop     │
└─────────────┘         └─────────────────┘       └─────────────┘
        │
        ▼
┌─────────────┐         ┌─────────────────┐       ┌─────────────┐
│  Positive   │────────▶│     DBPCFC      │──────▶│  Negative   │
└─────────────┘         └─────────────────┘       └─────────────┘
                               │                         │
                               ▼                         ▼
                        ┌─────────────────┐       ┌─────────────────┐
                        │    Postive      │       │Food hypersensitivity│
                        └─────────────────┘       │  not verified   │
                               │                  └─────────────────┘
                               ▼
┌─────────────┐Negative┌─────────────────┐Positive┌─────────────┐
│Food intolerance│◀───│  SPT, RAST, HR  │───────▶│Food Allergy │
└─────────────┘        └─────────────────┘        └─────────────┘
```

when fresh, standardized extracts are used, contrary to the findings when using commercial, unstandardized extracts.[23]

Elimination diets are needed in order to ensure that symptoms subside and thus serve to prepare the patient for provocations. Freedom from symptoms on an elimination diet does not imply food hypersensitivity *per se*, but must be followed by provocations.

No procedure can exclude the need for DBPCFC.[1,8] In patients with a history of severe systemic reaction, care should be taken and the provocations should be administered in a titrated fashion, beginning with small amounts of the offending food items, raising the dose with a fixed time interval until symptoms and signs occur, or until a normal daily amount has been reached. The food items can be administered freeze-dried in capsules or freshly prepared, masked in a vehicle.[4,8,22] The number of provocations depends on the patient's symptoms. If the patient demonstrates objective signs (e.g. sneezing, vomitus, asthma), one active and one placebo provocation will usually be sufficient, whereas three active and three placebo provocations are needed if the patient reports only subjective symptoms.[24]

Table 5.2. *In published reports DBPCFC induced nasal symptoms in a varying percentage of those with a positive test (0-80%). Patients reacting with symptoms from the nose invariably had symptoms from other organs as well.*

Author	Patient age (yrs)	No. patients	No. patients with a positive, DBPCFC test	No. patients with a positive test and nasal symptoms
Bock[6]	<3	43	16 (37%)	4 (9%)
Bock[6]	>3	25	13 (52%)	5 (20%)
Sampson[5]	<18	26	16 (62%)	5 (19%)
Novembre[10]	2-9	140	8 (6%)	3 (2%)
Høst[17]	<1	117	39 (33%)	8 (7%)
Bernstein[7]	Adults	22	10 (45%)	3 (14%)
Atkins[4]	28-51	25	10 (40%)	0 (0%)
Pastorello[9]	Adults	23	10 (43%)	8 (35%)
Our group[22, 24]	Adults	75	29 (39%)	12 (16%)

Food hypersensitivity and rhinitis

Rhinitis is one of the symptoms which can be elicited in patients during DBPCFC. The prevalence of rhinitis in DBPCFC-positive patients varies between 0 and 80% (Table 5.2). Food-induced rhinitis rarely occurs as a single symptom, except in gustatory rhinitis (rhinorrhea induced by hot spicy food).

Rhinitis symptoms most often occur within a few hours after oral provocation. Whether late-phase reactions in the nose after oral provocations exist remains unsettled, although Hill[25] reported a significantly higher proportion of rhinitis symptoms more than 24 hours after oral provocation with cow's milk in milk-allergic children than in milk-tolerant. Nasal symptoms also form part of the symptom complex in patients with verified food intolerance, reporting subjective symptoms only – in our study, by using DBPCFC (3 active and 3 placebo) we could verify 4 of 10 cases reporting nasal symptoms, and a total of 12 cases of food intolerance out of 42 patients investigated.[24] On the other hand, Parker found none of 23 patients with subjective symptoms only (but none reporting nasal symptoms) positive in DBPCFC.[11]

Treatment

The specific treatment of a verified food hypersensitivity is avoidance.

Adrenalin should be administered as soon as possible to patients with food anaphylaxis. Antihistamine therapy with H_1-antagonists may be useful in OAS,[26] but no data exist on their possible role in systemic reactions. Therapy with oral cromoglycate has shown varying results.[1]

Previous studies have shown effect of immunotherapy on baker's asthma, but no data exist on the effect of immunotherapy on classic food hypersensitivity.

Conclusion

Rhinitis is one of the symptoms elicited in food-hypersensitive patients but rhinitis is rarely the only symptom. Although food additives sometimes cause dermatological symptoms, rhinitis due to dyes and preservatives seems to be rare.

It is mandatory to establish the diagnosis by the use of a controlled program, finishing with DBPCFC,[27] in order to avoid dietary treatment of patients which is unnecessary in the vast majority of those with nasal complaints.

References

1. National Institute of Allergy and Infectious diseases. Adverse Reactions to Foods. US Dpt of Health and Human Services, NIH Publ No. 84-2442, 1984.
2. Ortolani C, Ispano M, Pastorello E, Bigi A, Ansaloni R. The oral allergy syndrome. *Ann Allergy* 1988; *61:* 47-52.
3. Pearson DJ. Psychologic and somatic interrelationships in allergy and pseudoallergy. *J Allergy Clin Immunol* 1988; *81:* 351-60.
4. Atkins FM, Steinberg SS, Metcalfe DD. Evaluation of immediate adverse reactions to foods in adult patients. II. A detailed analysis of reaction patterns during oral food challenge. *J Allergy Clin Immunol* 1985; *75:* 356-63.
5. Sampson HA. Role of immediate food hypersensitivity in the pathogenesis of atopic dermatitis. *J Allergy Clin Immunol* 1983; *71:* 473–80.
6. Bock SA, Lee WY, Remigio LK, May CD. Studies of hypersensitivity reactions to foods in infants and children. *J Allergy Clin Immunol* 1978; *62:* 327-34.
7. Bernstein M, Day JH, Welsh A. Double-blind food challenge in the diagnosis of food sensitivity in the adult. *J Allergy Clin Immunol* 1982; *70:* 205-10.
8. Sampson HA. Immunologically mediated food allergy: the importance of food challenge procedures. *Ann Allergy* 1988; *60:* 262-9.
9. Pastorello EA, Stocchi L, Pravettoni V, et al. Role of elimination diet in adults with food allergy. *J Allergy Clin Immunol* 1989, *84:* 475-83.
10. Novembre E, de Martino M, Vierucci A. Foods and respiratory allergy. *J Allergy Clin Immunol* 1988; *81:* 1059-63.
11. Parker SL, Leznoff A, Sussamnn GL, et al. Characteristics of patients with food-related complaints. *J Allergy Clin Immunol* 1990; *86:* 503-11.
12. May CD. Are confusion and controversy about food hypersensitivity really necessary. *J Allergy Clin Immunol* 1985; *75:* 329-33.
13. Sampson HA. Differential diagnosis in adverse reactions to foods. *J Allergy Clin Immunol* 1986; *78:* 212-9.
14. Anderson JA. The clinical spectrum of food allergy in adults. *Clin Exp Allergy* 1991; *21:* 304-15.
15. Reimann HJ, Ring J, Ultsch B, Wendt P. Intragastral provocation under endoscopic control (IPEC) in food allergy: mast cell and histamine changes in gastric mucosa. *Clin Allergy* 1985; *15:* 195-202.
16. Barrett KE, Metcalfe DD. The mucosal mast cell and its role in gastrointestinal allergic diseases. *Clin Rev Allergy* 1984; *2:* 39-53.
17. Høst A, Halken S. A prospective study of cow milk allergy in Danish infants during the first three years of life. *Allergy* 1990; *45:* 587-96.
18. Sampson HA, Scanlon SM. Natural history of food hypersensitivity in children with atopic dermatitis. *J Pediatr* 1989; *115:* 23-7.
19. Rosenhall L. Evaluation of intolerance to analgesics, preservatives and food colorants with challenge tests. *Eur J Resp Dis* 1982; *63:* 410-9.
20. Stevenson DD, Simon RA, Lumry WR, Mathison DA. Dyes, preservatives and salicylates in the induction of food intolerance and/or hypersensitivity in children. *J Allergy Clin Immunol* 1986; *78:* 182-91.
21. Lessof MH. Medical aspects of food intolerance. A group of papers sponsored by the Ministry of Agriculture, Fisheries and Food. *J Royal Coll Phys* 1987; *21(4):* 1-30.
22. Norgaard A, Bindslev-Jensen C. Allergy to milk and egg in adults. Diagnosis and characterization. *Allergy* 1992 (in press).
23. Norgaard A, Skov PS, Bindslev-Jensen C. Egg and milk allergy in adults. Comparison between fresh foods and commercial allergen extracts in SPT and HR. *Clin Exp Allergy* 1992 (in press).
24. Bindslev-Jensen C, Madsen F. Food intolerance in adults. (Manuscript in preparation).
25. Hill DJ, Ball G, Hosking CS. Clinical manifestations of cow's milk allergy in childhood. I. Association with in vitro cellular immune responses. *Clin Allergy* 1988; *18:* 469-79.
26. Bindslev-Jensen C, Vibits A, Skov PS, Weeke B. The oral allergy syndrome – effect of Astemizole. *Allergy* 1991; *45:* 610–3.
27. Metcalfe DD, Sampson HA. Workshop on experimental methodology for clinical studies of adverse reactions to food and food additives. *J Allergy Clin Immunol* 1990; *86:* 421-42.

CHAPTER 6

Rhinoscopy

HEINZ STAMMBERGER

From a rhinoscopist's view, the "truly" allergic nose is a very boring one, especially when dealing with a seasonal allergy. If not exposed to allergens, the mucosa usually cannot be differentiated from a healthy non-allergic individual's nose. In case of allergen exposure, little else but watery secretions and a swollen mucosa with increased vascularity, sometimes presenting with a purplish color, can be noted. At the extreme, the nose is totally blocked, allowing no insight at all.

But even in an allergic nose, factors predisposing to early manifestations of allergic symptoms can be identified endoscopically, as will be described below.

The non-allergic rhinosinusitis, in contrast, is a demanding challenge for the nasal endoscopist. Using rigid endoscopes for diagnosis, it becomes evident that anterior and/or posterior rhinoscopy with speculum and mirror provide very limited information only, not enough in any case to understand more of the pathophysiology of the nose and its sinuses. Augmented by modern imaging techniques like CT, the endoscope may help the diagnostician, the surgeon and the scientific researcher and thus serve the patient.

Endoscopic investigations of the lateral nasal wall over the last decades have demonstrated that most infections of the larger sinuses are rhinogenic: disease spreads from the nose to the paranasal sinuses. At the beginning of a non-allergic inflammatory process, the nasal mucosa usually is affected in a very limited and circumscribed area only: at the entrance of the middle nasal meatus, where the clefts of the anterior ethmoidal labyrinth form a complex system of cells and pathways, through which frontal and maxillary sinuses are ventilated and drained. It is here where changes occur first, making it evident that the nasal mucosa does not react uniformly as an entity but that there are predilection sites from which disease spreads through the nose and eventually to the larger sinuses.

The normally already very narrow clefts of the anterior ethmoid hold the key position for normal function and the pathophysiology of the larger sinuses. These clefts can be seen as prechambers,

Table 6.1. *Frequent anatomical variations predisposing to acute and recurrent rhinosinusitis.*

Septal deviation / spurs	
Agger nasi cells:	large, narrowing frontal recess
Uncinate process:	medially bent, laterally bent, curved anteriorly ("double middle turbinate"), fractures (trauma, iatrogenic), contacting turbinate, pneumatized
Middle turbinate:	concha bullosa, paradoxically bent, framing lateral nasal wall
Ethmoidal bulla:	large, filling turbinate sinus, contact areas, anterior growth, overlapping hiatus semilunaris, protruding out of middle meatus
Haller's cell:	narrowing maxillary ostium
Combinations of all the above	

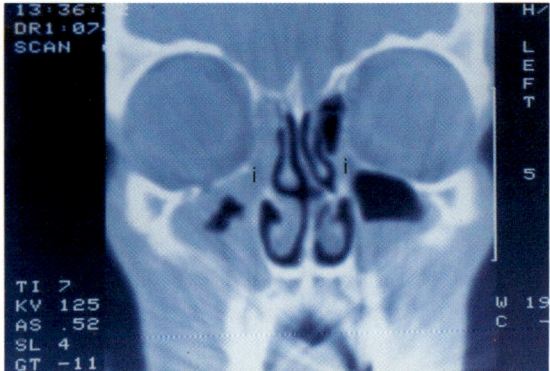

Fig. 6.1a. Coronal CT-scan of a bilateral non-allergic rhinosinusitis. On anterior rhinoscopy, the nose was unremarkable except for the septal spur to the left. Endoscopically, however, the disease in the anterior ethmoids on both sides clearly could be identified. Both sides present with considerable disease in the maxillary sinus due to blockage of the ethmoidal infundibulum (i). This patient responded well to functional endoscopic sinus surgery and required no further medication.

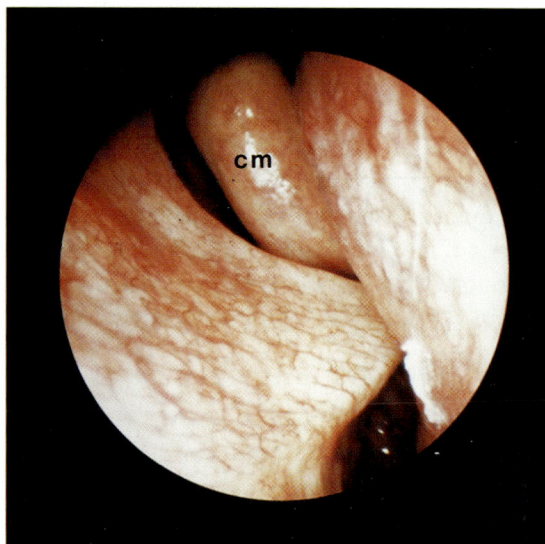

Fig. 6.1b. Endoscopic view of the patient in Fig. 6.1a. Clearly the septal spur can be identified, piercing into the inferior turbinate (cm = middle turbinate). Note the normal appearance of the nasal mucosa despite the presence of considerable disease in the lateral nasal wall.

neath the middle turbinate may constrict or completely block another physiologically important cleft in the vicinity, or at least bring opposing mucosal areas in close proximity. Here, a minimal mucosal swelling – whatever the underlying cause may be – can bring opposing mucosal areas into contact and their ciliary activity can be impeded. The secretion in between such contact areas cannot be transported away anymore and lesions – caused by allergens, noxious substances, bacteria, viruses or other immunologically active agents – are prone to start here. Under certain conditions infection can spread to adjacent sites, affecting the entire lateral nasal wall and eventually the dependent larger sinuses. Even a relatively limited disease in the ethmoidal infundibulum – the prechamber to the maxillary sinus – or the frontal recess – the prechamber to the frontal sinus – may severely affect the respective sinus. This may result in the retention of secretions, poor ventilation of the sinus and inflammation if superinfection occurs. The symptoms of this diseased sinus may dominate the clinical picture. The underlying cause of the disease, however, in most of the cases will be found in the lateral nasal wall and not in the sinus itself.

The patient can have massive symptoms long before diseased mucosa or free polyps appear in the common nasal meatus protruding out of the ethmoid. The key symptom of even mild ethmoiditis is *nasal obstruction*[2] (Fig. 6.1).

The preferred areas of contact sites in the nose

Table 6.2. *Origin of polyps in 200 consecutive patients.**

Uncinate – turbinate – infundibulum	80%
Face of bulla – hiatus – infundibulum	65%
Frontal recess	48%
"Turbinate sinus"	42%
Inside bulla	30%
"Lateral sinus"	28%
Posterior ethmoid (superior meatus)	27%
Middle turbinate	15%
Secondary sinuses affected:	
Maxillary sinus (mucosal swelling)	65%
Frontal sinus (mucosal swelling)	23%
Sphenoid sinus	8%

* Not including diffuse polypoid rhinosinopathy (NARES)

on which frontal and maxillary sinuses are dependent. Many an anatomical variant here can stenose these clefts and prechambers even more and thus predispose this area to recurring or persistent infections.[1]

The space between the middle turbinate and the lamina papyracea is very limited. An anatomical variation of one of the structures hidden under-

– apart from septal deviations – include the frontal recess and the ethmoidal infundibulum, the cleft between the uncinate process and the middle turbinate, between the ethmoidal bulla and the middle turbinate, the so-called lateral sinus above and behind the ethmoidal bulla. Many anatomical variants of these structures and the clefts between them may constrict the pathways of mucociliary transport even more, thus apparently predisposing patients to recurring disease, especially if combinations of the anatomical variations exist.

Once a localized problem is established in one of these clefts, a cascade effect may start: the hiatus semilunaris can be affected from an infected area between the uncinate process and the middle turbinate. This in turn may lead to inflammation of the infundibulum and/or the frontal recess from where maxillary or frontal sinuses may be affected.

Table 6.1 lists some of the more frequent anatomical variations that we have encountered in patients with chronic or recurrent rhinosinusitis. The endoscope furthermore reveals that nasal polyps usually do *not* start *inside* the sinuses or cells, but from contact areas in ethmoidal clefts in the middle meatus. Table 6.2 displays the findings that we have gathered in 200 consecutive patients during endoscopic examination or surgery. The majority of polyps originate in the anterior ethmoid, the most frequent sites being contact areas of the uncinate process and the middle turbinate and the ethmoidal infundibulum as well as the ethmoidal bulla and its vicinity in almost $2/3$ of our patients. From here polyps obstructed the hiatus semilunaris, invaded the ethmoidal infundibulum or protruded anteriorly between the middle turbinate and the uncinate process into the middle meatus (Fig. 6.2).

In about 50% of all patients, polyps were found in the frontal recess. This is particulary of interest since in this area polyps may not be visible in many cases, even through the endoscope. In this situation the combination of endoscopy and tomography is particulary valuable. Less than $1/3$ of the patients had their posterior ethmoid affected and less than 8% had polyps or mucosal thickening in the sphenoid sinus.

The air-flow through the nose apparently plays an important role: due to the direction of the nasal valve, it is aimed at the head of the middle turbinate. When passing through the middle meatus, the air stream here meets frontally with structures like the uncinate process, the anterior face of the ethmoidal bulla and particles and other matter preferably are deposited here. It is not by chance that the adenocarcinoma of the woodworkers starts in

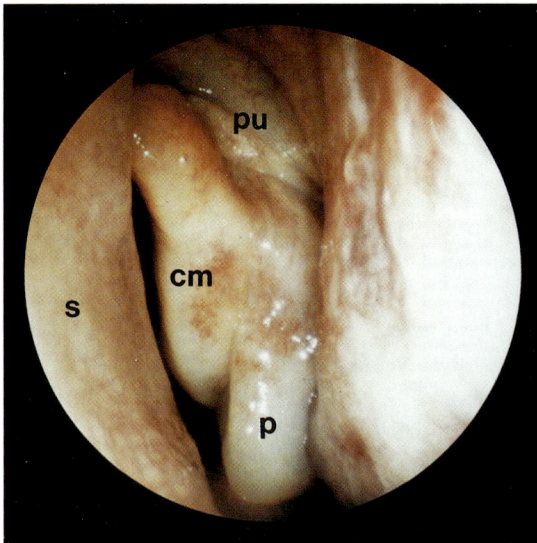

Fig. 6.2a. Large polyps are protruding out of the middle meatus on the left side of the nose. The uncinate process is bent medially and curved anteriorly (so-called doubled middle turbinate, according to Kaufmann). The polyps originated from the contact area between uncinate process, anterior face of the ethmoidal bulla and the middle turbinate (s = septum, cm = middle turbinate, p = polyp, pu = uncinate process).

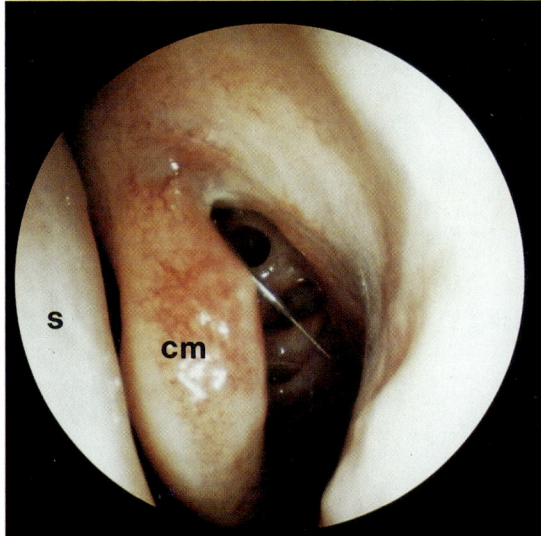

Fig. 6.2b. Situation a few weeks after endoscopic surgical approach: free passage into the middle meatus, the ethmoidal mucosa has normalized after resection of the uncinate process and most of the ethmoidal bulla (s = septum, cm = concha media).

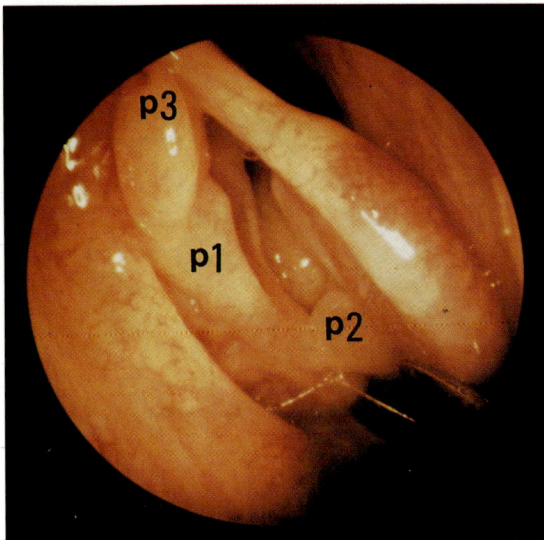

Fig. 6.3. After the middle turbinate was luxated medially with Freer's instrument, in this right middle meatus the origin of polyps that had protruded into the nose becomes evident: polyps rise from the anterior face of the ethmoidal bulla (p1), from the middle turbinate where this contacted the medial lamella of the bulla (p2) and from superiorly, where middle turbinate, bulla lamella and uncinate process constricted the passage into the frontal recess and were in contact (pe).

this part of the anterior ethmoid, as it is here that the carcinogens are deposited by the air stream. Contact areas apparently allow noxious substances to adhere longer locally and thus develop their potentially irritating, noxious or allergic and immunologic activity, resulting in mucosal irritation and/or lesions or triggering other cascade effects.

It is fascinating to see polyps rise from contact areas (Figs. 6.2 and 6.3). They are easily detectable at the entrance of the middle meatus or – more challenging for the endoscopist – hidden in the narrow clefts of the ethmoid. Those changes cannot be detected with the microscope, let alone the unaided eye. But it can be "hidden" lesions that irritate the nasal function, give the patient the feeling of nasal obstruction and may even mimic allergic symptoms.

It is with the identification of this kind of "hidden disease", that the functional endoscopic sinus surgery concept can achieve a sometimes dramatic improvement of a patient's symptoms.

It is, however, not exclusively to the surgical approach that the endoscope is of great value. In patients who are treated medically we now are able to much better evaluate the efficacy of our therapy as we can actually watch the response of the nasal mucosa. This holds especially true for the response of polypoid changes to either systemic or topical steroid therapy. No longer do we have to rely on the patient's symptoms alone or on the results of rhinomanometry/rhinometry. The endoscope therefore is the tool that helps to avoid unnecessary surgery by allowing for better diagnosis and therapeutic evaluation.

If, in an otherwise typical allergic rhinitis patient, antiallergic and/or immunotherapy does not improve the nasal symptoms as expected, an endoscopic approach may help to identify an anatomical variation in the lateral nasal wall, like a concha bullosa or an overpneumatized ethmoidal bulla or a deflected uncinate process (Figs. 6.4-6). A surgical correction of these variations usually is a minimal procedure with little risk involved in the hands of an experienced surgeon. Naturally, an IgE-mediated allergy cannot be cured by surgery. But in the situation mentioned above, a functional endoscopic approach can be a very helpful adjunctive therapy by eliminating contact areas and stenotic clefts, where, under allergen exposure, symptoms would occur first. Thus, a better threshold may be reached when the mucosa is exposed to allergens. We have seen that antiallergic medication could be significantly reduced or fully omitted after such a therapy in selected cases.[4]

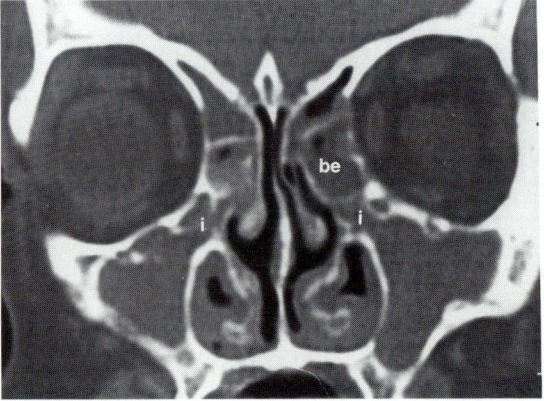

Fig. 6.4. Coronal CT-scan of a chronic rhinosinusitis in a non-allergic patient. Clearly, the diseased ethmoidal bulla on both sides (be) is visible. The ethmoidal infundibulum is blocked (i) and there is retention in both maxillary sinuses. Some secretion can be seen on the nasal floor near the inferior turbinate.

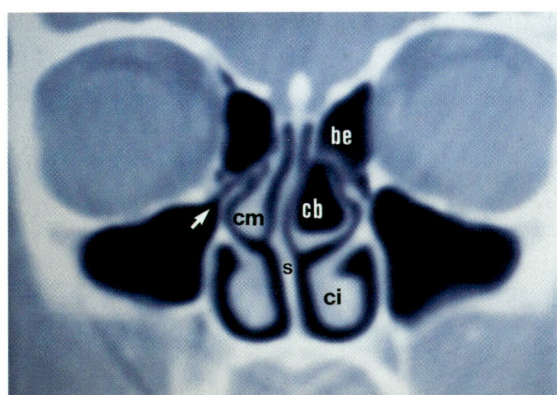

Fig. 6.5. Coronal CT-scan of a patient with nasal obstruction. Clearly the pneumatisation of the middle turbinate on the patient's left side can be seen (cb = concha bullosa). There is extensive contact between the concha bullosa and the septum medially as well as with the ethmoidal bulla (be) lateral superiorly (s = septum, ci = concha inferior, arrow = ethmoidal infundibulum).

Of course, differential diagnosis should not be forgotten: not infrequently, malignant diseases of the nose have rhinitis symptoms as their only manifestation for a considerable time and/or such disease may be hidden behind reactive polyps. Especially unilateral disease should always be investigated with this possibility in mind.

The endoscopic findings might provide a new stimulus to researchers: What goes wrong in those contact areas? What lesions do occur here? What triggers the cascade of disease spreading into the surroundings? How can such small lesions interfere with the nasal cycle and the nasal function?

Clinical experience has shown that, after relatively limited removal of such contact areas and diseased clefts, patients can be cured and nasal function as well as the appearance of the mucosa completely normalized again. We do not, however, know and understand how we achieve what we are achieving: what pathophysiological cycle are we able to break by surgical intervention and why does it not work to the same degree in the NARES (non-allergic rhinitis with eosinophilia) syndrome? What makes this clinical entity, which is characterized by a more diffuse swelling of the entire nasal mucosa, or at least the larger part of it, the mucosa presenting with the dense eosinophilic infiltration, behave so differently? Why is this disease group so frequently associated with asthma? Apparently we are facing at least two entirely different groups of "nasal polyposis", one of which is extremely therapy-resistant, frequently requires long-term corti-

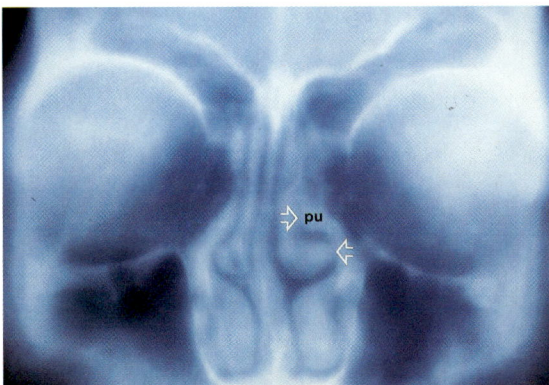

Fig. 6.6. This conventional tomography demonstrates an uncinate process (pu) which as an anatomical variant is extremely curved medially, creating two areas of contact with the middle turbinate (arrows). The patient suffered from nasal obstruction, feeling of fullness, postnasal discharge and episodes of sneezing. After resection of the uncinate process and the diseased ethmoidal bulla (not visible in this tomographic cut) the symptoms disappeared.

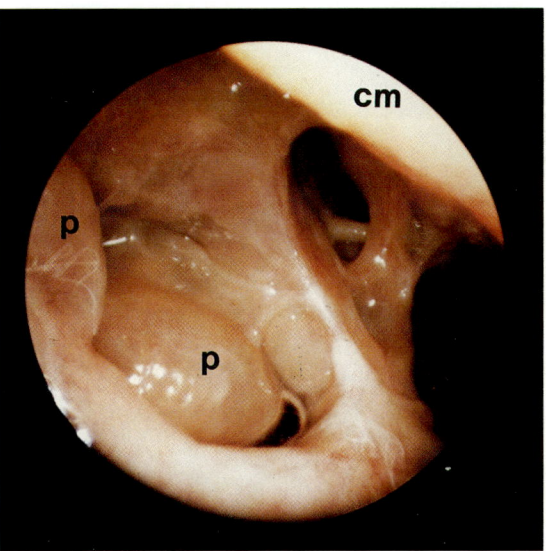

Fig. 6.7. NARES (non-allergic rhinitis with eosinophilia syndrome): polyp recurrence in the maxillary sinus ostium on the right side of a patient 6 months after endoscopic surgery. Topical corticosteroid therapy was applied and the mucosa almost normalized after 3 weeks. The patient had to continue this therapy to prevent regrowth of polyps.

costeroid therapy and despite this accounts for the majority of surgical failures. Do we have criteria to differentiate those different kinds of nasal polyps before choosing a therapy, thus limiting our frequency of indication for surgery?[5-11] (Figs. 6.7–6.9).

There are many more questions to hand than we can answer for the time being. Does the endoscope have the answer? For sure it does not, but its use may help in several respects:

1. There is more in the allergic and non-allergic nose than can be seen with the speculum, the unaided eye and standard x-rays. Especially in chronic and/or therapy-resistant cases, anterior and posterior rhinoscopy simply are not sufficient means to evaluate a nose.

2. In addition to evaluating the patients symptomatic improvement under any given therapy, the endoscope allows for visual evaluation of mucosal changes in areas otherwise hidden from the unaided eye and even from the microscope.

3. The endoscope may help to direct researchers' interest to the sites where the problems (and most

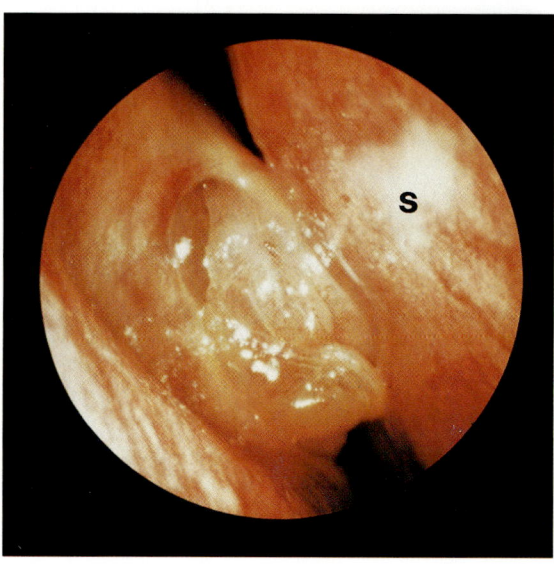

Fig. 6.9. Endoscopic view of a diseased middle meatus on the right side: note the profuse protrusion of polyps between uncinate process and middle turbinate, whereas the entire mucosa of the septum, the inferior turbinate and the rest of the nose appears healthy and normal.

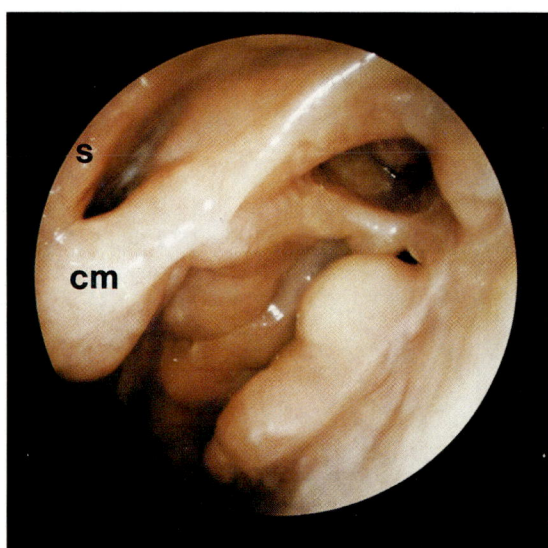

Fig. 6.8. NARES: view into the middle nasal meatus on a left side, demonstrating the situation following numerous surgical procedures – including radical ethmoidectomy – for a diffuse polypoid disease. The symptoms had improved; the mucosa, however, is far from normal. Despite continuous topical and systemical corticosteroid therapy this was the best condition that could be reached over the years.

of the polyps) start: biopsies of those areas might provide useful additional information that may not be present in biopsies or smears from mucosal areas that are only secondarily involved – like the inferior turbinate or the maxillary sinus.

4. When discussing the problem of "nasal polyposis" we should be aware that we are not talking about one disease entity, but are dealing with a mucosal reaction to various, apparently quite different stimuli, which may well require different therapeutic approaches.

5. Finally, the endoscope might be a tool to bring the two groups of people who "work" in the nose, but have talked so little to each other closer together: the allergologists/immunologists and the surgeons. For the latter group this could mean being more selective with their indications for surgery by trying to exclude those cases that could better be approached with anti-allergic or immunotherapy. The immunologists should consider the fact that the mucosa is not lining a simple box with plane walls in the nose with allergic/immunologic reactions taking place anywhere, but that the ethmoidal labyrinth in the lateral nasal wall holds a key position, with its clefts, meatus and cells. Here,

mechanistic (anatomical variations causing stenosis and contact areas) and aerodynamic principles must be considered as well. In a multifactorial disease complex, a closer cooperation between those involved in research and those in therapy is required to meet the challenge.

References

1. Messerklinger W. *Endoscopy of the Nose*. Baltimore: Urban & Schwarzenberg, 1978.
2. Stammberger H. *Functional endoscopic sinus surgery*. Philadelphia: BC Decker-Mosby Year Book Publ. 1991.
3. Kleinsasser O, Schroeder H-G. Adenocarcinomas of the inner nose after exposure to wood dust. *Arch Oto-Rhino-Laryngol* 1988; *245:* 1-15.
4. Posawetz W, Stammberger H. Chirurgische Massnahmen im Rahmen einer Inhalationsallergie. *Allergologie* 1991; *14:* 440-5.
5. Ogava H. Atopic aspect of eosinophilic nasal polyposis and a possible mechanism of eosinophil accumulation. *Acta Oto-Laryngol* (*Stockh*) 1986; *(suppl 430):* 12-7.
6. Ogino S, Harada T, Okawachi I, Irifune M, Matunaga T, Nagano T. Aspirin induced asthma and nasal polyps. *Acta Oto-Laryngol* (*Stockh*) 1986; *(suppl 430):* 21-7.
7. Hsieh V. Nonallergic rhinitis with eosinophilia (NARES): a precursor of the triad nasal polyposis – intrinsic asthma – intolerance to Aspirin. *Rhinology* 1988; *(suppl 1):* 129.
8. Barnes PJ. Asthma as an axon reflex. *Lancet* 1986; *1:* 242-5.
9. Mygind N, Winter B. Immunological barriers in the nose and paranasal sinuses. *Acta Oto-Laryngol* (*Stockh*) 1987; *103:* 363-8.
10. Amr Ali Sobieh. Endoscopic study and surgery of paranasal sinus disease in asthmatic patients. Thesis. Cairo, Egypt: Alahzar University Press, 1990.
11. Wolf G, Saria A, Gamse R. Neue Aspekte zur autonomen Innovation der menschlichen Schleimhaut. *Laryngol Rhinol Otol* 1987; *66:* 149-51.

CHAPTER 7

X-ray, CT-scan, MR-imaging

P Clement
P Van der Veken
P Iwens
Th Buisseret

Introduction

The development of computerized tomography (CT) in the early seventies by Ambrose[2] and by Hounsfield[9] introduced a revolution in radiological technique. The paranasal sinuses and their surrounding structures are very appropriate for this type of examination,[8,15] since there is such a large variety of contrast difference in this milieu[4] with bone, mucous membrane, muscle, fat and air. Due to the fact that the number of CT-scanners in most countries has increased dramatically, access to this type of examination has become easier and the cost has dropped considerably. Furthermore, the latest generation of CT-scanners is much faster (1 second per scan) than the first generation, and they now have an increased degree of resolution (structures down to 0.6 mm can be visualized). For these reasons, the scanner can now fully obviate the need for ordinary X-ray examination of the paranasal sinuses. Even when using multiple projections, a standard X-ray examination does not permit an accurate delineation of the ethmoid region and does not provide good visualization of the structures of the lateral wall of the nasal cavity. As to radiation, exact dosimetric studies are lacking, but the total dose of a CT-scan is presumed to be equal to, or slightly higher than the dose of four standard projections.

Magnetic resonance (MR) imaging, especially T2-weighted images, shows very clearly the extent of mucosal swelling, but does not visualize the bony structures, which are important for the diagnosis of sinus disease (Fig. 7.1). Also, access to MR-imaging is still limited. Therefore, it is the opinion of many authors that CT-scanning is the examination of choice in inflammatory sinus disease.

During childhood, the nose and the paranasal sinuses undergo a tremendous development.[13,18] The anatomy changes considerably, and the local immune system matures. For these reasons, the growing child runs a risk of developing sinusitis, which may differ considerably from that of an adult with completely developed anatomy and a fully mature immune system.[1,7,10,18] The occurrence of sinusitis in childhood has in the past been studied using ordinary X-ray examination.[3,11,14,16] Today, CT-scans can provide much more information.[12]

In the studies presented below, it has been our main aim to examine the frequency and extent of sinusitis, as visualized by CT-scanning, in adults and in children with chronic nasal complaints.

Methods and patients

For the CT-scanning, a high-resolution technique was used (Siemens, Somatom DRG or DRH). One total CT-study consisted of a scout view, and of 18 sections for an adult, and 6 to 12 sections for a child, in order to cut down the radiation dose. Scan time per section was 5 seconds, and the total time for the examination was about 15 minutes. Normally, the sections were taken at 4-mm intervals and had a 4-mm thickness. Whenever the patient was able to lie in ventral decubitus with the head in hyperextension (more than 40%), coronal sections were taken. A coronal section gives better infor-

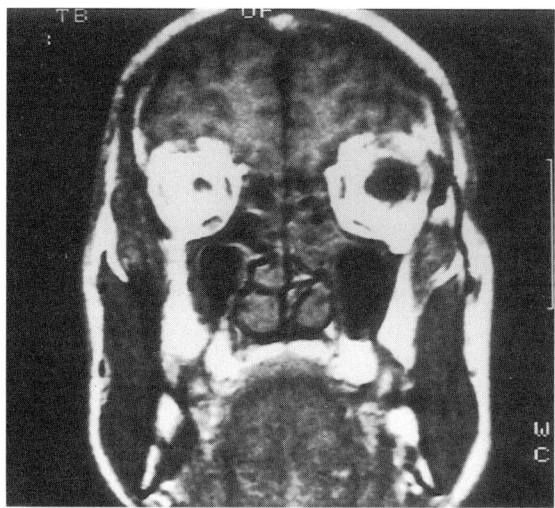

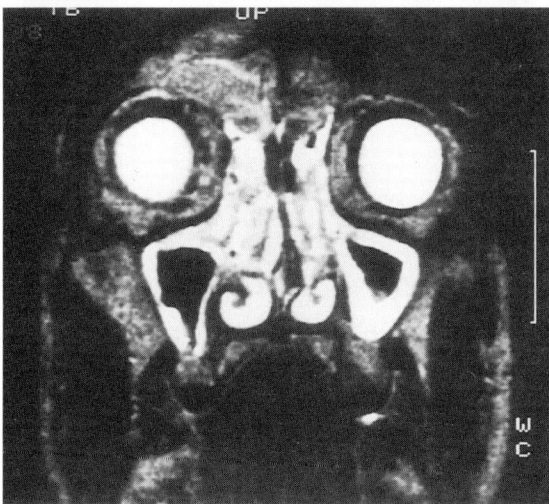

Fig. 7.1. Magnetic resonance imaging of a patient with polyposis and involvement of ethmoidal and maxillary sinuses. The mucosal swelling is less clear in T1- (upper photo), as compared to T2-weighted image (lower photo). Bone structures are not visible in MR imaging.

Table 7.1A. *CT-scan findings of mucosal sinus disease in a population of 350 adult patients with chronic nasal complaints.*

No CT signs of mucosal disease	149 (42%)*
CT signs of mucosal disease	201 (58%)

* Anatomical abnormality shown in 100 of these patients.

Table 7.1B. *Number of patients with CT-scan signs of anatomical abnormalities in a population of 350 adult patients with chronic nasal complaints.*

Signs of mucosal sinus disease	No (n=149)	Yes (n=201)
Septal deviation	45%	75%
Concha bullosa	44%	33%
'Haller cell'	10%	1%
Processus uncinatus bullosa	2%	1%

Table 7.1C. *CT-scan signs of involvement of different sinuses in patients with sign of mucosal sinus disease at CT-scan (our study) or at endoscopy (study of Zinreich et al[15]).*

Per cent of all patients	Our study (n=201)	Zinreich study (n=100)
Maxillary	73%	65%
Anterior ethmoidal	35%	72%
Posterior ethmoidal	19%	40%
Frontal	13%	34%
Sphenoidal	13%	21%

Table 7.1D. *Gradation (see Fig. 7.5) of maxillary sinus involvement in 201 patients with chronic nasal complaints and CT-scan signs of mucosal sinus disease.*

	Opacity	Polyp
Grade 1	23%	4%
Grade 2	12%	22%
Grade 3	4%	3%
Grade 4	3%	

mation about the nasal lateral wall and makes it much easier to differentiate between anterior and posterior ethmoidal cell involvement than do transversal and axial sections.

We examined 4 series of consecutive patients referred to our university ENT clinic for chronic nasal complaints. Their complaints consisted mainly of nasal obstruction and/or discharge, sometimes associated with 'post-nasal drip', anosmia, sinus tenderness and, in children, middle ear problems, cough (especially at night), fever, and fetor ex ore. Most patients, in particular when they had purulent nasal discharge, were treated with antibiotics and decongestants before the examination.

We studied 2 groups of adults (20 to 79 years) and 2 groups of children (3 to 14 years). Group 1 consisted of 350 adults, studied with attention focused on the presence of polyps and their relationship to chronic rhinosinusitis. Group 2: 258 adults in a study with special attention paid to anatomical abnormalities and to the extent of the sinusitis.

Group 3: 196 children with chronic nasal complaints. Group 4: 57 children with both chronic nasal complaints and a known positive allergy test (skin test and RAST) to grass pollen (n = 17), house dust mite (n = 29) or both (n = 11). In the pollen-allergic patients, the CT examination was performed during the pollen season.

Results

CT-scan signs of sinusitis were found very frequently in all 4 groups of adults and children with chronic nasal complaints. There was involvement of the sinuses in 56% to 70% of all patients.

Group 1: adults

In Group 1, 42% of the adults with chronic nasal complaints did not have any CT-scan signs of sinusitis, although two-thirds of them had clear-cut anatomical abnormalities (septal deviation, concha bullosa, 'Haller cells') (Table 7.1A) (Fig. 7.2-4). A septal deviation was more common in patients with sinus disease than in patients without (75% and 45% respectively) (Table 7.1B), suggesting that this anatomical abnormality predisposes to sinusitis.

In the adults, we found CT-scanning signs of sinusitis most frequently in the maxillary sinuses, followed by the anterior ethmoidal cells, the posterior ethmoidal cells, the frontal sinuses, and the sphenoidal sinus (Table 7.1C). These figures are different from those published by Zinreich et al.[16] But the selection criteria used in these two studies were also different. The series of Zinreich and coworkers consisted of patients with clinical and endoscopic signs of sinusitis, while our patients had chronic nasal complaints and CT-signs of sinus disease.

We were able to determine the prevalence of polyps (or cysts) in the maxillary, frontal and sphenoid sinuses, as these sinuses have a size that is sufficient for the recognition of a rounded mucosal swelling. Polyps were found in 31% of all patients with sinusitis, in 42% of those with maxillary sinusitis, and in 11% and 10% of those with frontal and sphenoid sinusitis, respectively.

A gradation scale was used for evaluation of the degree of opacity (mucosal swelling and secretion) and of polyp formation in the maxillary sinus (Fig.

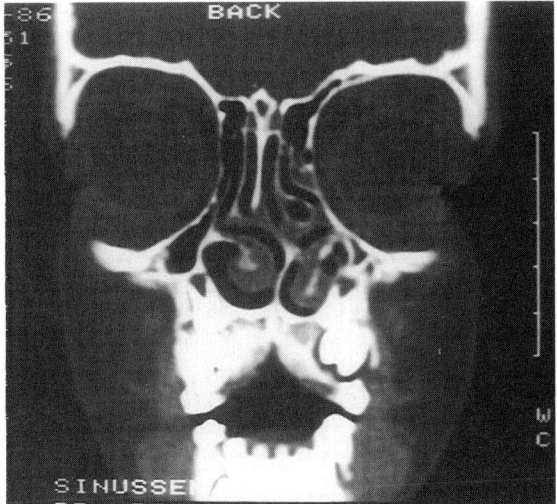

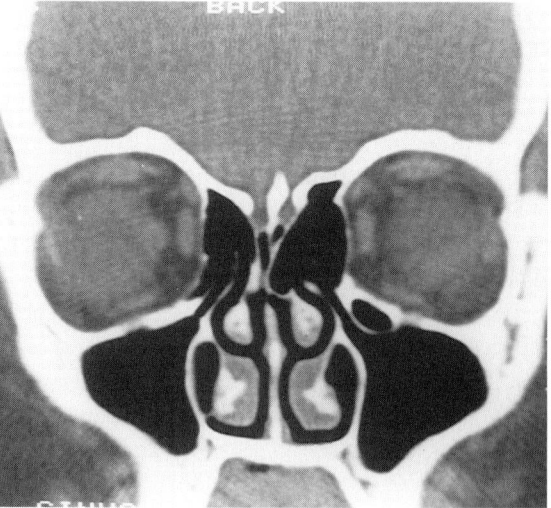

Fig. 7.3. Upper part. Significant septal deviation and concha bullosa (middle turbinate). CT-scan, coronal plane in child. *Lower part.* "Haller cell" (pneumatization of orbital floor). CT-scan, coronal plane in adult.

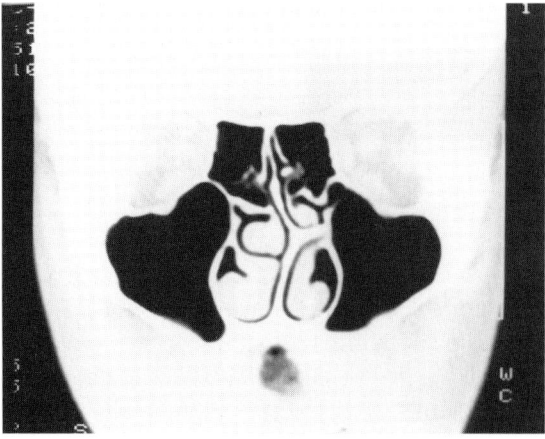

Fig. 7.2. Extreme septal deviation with impaction but without signs of sinusitis. CT-scan, coronal plane in adult.

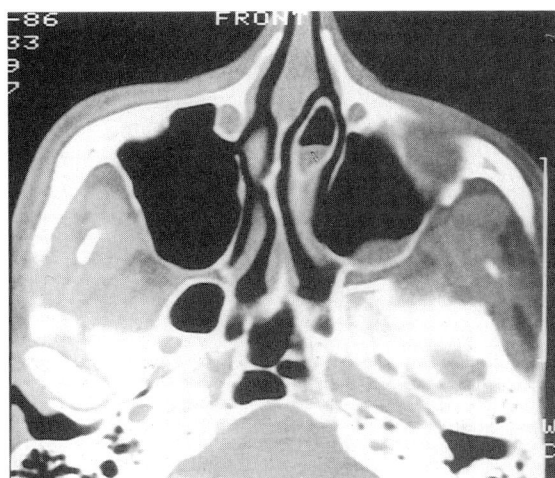

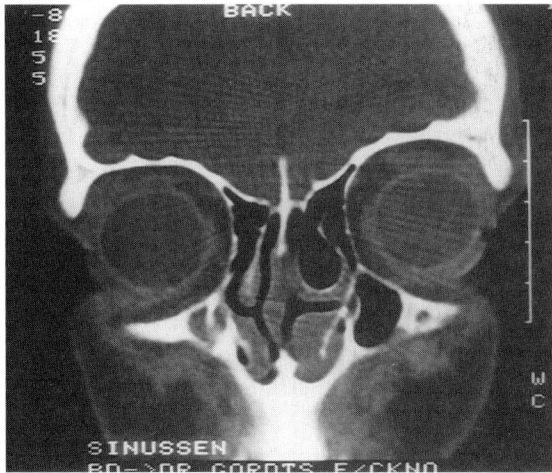

Fig. 7.4. Upper part. Concha bullosa (middle turbinate) with fluid level and with light mucosal thickening in the maxillary sinus on the same side. CT-scan, axial plane in adult. *Lower part.* Big concha bullosa (middle turbinate) with moderate septal deviation. CT-scan, coronal plane in child.

Table 7.2. *CT-scan signs of mucosal sinus disease, related to age, in a population of 258 adult patients with chronic nasal complaints.*

Years	20-49	50-79
Maxillary	59%	72%
Anterior ethmoidal	26%	35%
Posterior ethmoidal	11%	23%
Frontal	9%	18%
Sphenoidal	12%	18%

7.5). Using this gradation scale in patients with CT-scan signs of sinusitis, we found that the majority of patients had minimal or moderate changes. Only 7% had opacification of 75% or more of the maxillary sinus, and only 3% had multiple polyps (Table 7.1D).

Sixteen of the polyp patients showed massive polyposis with intranasal polyps identified by rhinoscopy. The maxillary sinuses were involved in 100%, the ethmoidal cells in 93%, the sphenoidal sinus in 69%, and the frontal sinuses in 53%.

Group 2: adults

In this group, consisting of 258 adults with chronic nasal complaints, the CT-scan showed sign of mucosal disease in 70%. Fig. 7.6 shows that, although most of the patients presenting with chronic nasal complaints were young, the elderly had the highest percentage of concomitant involvement of the paranasal sinuses. This applied to all sinuses, in particular the posterior ethmoidal, frontal and sphenoidal (Table 7.2).

Whenever sinus pathology was shown, the maxillary sinuses were involved in more than 90% of the cases for all age groups; that is, at least twice as frequently as any other sinus.

While the frequency of CT-signs of frontal recess disease exceeded or equaled that of frontal sinusitis in all age groups, the number of patients with infundibulum ethmoidale disease was lower for all ages than that of maxillary sinusitis. These findings indicate that frontal sinusitis is practically always an extension of frontal recess pathology, while this is not the case with maxillary sinusitis and infundibulum ethmoidale pathology. In other words, pathology of the maxillary sinuses is often, but not always, caused by extension of ethmoidal infundibulum pathology.

Group 3: children

In this group, consisting of 196 children with chronic nasal complaints, 64% had CT-signs of mucosal sinus disease. The proportion presenting with chronic nasal complaints was higher in the young children (aged 3 to 8 years) than in the older children (Table 7.3A). The percentage of children having maxillary sinusitis, shown at CT-scan, was rather constant, around 50%, in all age-groups (Table 7.3A) but in small children (3 to 8 years) the disease was more severe, with a higher degree of opacity and more frequent bilateral disease. The relative frequency of sinusitis in the ethmoidal and

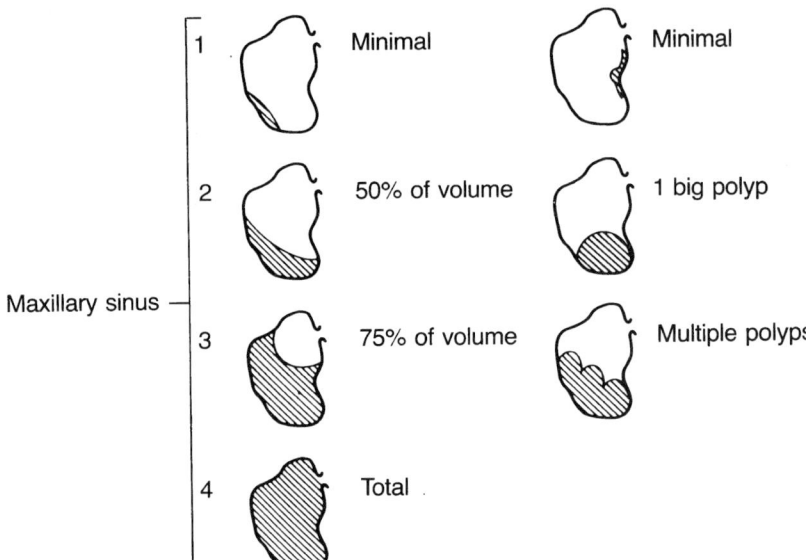

Fig. 7.5. Scale for grading mucosal thickening or opacity (4-step scale) and polypous transformation (3-step scale) in the maxillary sinus.

the sphenoidal sinuses tended to fall with increasing age (Table 7.3A).

In all age-groups, the anterior ethmoidal cells were more frequently involved than the posterior, and boys more often had sinus pathology than girls.

Sinusitis in children usually involves more than one type of sinus. Isolated maxillary sinusitis occurred in only 5% of the young children, but in 31% of the oldest children, probably as a result of an increasing frequency of septal deviations with age (see below). Isolated sinusitis was found in the ethmoidal cells in 1.5%, the sphenoidal sinus in 1%, and the frontal sinus in 0.5%.

Anatomical abnormalities were also studied in the children, and Table 7.3B shows a dramatic increase from 16% to 72% in the occurrence of septal deviation with age. A similar trend, although less pronounced, was found for other anatomical abnormalities (Table 7.3B).

Allergy testing showed allergy to seasonal and/or perennial allergen in 15% of the children. The sinus involvement did not differ between allergic and non-allergic children.

Group 4: allergic children

Finally, we studied 57 children who were known to have seasonal and/or perennial allergic rhinitis, and who also had chronic nasal complaints. They did not differ from the other 3 groups with regard to percentage of positive sinus CT-scans (56%), in involvement of specific sinuses (Table 7.4A), or the severity of the sinus involvement. There did not appear to be any difference between results in children with seasonal and with perennial allergic rhinitis (Table 7.4B).

Discussion

Our studies have indicated that sinusitis is more frequent in patients with chronic nasal complaints than has been generally assumed. However, the sinus affection, seen on CT-scan, was in most cases mild, and may not necessarily require treatment.

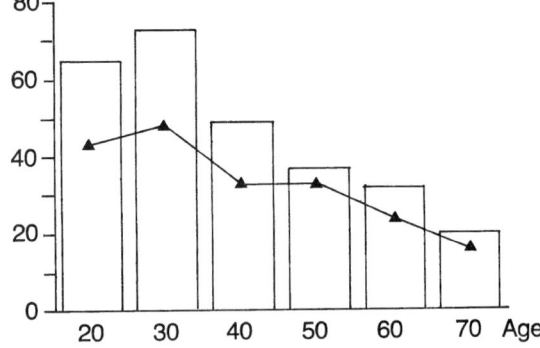

Fig. 7.6. Age distribution of 258 adults with chronic nasal complaints (open bars) and of those with a positive CT-scan of paranasal sinuses (black triangles).

Table 7.3A. *CT-scan signs of sinus involvement, related to age group, and to specific sinus, in a population of 196 children with chronic nasal complaints.*

Age group (years)		Sinus disease	Maxillary	Frontal	Ethmoidal	Sphenoidal
3-4	(n = 38)	72%	63%	—*	58%	29%
5-6	(n = 46)	50%	39%	—*	35%	13%
7-8	(n = 42)	70%	52%	7%	35%	13%
9-10	(n = 21)	62%	33%	5%	23%	19%
11-12	(n = 20)	65%	45%	15%	20%	10%
13-14	(n = 29)	66%	65%	0%	10%	0%

* not yet developed.

Table 7.3B. *Percentages of CT-scans showing nasal anatomical abnormalities, related to age group, in a population of 196 children with chronic nasal complaints.*

Age group (years)	Septal deviation	Concha bullosa	'Haller cell'
3-4	16%	0%	6%
5-6	37%	8%	3%
7-8	55%	6%	2%
9-10	48%	2%	2%
11-12	65%	15%	10%
13-14	72%	23%	3%

The high frequency of sinus involvement in the younger children, and the fact that they often have bilateral disease and severe involvement of many sinuses, all speak in favor of a major role played by an immature immune system in the pathogenesis of sinusitis at this age. We believe that this is more important than allergy for the majority of children with sinusitis. In favor of this statement are two observations. First, the prevalence of allergy increases considerably with age during childhood, while than of sinusitis clearly decreases. Second, we found that 15% of the children with sinusitis were allergic, and this cannot be considered a significant overrepresentation of allergy in this group as compared to the background population.

A CT-scan of the paranasal sinuses is abnormal in less than 10% of children examined for neurological symptoms (D'Hondt, personal communication). It was therefore astonishing that 50% of our children with both seasonal and perennial allergic rhinitis showed CT-signs of sinusitis. However, as all these children also suffered from chronic nasal complaints, this is a likely cause of most cases of sinusitis. It is striking (Fig. 7.7) that children with allergic rhinitis can have a markedly swollen mucous membrane in the nose, and normal conditions in the sinuses.

In conclusion, we cay say that the prevalence of sinusitis in patients with chronic nasal complaints depends on several factors. Two important factors

Table 7.4A. *Involvement of different sinuses in 32 allergic children with CT-scan signs of sinusitis.*

Maxillary	64%
Anterior ethmoidal	39%
Posterior ethmoidal	20%
Frontal	14%
Sphenoidal	26%

Table 7.4B. *Percent CT-scan signs of involvement of maxillary sinuses, related to allergen, in 57 allergic children.*

	Signs of sinusitis	Mild	Severe
Pollen (n = 17)	59%	60%	40%
House dust mite (n = 29)	48%	71%	29%
Both (n = 11)	73%	63%	37%

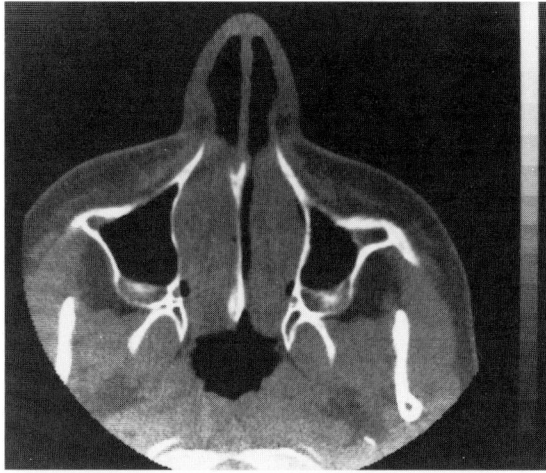

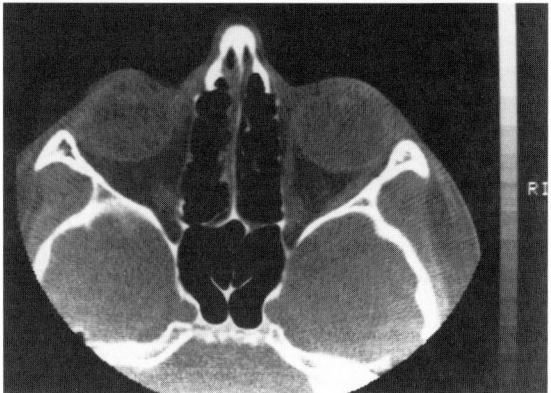

Fig. 7.7. Example of CT-scan from a child with allergic rhinitis and massive mucosal thickening in the nose (upper photo) but without involvement of maxillary (upper photo) or ethmoidal (lower photo) sinuses.

seem to be age and the presence of anatomical abnormalities. During childhood, rhinosinusitis is very common, but seems to be self-limiting in most cases, and there is a sharp drop in prevalence at the age of 7-8 years. The course of childhood sinusitis looks very similar to that of chronic otitis media with effusion. Maybe both diseases have a common etiology, which could be immaturity of the immunological defence system. Therefore one should refrain from aggressive surgical therapy as much as possible in this age group.

In adulthood, the presence of anatomical abnormalities of the septum and of the lateral wall of the nasal cavity seems to predispose to chronicrhinosinusitis, and therefore surgery can be very beneficial.

Allergy does not seem to play an important role in the etiology of chronic rhinosinusitis in either childhood or adulthood. However, as perennial rhinitis induces a condition of chronic inflammation (accompanied by chronic nasal complaints), one will find in these patients a higher prevalence of rhinosinusitis than in a normal population. It is the authors' opinion that any condition of chronic inflammation of the nasal mucosa, whatever etiology (allergy, infection, anatomical variations) can induce chronic rhinosinusitis.

Conclusion

A CT-scan gives a much better visualization than does a plain X-ray examination of the anatomy of the bone and mucous membranes of the nose and the paranasal sinuses. With modern scanners, the irradiation, the time and the cost have all been considerably reduced, and a CT-scan can now offer a considerably improved relationship between information and irradiation/time/cost. Obviously, the use of CT-scans depends upon the local situation, *i.e.* access to a modern scanner and cost of the examination. Our recommendations may therefore not be valid for all hospitals, but in our opinion a CT-scan is the preferred examination, and ordinary X-ray is an outdated examination: a waste of time and money.

We perform a CT-scan when there is a suspicion of chronic rhinosinusitis, *i.e.* all patients with long-standing, severe complaints of nasal blockage and/or discharge, and also when nasal endoscopy shows clearcut signs of inflammation of the lateral nasal wall, especially of the structures of the middle meatus. To limit the number of CT-scans, the examination should only be performed after attempted medical therapy. In children under the age of 8 years, CT-scans should only be performed when serious complications are suspected.

References

1 Albegger K. Zur Rhinosinusitis des Kindes aus HNO-ärtzlicher Sicht. *HNO* 1980; *28:* 321-8.
2 Ambrose J. Computerized transverse axial scanning (tomography). II. Clinical application. *Br J Radiol* 1973; *46:* 1023-47.
3 Caffey J. *Pediatric X-ray diagnosis*, 7th edn. Vol 1, section 1. The skull. Chicago: Year Book Medical Publishers, 1977: 111-7.
4 Carter BL. Computed tomographic scanning in head and neck tumors. *Otolaryngol Clin N Am* 1980; 449-57.
5 Clement PAR, Van der Veken P, Verstraelen J, et al. Some remarks on nasal polyposis. *Acta Otolaryngol (Belg)* 1989; *3:* 267-78.
6 Clement PAR, Van der Veken P, Verstraelen J, et al. Recurrent polyposis nasi. *Rhinology* 1989; *suppl 8:* 5-14.
7 Flock H. Sinusitis maxillaris im Kindesalter und ihre Behandlung. *HNO* 1957; *6:* 165-7.
8 Hesselinck JR, New FJ. Computed tomography of the paranasal sinuses and face. Part I and II. *Comput Assist Tomogr* 1978; *5:* 559-76.
9 Hounsfield GN. Computerized transverse axial scanning (tomography). Description of system. *Br J Radiol* 1973; *46:* 1016-22.
10 Jazbi B. Sinusitis in infants and children. In: Jazbi B, ed. *Pediatric otolaryngology*. New York: Appleton-Century-Crofts 1980; 143-57.
11 Kovatch AL. Maxillary sinus involvement in children with non-respiratory complaints. *Pediatrics* 1984; 306-8.
12 Messerklinger W. Die Rolle und Therapie der recidiverenden und chronischen Rhinosinusitis. *Laryngol Rhinol Otol* 1987; *66:* 293-9.
13 Pirsig W. Phasen des postnatalen Nasenwachstums. Eine kritische Übersicht. *Laryngol Rhinol Otol* 1986; *65:* 243-9.
14 Shurin PA. Inflammatory disease of the nose and paranasal sinuses. In: Bluestone CD, Stool SE, Arjona SK, eds. *Pediatric otolaryngology*. Philadelphia: WB Saunders Co, 1983; vol 1: 781-90.
15 Tadmor R, New PFJ. Computed tomography of the orbit with special emphasis on coronal sections. II. Pathological anatomy. *J Comput Assist Tomogr* 1978; *2:* 35-44.
16 Unger JM. The nose and paranasal sinuses. In: Eisenberg RL, ed. *Head and neck imaging. Handbooks of diagnostic imaging*. Edinburgh: Churchill Livingstone, 1987: 3-45.
17 Van der Veken PJV, Clement PAR, Buisseret T, Desprechins B, Kaufman L, Derde MP. CT-scan study of the incidence of sinus involvement and nasal anatomic variations in 196 children. *Rhinology* 1990; *28:* 177-84.
18 Wald ER. Sinusitis and its complications in the pediatric patient. *Pediat Clin N Am* 1981; *28:* 777-95.
19 Zinreich SJ, Kennedy DW, Rosenbau AE, Gayler BW, Kumar AJ, Stammberger H. Paranasal sinuses: CT imaging requirements for endoscopic surgery. *Radiology* 1987: *163:* 769-75.

CHAPTER 8

Cytology

ELI O MELTZER
H ALICE ORGEL
ALFREDO A JALOWAYSKI

Introduction

A series of diagnostic modalities can help to classify nasal disorders (Table 8.1).[1] These include history, physical examination, rhinoscopy, rhinomanometry, provocation challenges, biochemical determinations, immunologic studies, *in vivo* and *in vitro* testing for specific IgE, imaging, blood flow and ciliary function analyses, and examination of nasal cytology.

This chapter is organized to present 1) techniques for obtaining, processing and interpreting cytologic specimens, 2) findings in various rhinopathies, and 3) findings in the nasal cytology consequent to various therapeutic agents. It is hoped that this review will document that evaluating nasal cytology can assist in: 1) distinguishing inflammatory from non-inflammatory rhinopathies; 2) distinguishing between allergic, non-allergic, and infectious rhinitis; 3) distinguishing between viral and bacterial infections; 4) classifying the cellular response to an infection; 5) following the course of a disease; 6) following the response to treatment.

Morphological changes in the nasal mucosa may reflect reactions which are also valid for other parts of the airways.

Table 8.1. *Classification of chronic rhinopathies.*

Inflammatory rhinitis

Allergic rhinitis
   Seasonal
   Perennial

Eosinophilic nonallergic rhinitis

Basophilic nonallergic rhinitis

Infectious rhinitis
   Viral
   Bacterial
   Fungal

Nasal polyposis

Atrophic rhinitis

Noninflammatory rhinitis

Vasomotor rhinitis
   Autonomic dysfunction
   Associated with systemic conditions, e.g. pregnancy or thyroid disease

Rhinitis medicamentosa
   Local sympathomimetic overuse
   Systemic medications, e.g. antihypertensives or contraceptives

Structure-related rhinitis

Anatomic deformities, e.g. septal deviations, ciliary disorders

Obstruction, e.g. adenoidal hypertrophy, foreign body or tumor

Methods

Various techniques have been used for obtaining, processing, evaluating and interpreting nasal cytology specimens.[2]

Sampling methods

The selection of a sampling method depends in part on the requirements of the specimen. Some of the considerations are: the age of the patient, the need for repeated samples, the position or site or depth or thickness of the nasal mucosa of interest, the requirement for simultaneous biochemical studies.

Blown secretions. In this method, secretions in the nasal airways are blown onto wax paper or a plastic wrap and then placed onto a glass slide.[3,4] The cells are only those contained in the secretions and may thus reflect a different population from that collected from the epithelium. Another disadvantage is that many children and patients with some nasal disorders cannot produce an adequate secretion specimen.

Smears taken with cotton wool swabs. This is a simple procedure for obtaining cells from the adherent secretions and epithelial layer. As with blown specimens, the cell count varies considerably. However, this method can be used to determine the presence or absence of a specific cell population in terms of a relative proportion of total cells.[5]

Imprints. These involve the use of thin plastic strips painted with 1% albumin to produce a sticky surface. These are gently pressed onto the mucosal surface, usually the septum. A reasonably good cell yield is obtained and the number of different cells can be counted. Disadvantages of this method include the need to be manually dexterous and the presence of a considerable quantity of secretions on the strip.[6]

Brush method. This employs small plastic-coated steel-wire brushes with nylon bristles. The brush is placed between the septum and inferior turbinate and rotated while being removed. The total number of cells can be estimated, as the volume in which the cells are suspended is known. The cells obtained include those from secretions and those from the epithelial surface layer. A useful features of the brush method is that cell samples can be used for biochemical analysis studies as well as for morphological studies.[7] Local discomfort is a disadvantage.

Nasal scraping. A nasal specimen of both the secretions and surface epithelium can, with minimal trauma, be easily obtained by scraping the surface in the middle third of the inferior turbinate. After excess secretions are cleared, the more patent side is sampled using a plastic curette (Rhino-Probe, Apotex Scientific, Arlington, TX) under direct visual inspection.[8,9] The cells harvested from the epithelial lining are well-preserved and permit differential grading of specific cell elements. Advantages of this method include specificity of sampling site, minimal trauma with no need for anesthesia, ease of repetition, adequacy of specimens at any age in all nasal conditions. Cell samples can also be used for rapid viral and bacterial diagnostic studies as well as biochemical analysis.[10] The main disadvantage is that the superficial quality of the specimen does not permit evaluation of changes in the deeper mucosal layers.

The sampling methods of nose blowing and mucosal scraping have been compared in several studies in adults and children.[11,12,13] In adults with allergic rhinitis, a specimen adequate for microscopic grading could be obtained 100% of the time by the scraped technique, but in only 60-66% of the patients by the blown method. In children and in patients with rhinopathies not characterized by an increase in anterior discharge, the yield of evaluable specimens is even lower with the nose blowing technique. There was no difference between the two techniques as to the presence of neutrophils and the concordance for the presence of eosinophils was fair (67%). However, eosinophils were found more often in the nasal scraping sample when they were absent in the blown secretion than vice versa (28% vs 5%). Basophils were much more frequently noted in the scrapings than in the blown specimens (70% *vs* 4%).

Nasal lavage. This is performed by introducing 5 ml of saline solution in each nasal cavity with the patient's head bent backwards during closure of the soft palate. The volume of the return lavage fluid is known and the total number of cells harvested can be calculated. The cells are counted in a hemocytometer and the cell differential determined on a cytospin slide.[14]

The cytologic findings from nasal mucosal scrapings and nasal lavages have been studied to examine their correlation.[15] In patients with allergic rhinitis challenged with relevant allergens, scrapings and lavages correlated significantly for increased eosinophil number and percentage and for increased neutrophil count and percentage. In non-allergic patients or allergic rhinitis patients provoked by an irrelevant allergen, the correlation was not good, although the neutrophils increased in response to the non-specific stimulus. These data indicate that there is generally a positive correlation between mucosal scrapings and lavages for cell number and percentage.

Biopsy. The most common site of biopsy is the lower edge of the inferior turbinate. It is important to know the site of the biopsy since the mucosal lining changes from the squamous type anteriorly to the ciliated, columnar epithelium in the middle and posterior parts of the nasal cavities. Anesthesia is necessary and a vasoconstrictor agent is often required. A disadvantage of the biopsy procedure is that it is too traumatic to repeat in a serial fashion. The major advantage is that it allows examination of not only the superficial epithelium, but also the basement membrane and the submucosal components.

The leukocytes found in nasal lavage fluid have been compared to those in biopsies following antigen challenge. In allergic patients after challenge, in both the lavage fluid and the biopsy tissue, eosinophils and mononuclear cells increased although the cell counts did not correlate. Neutrophils increased more in the lavage samples than in mucosal biopsies in both allergic and non-allergic subjects, possibly reflecting nonspecific irritation.[16]

Processing methods

The specimen is transferred to a slide. In the case of the Rhinoprobe specimen, the cupped tip is tilted onto the glass and the wet contents of the sample spread over a small area. The specimen should be visible to the naked eye on the microscope slide.

Fixatives for the specimen on the slide include: air drying – not recommended: acetone; unscented hair sprays; Mota's basic lead acetate; buffered formalin; methyl alcohol; ether – 95% ethyl alcohol (1:1); and 95% ethyl alcohol. The latter preparation gives excellent results.

Histological stains have variable advantages: Hansel's – eosinophils; Wright's – basophils; Wright-Giemsa – eosinophils, neutrophils and basophilic cells; Papanicolaou – epithelial cells, nuclear and cytoplasmic changes; toluidine blue – basophilic cells; Leishman's – eosinophils; alcian yellow – mast cells; Randolph's – eosinophils; alcian blue – basophilic cells; May-Grünwald – neutrophils.

Staining may be achieved with the Wright-Giemsa Dip method as follows: a) Remove the slide(s) from the jar containing 95% ethyl alcohol and drain the excess alcohol. Do not allow the cells to air-dry; b) Dip the slide(s) in Wright-Giemsa (Volu-Sol) stain for 10-15 seconds; c) Drain the excess stain, then dip the slide(s) in Volu-Sol buffer for 10-30 seconds; d) Drain the excess buffer, then dip the slide(s) in Volu-Sol hematology rinse for 4-5 seconds, using quick dips, or flood slides with rinse contained in a squeeze bottle; e) Drain the excess rinse and air-dry the specimens.

Modes of evaluation

Light microscopy. Add a drop of immersion oil to the specimen and scan at low power ($\times 100$) to determine if the specimen has an adequate number of nonsquamous epithelial cells and a good-quality stain.

The nasal cytogram should then be viewed at high power (oil immersion, $\times 1000$). The various cell types seen in the stained specimen are described in Fig. 8.1.

Two evaluation methods of the cytogram can be used. One is to make a semiquantitative assessment of the specimen, graded as a mean of cells per 10 high power fields, or qualitatively on a scale of 0-4+ as suggested in Table 8.2. The other method involves making a percentage calculation of specific leukocytes, e.g., 10% eosinophils. The finding of 10% eosinophils in blown secretions generally corresponds to a 1+ grading seen in the nasal scraping cytogram. However, as previously stated, inadequate specimens for microscopic evaluation are often obtained by the blown method. The semiquantitative method is generally more informative.

A guide for interpreting the nasal cytogram is presented in Table 8.3.[9]

Cytology findings in clinical conditions

Normal subjects

The normal nasal mucosal cytology of infants, children, and adults consists of numerous epithelial

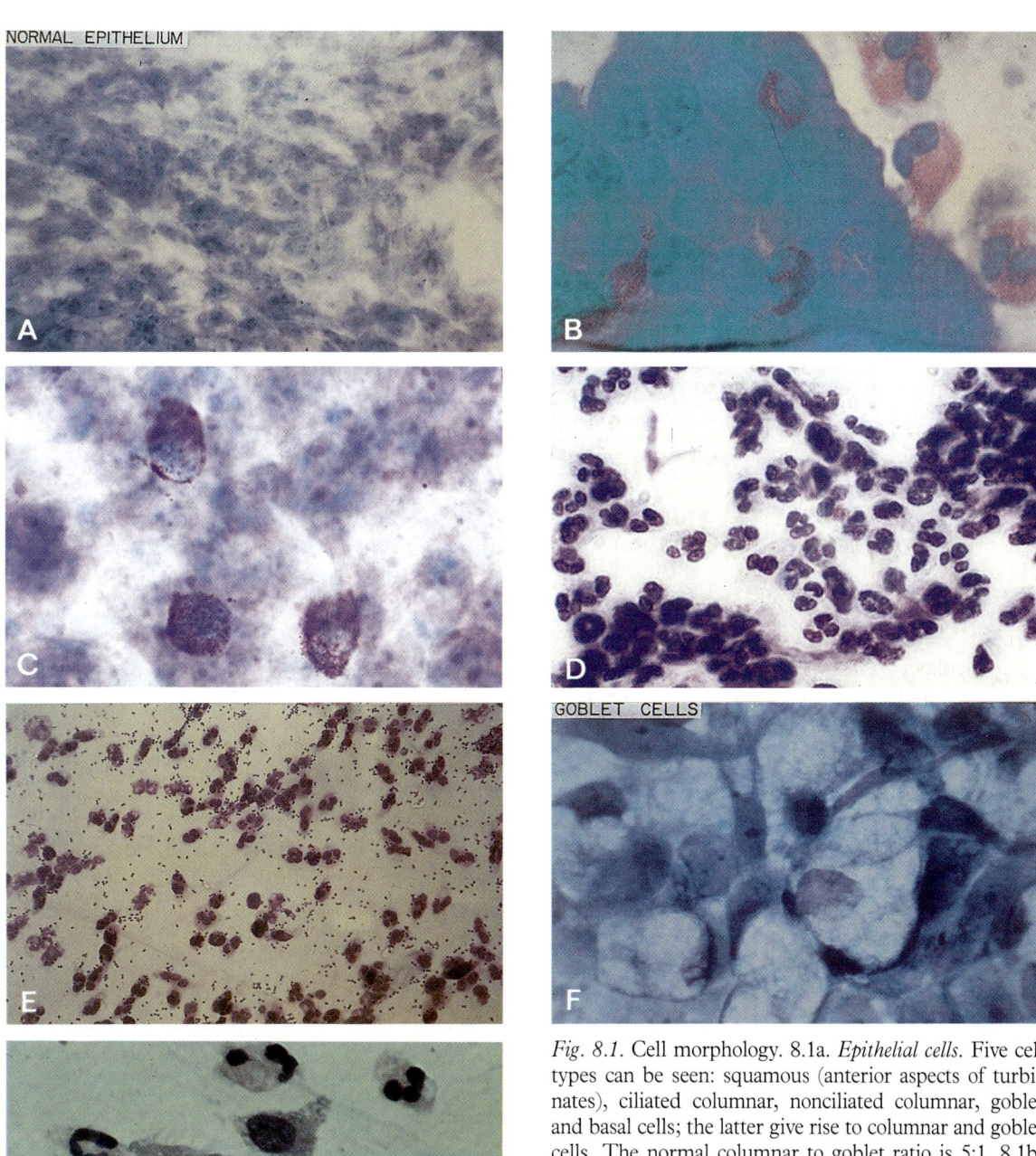

Fig. 8.1. Cell morphology. 8.1a. *Epithelial cells.* Five cell types can be seen: squamous (anterior aspects of turbinates), ciliated columnar, nonciliated columnar, goblet and basal cells; the latter give rise to columnar and goblet cells. The normal columnar to goblet ratio is 5:1. 8.1b. *Eosinophils.* Slightly larger than neutrophils. Usually have bilobed blue-staining nucleus. Cytoplasm filled with distinct large granules, which are eosinophilic and stain reddish-orange in this procedure. Not common in epithelium and nasal secretions under normal conditions. 8.1c. *Basophils.* Contain conspicuous, large or coarse, densely purple-staining basophilic granules. These cells have bilobed nucleus and are on average smaller than the mast cells described below. 8.1d. *Neutrophils.* Similar in appearance to those in blood smear. They have multilobed blue-purplish nuclei with clear or lightly pink-stained and finely granulated cytoplasm. Polymorphonuclear leukocytes are classified as neutrophils. A small number can be found in normal nasal mucosa. 8.1e. *Bacteria.* Stain dark blue. A small number of bacteria, which may be rods or cocci, is normal. When bacteria are seen with many squamous epithelial cells, the sample was taken too far anteriorly and has no clinical relevance. During a bacterial infection, intracellular bacteria may be seen. 8.1f. *Goblet cells.* Have foamy, vacuolated appearance with the nucleus displaced toward the basal part of the cell. 8.1g. *Ciliocytophthoria.* Epithelial cells infected by virus may demonstrate clumping of chromatin material, appearance of clear area (halo) surrounding nuclear material, or splitting of cells into ciliated portions (tufts) and nuclear portions.

Table 8.2. *A guide for grading nasal cytograms.*

Quantitative analysis	Semi-quantitative analysis	Grade
Epithelial cells		
N/A	Normal morphology	N
N/A	Abnormal morphology	A
N/A	Ciliocytophthoria	CCP
Eosinophils, neutrophils		
0*	None	0
0.1-1.0*	Occasional cells	1/2+
1.1-5.0*	Few scattered cells or small clumps	1+
6.0-15.0*	Moderate number of cells and larger clumps	2+
16.0-20.0*	Larger clumps of cells which do not cover the entire field	3+
>20*	Large clumps of cells covering the entire field	4+
Basophilic cells		
0*	None	0
0.1-0.3*	Occasional cells	1/2+
0.4-1.0*	Few scattered cells	1+
1.1-3.0*	Moderate number of cells	2+
3.1-6.0*	Many cells easily seen	3+
>6.0*	Large number of cells, as many as 25 per high power field	4+
*Bacteria***		
N/A	None seen	0
N/A	Occasional clump	1+
N/A	Moderate number	2+
N/A	Many easily seen	3+
N/A	Large numbers covering the entire field	4+
*Goblet cells****		
0	None	0
1-24%	Occasional to few cells	1+
25-49%	Moderate number	2+
50-74%	Many easily seen	3+
75-100%	Large number, may cover the entire field	4+

* Mean of cells per 10 high power fields ($\times 1000$).
** Note presence of intracellular bacteria.
*** Ratio of goblet cells to epithelial cells, expressed as percentage.

cells including ciliated columnar, non-ciliated columnar, goblet and basal cells. An adequately sampled specimen will always contain some ciliated cells and goblet cells. There are ususaly no eosinophils or basophilic cells (<1+) within the superficial layer above the basement membrane. A moderate number of neutrophils (≤2+) and a few bacteria (≤1+) can be seen, especially if the specimen is taken from the anterior portion of the inferior turbinate.[17-22]

Allergic rhinitis

Allergen challenge. In allergic rhinitis after exposure to an allergen, the immunologically-sensitized patient develops an immediate nasal response and, in over 50% of patients, a late-phase response. Pelikan[23] studied the cytology of these responses. The cells seen in the blown secretions of 102 patients were evaluated for their immediate nasal response as defined by a period of 0 to 120 minutes

Table 8.3. *A guide for interpreting the nasal cytogram.*

Cellular type	Diagnostic classification
Increased eosinophils (1-4+)	Allergy Nonallergic rhinitis with eosinophilia Aspirin sensitivity
Increased basophilic cells (1-4+)	Allergy Nonallergic rhinitis with eosinophilia Aspirin sensitivity Nonallergic rhinitis with basophilia
Increased neutrophils (2-4+)	
With intracellular bacteria	Nasopharyngitis or sinusitis
With ciliocytophthoria	Viral upper respiratory infection
With fungi	Fungal upper respiratory infection
With no bacteria	Irritant reaction
Bacteria (2-4+) (diagnostic if intracellular)	Nasopharyngitis or sinusitis

after allergen challenge. The positive symptom responses were accompanied by significant changes in the count of eosinophils (increase followed by decrease) in 67%, of basophilic cells (decrease) in 13%, and of neutrophils (decrease followed by increase) in 40%. No significant changes in the count of individual cell types in nasal secretions were found during most cases of 68 negative immediate nasal responses, or during any of the 102 saline control challenges. Increase in eosinophils immediately following allergen challenge has also been described by other investigators.[24,25]

The cells of nasal secretion were also examined 4 to 12 hours following antigen challenges in 164 allergic rhinitis patients for their late nasal response. The 104 positive late nasal responses were accompanied by significant changes in the count of eosinophils in 58% of the cases (increase immediately before and decrease during appearance of the late response), in basophils in 8% (slight increase during appearance of the late response), and in neutrophils in 84% (increase immediately before and decrease during appearance of the late response and increase again during resolution of the late response). Most of the 60 cases of negative allergen response were not accompanied by significant changes in the count of individual cell types and no changes were recorded during saline-control challenges.[26]

Nasal lavage studies have also confirmed the changes of inflammatory cells during the late-phase reaction. The pattern of influx varied among individuals, but in general eosinophils increased within 1-2 hours after challenge and peaked (in contrast to Pelikan's work) at 7-10 hours, neutrophils increased somewhat later than eosinophils and represented the greatest number of infiltrating cells in the late response, basophilic cells also increased significantly but did not exceed 1% of the total cells.[27]

Natural allergen exposure. The cellular response of the allergic mucosa to natural allergen exposure has also been studied. Pipkorn and coworkers[28] studied 10 patients with isolated birch-pollen allergy from a symptom-free state before, and then in the symptomatic state during the birch-pollen season. As the birch pollen increased, and the symptoms increased, the percentage and total number of eosinophils from the nasal lavages increased. The number of eosinophils increased 20-fold. The total number of basophilic cells found imprinted on plastic strips also significantly increased during the pollen season, but did not start to appear until 4 to 5 days of pollen exposure. A tendency toward an increase of the number of neutrophils was noted at the peak of the pollen season (Fig. 8.2).

In contrast to Pelikan's challenge data, Karlsson & Pipkorn[29] have noted no change following natural pollen allergen exposure in the number of goblet cells in the nasal mucosa.

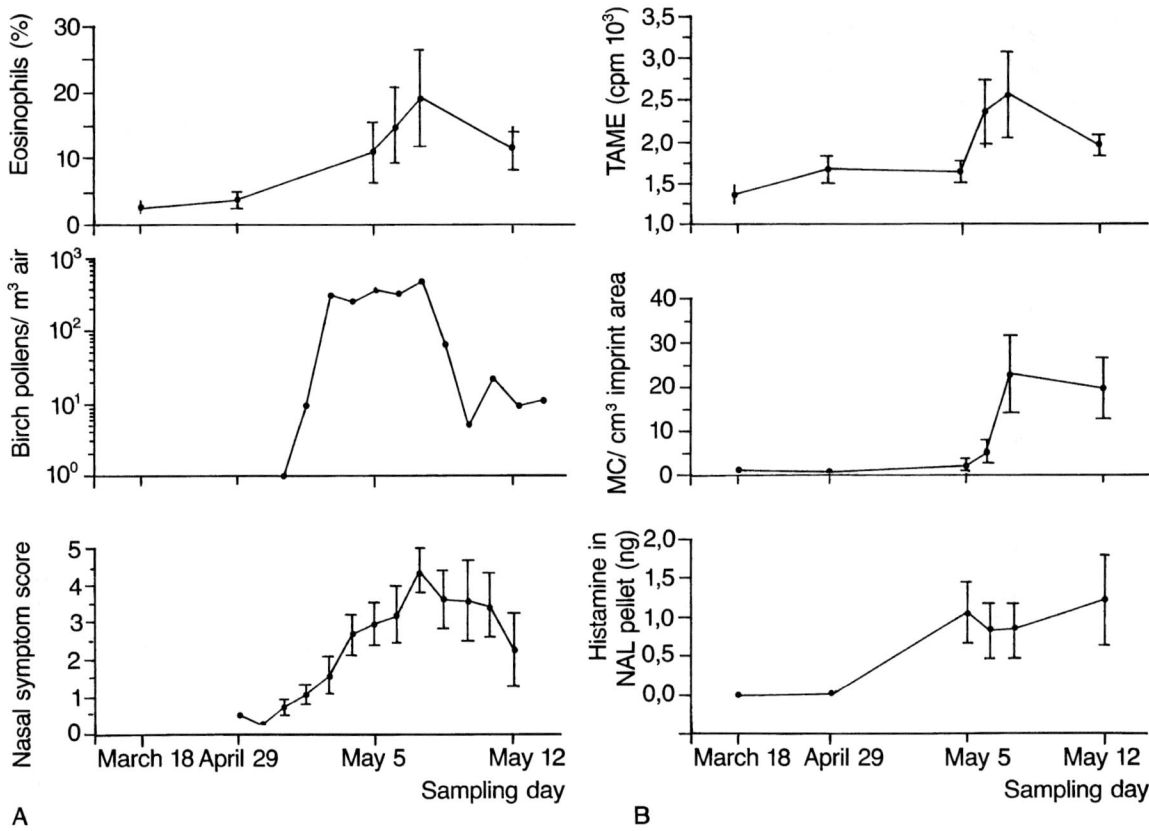

Fig. 8.2. Natural allergen exposure. *A.* The mean percentage of eosinophils found in the nasal lavages. Birch-pollen counts expressed as pollen grains per cubic meter of filtered air, and the nasal symptoms experienced by the patients. *B.* TAME-esterase levels in the nasal lavages, the mean number of mast cells per square centimeter imprint area, and the histamine content of the lavage cell pellet. Mean values and standard errors are vertical bars. Significance levels denote changes in relation to preseasonal values. From Pipkorn U, Karlsson G, Enerbäck L. The cellular response of the human allergic mucosa to natural allergen exposure. *J Allergy Clin Immunol* 1988; *82:* 1046-54.

Clinical findings. Increased numbers of eosinophils are found in the nasal mucosa in active allergic disease.[3, 18, 19] In university students, schoolchildren, and infants, a highly significant correlation has been shown with nasal secretion eosinophilia and evidence of allergy such as nose rubbing, sneezing, sniffing, runny nose, and wet and swollen turbinates.[30, 31] The degree of nasal eosinophilia appears to correlate with the extent of allergen exposure and with symptoms in allergic rhinitis.[32] The presence of eosinophilia also correlates with the presence of positive allergy skin tests and, along with basophilic cells, to the serum IgE level.[22, 33, 34]

Regional differences in the presence of eosinophils in the nose of patients with rhinitis have been observed. Gristwood[35] noted eosinophils in 100% of adult patients with perennial allergic rhinitis in specimens from both the middle and inferior turbinates. However, more cells were found in the middle turbinate specimens. Adult allergic rhinitis patients in another study had eosinophils in 90% of the specimens obtained from the ethmoid region and maxillary sinus mucosa, 80% and 40% of specimens from the middle and inferior turbinates, respectively, and 50% of nasal secretions.[36]

Surveying for possible variability of eosinophil detection from each nostril, Kaufman et al[37] found a concordance between nostrils for the absence or presence (>8%) of nasal secretion eosinophils in 90% and 80%, respectively, but with an overall detection rate for eosinophils >90%.

Eosinophils are found in allergic disease at all ages. In 186 children under 6 years of age referred to a group of pediatric allergists, 42% of blown secretions were positive (≥10% of leukocytes). Ninety-five percent of the positive nasal smears were obtained in children determined to be atopic, 5% in an undecided group and none in the non-atopic group.[33]

In recent unpublished work,[38] 50 children (10 per each of 5 groups) 2-7 years old, were clinically categorized as being healthy or as having allergic rhinitis or non-allergic rhinitis. By nasal scraping, at least 1+ eosinophils and basophilic cells were found in 70% of the 20 allergic children. None of the 10 healthy children had eosinophils and only 1 had a 1+ basophilic specimen.

Miller et al[21] confirmed the diagnostic usefulness of the nasal smear for eosinophilia in 177 children aged 4-15 years. Significant nasal smear eosinophilia ($\geq 4\%$) was observed by either nose-blowing or scraping techniques in 69% of children with seasonal allergic rhinitis (n=65), 12% with non-allergic rhinitis (n=42) and 7% of non-allergic controls (n=70). In their study, although the nose-blowing and scraping techniques evidenced an equal sensitivity of 70% and specificity of 94%, almost 40% of children could not provide blown specimens.

In a study of adults, 19-72 years of age, Lans and coworkers[22] reported that with Rhinoprobe scrapings 43% of patients with allergic rhinitis had over 20% of sampled cells that were eosinophils. No nasal eosinophilia of this magnitude was seen in a control population or in patients with non-allergic rhinitis. Thus, in their study, the sensitivity of finding increased eosinophils in allergic rhinitis was 43%; the specificity was 100%. In another study of 210 adults with seasonal allergic rhinitis using the Rhinoprobe scraping technique, eosinophils were present in 81%, basophilic cells in 42%, neutrophils in 64% and bacteria in 28% with at least 1+ grading[39] (Table 8.4). The frequency of neutrophil-positive and bacteria-positive specimens in patients with pollen allergy is noteworthy. Whether this represents low-grade inflammation, infection or artifact and how this compares with controls with no rhinopathy requires further investigations.

The normal basophilic cell content of the nose is about 200-400 cells/mm^3 of mucosa.[40] The great majority of these cells are located in the lamina propria. Some patients with chronic rhinitis have more than 2,000 basophilic cells/mm^3 as the only histologic abnormality. They have been referred to as having "nasal mastocytosis."[41]

There are three populations of basophilic, metachromatic cells in the nose: basophil leukocytes and two histochemically distinct populations of mast cells. The basophils are recognized by their small size (5-6.5 µm), limited number of granules of different size, lobed nucleus which tends to be located at one edge of the cell, and peripherally condensed chromatin. Mast cells range in size form 5 to 12 µm in diameter. They have an abundance of small granules which often obscure an oval nucleus that is generally centrally located within the cell.

Basophilic cells have been identified as being biologically active in allergic reactions. As the number of basophilic cells increases, the nasal symptoms become more severe and provocative challenge responses usually become stronger.[42] However, nasal reactivity to allergen challenge can also increase without a concomitant increase in the number of surface basophilic cells.[43] The number of basophilic cells also correlates with nasal eosinophilia in allergic rhinitis.[44] The finding of these cells and/or eosinophils increases the sensitivity of the test for confirming an allergic diagnosis to nearly 80%.[45]

Some workers have found that, in allergic rhinitis, basophils are the predominant basophilic cell in nasal secretions and "connective tissue mast cells" are the most abundant basophilic cell in the submucosa. They also have determined that "mu-

Table 8.4. *Nasal cytology. Percent of patients with specific cell type present in nasal scraping.*

	Seasonal allergic rhinitis (n=210)	Perennial allergic rhinitis (n=88)	Nonallergic rhinitis (n=78)	Chronic sinusitis (n=51)
Eosinophils	81%	89%	25%	78%
Basophilic cells	42%	31%	9%	41%
Neutrophils	64%	67%	47%	90%
Bacteria	28%	29%	10%	24%

cosal mast cells" are the major cell type in nasal scrapings in the epithelium and lamina propria of patients with allergic rhinitis.[46]

In contrast, other researchers have asserted that basophil leukocytes, not "mucosal mast cells", constitute the majority of the basophilic cells in mucosal scrapings and nasal lavages. In studies using either a specific staining procedure (naphthol-ASD-chloroacetate esterase reaction)[47] or by direct morphological examination,[48] it was found that only 6-8% of the metachromatic cells are mast cells.

In Bascom's study[48] of allergic rhinitis patients, allergen challenge produced a 12-fold increase in the number and a three-fold increase in the percentage of basophilic cells in nasal lavage fluid during the late-phase response. At least two-thirds of these cells were observed to be basophils.

In biopsies of nasal mucous membranes from 8 patients with allergic rhinitis both during and after a pollen season there was an eight-fold increase in the number of basophilic cells seen in the superficial epithelium and deeper lamina propria during the pollen season. In the surface epithelial layer, counts increased from almost totally absent out-of-season to between 2,000 and 28,000/mm^3 in-season.[49]

Nonallergic rhinitis

Of patients undergoing evaluation for chronic perennial rhinitis, approximately 50% have history and skin reactivity consistent with allergic rhinitis. In the remaining 50%, who are nonallergic, over two-thirds are characterized by the absence of eosinophils on nasal smear. They have been classified as having vasomotor rhinitis. This term is used to describe a non-immunologic, non-infectious, chronic rhinopathy. There is a history of nasal congestion and/or rhinorrhea with no history of allergen exacerbation and with negative skin tests. The majority of these patients identify physical irritants and climatic changes as precipitants.[50] In addition to the scarcity of eosinophils in patients with vasomotor rhinitis there is also no increase in degranulated basophilic cells or plasma cells.[51]

About one-fourth of nonallergic patients with chronic rhinitis have eosinophilic nonallergic rhinitis or the nonallergic rhinitis with eosinophilia syndrome (NARES) (Table 8.4). Nonallergic rhinitis with eosinophilia can present at any age and symptoms are similar to those of patients with allergic rhinitis and vasomotor rhinitis. As with allergic rhinitis, nasal cytology during symptomatic periods reveals marked eosinophilia. In Jacobs' study,[52] eosinophil percentages varied from 19% to 66% in spontaneously collected nasal secretions and 7% to 74% in nasal wash specimens. According to Mullarkey and coworkers,[50] sinusitis and nasal polyps are more common in this rhinopathy than in allergic rhinitis or vasomotor rhinitis. This may be the result of damage to the mucosal epithelium induced by eosinophils and their products.[53] A subset of patients with increased nasal eosinophils also have increased blood eosinophils.[54]

Another form of non-allergic rhinitis is the rhinitis of pregnancy. Studies have suggested that estrogen and progesterone cause both an increased acitivity of nasal mucosal glands and mucosal swelling. Increased circulating blood volume probably also leads to increased airway resistance.[55] Unless there is an associated allergic rhinitis or bacterial rhinosinusitis, nasal cytology is normal.

Irritant rhinitis

Nasal cytology has been studied following exposure to various intranasal stimuli. Some observations include: saline (n = 7), no change in number or types of cells in nasal lavage fluid; distilled water (n = 7), no change in number or types of cells in nasal lavage fluid;[56] formaldehyde, occasional epithelial metaplasia and dysplasia;[57] cold air, no change in number or types of cells in nasal lavage fluid;[58] Excessive alpha adrenergic agents resulting in rhinitis medicamentosa, no change in number or types of cells in nasal lavage fluid; non-atopic or atopic individuals receiving irrelevant allergen challenge, increased neutrophils possibly induced by repeated scraped nasal sampling.[15]

Infectious rhinitis

Upper respiratory tract infections are frequently observed in children and less often in adults. With bacterial infections such as rhinosinusitis, especially if they have been recurrent, a number of histopathological abnormalities have been noted. These include fewer ciliated cells causing decreased mucus transport; abnormal cilia causing impaired ciliary movement; disruption of epithelial lining causing increased leakage of tissue fluid; thickened basement membrane causing impairment of transport of fluid and nutrients between the epithelial cells and the mucosal layers; increased vascularity causing increased tissue fluid; increased inflammatory cells such as lymphocytes and plasma cells causing inflammation; increased microabscesses with bacteria and leukocytes causing purulent drainage; and increased mast cells causing increased mediator release.[59]

Nasal cytology is also useful in evaluating patients for bacterial infections. In a study of acute and chronic sinusitis, Wilson et al[60] compared cytograms with radiologic findings. A nasal scraping, obtained by the Rhinoprobe, was considered positive if there was greater than 1.1 neutrophils per high power field ($\geq 1+$) with bacteria present. An x-ray was positive if the radiologist saw asymmetry, mucoperiosteal thickening, opacification, or air-fluid levels. Unfortunately, no asymptomatic control patients were included in this study. Correlation between the nasal cytology and the sinus x-rays was 79%. Ninety percent of the sinus x-rays were positive in those patients with $2+$ or greater neutrophils and bacteria present on nasal cytograms. Although small numbers of bacteria and neutrophils may be normal, large numbers of bacteria, especially intracellular bacteria, support the diagnosis of infections.

Gill & Neiburger[61] also found nasal cytology to be informative in the diagnosis of sinusitis. In their study of 300 children and adults, sinus radiographs were significantly more likely to be positive when there were >5 neutrophils/HPF ($\geq 2+$). The presence of 25 neutrophils/HPF was 86% sensitive and 40% specific in predicting radiographic pathology.

The observations made in a recently completed study are not as conclusive as to the usefulness of nasal cytology as an aid in the diagnosis of bacterial infections. Nasal cytology was evaluated in 51 patients, 14 years of age and older, with sinusitis. The diagnosis was defined by symptoms and an x-ray demonstrating at least 6 mm of maxillary mucosal thickening, opacification or an air-fluid level. In this population of patients, culled from an allergy medical practice, nasal scraping specimens revealed eosinophils in 78%, basophilic cells in 41%, neutrophils in 90%, and bacteria in 24% of the patients. The eosinophil, basophilic cell and bacteria percentages noted were similar to those observed in studies of patients with both seasonal and perennial allergic rhinitis[39] (Table 8.4). Only the frequency of neutrophils seen in these sinusitis patients (90%) was different from the percentages usually seen in allergic rhinitis (60-70%).

Although not all the study patients were allergic, many were, and this may account for the high incidence of eosinophils and basophils. Increased eosinophilia has also been seen in surgical sinus mucosal specimens from patients with nonallergic, chronic sinusitis. This may represent an extension of the NARES process into the adjoining sinuses. Certainly the high frequency of eosinophils in our sinusitis patients' nasal cytology is in contrast to previous observations that, in the presence of infection and increased numbers of neutrophils, eosinophils decreased.[3, 30] Basophilic cells have not been shown to increase with infectious rhinosinusitis.[62] Neutrophils have been shown to be increased in the nasal cytology of patients with allergic rhinitis and from non-specific stimulation.[15] Because of these findings, the previously described relationship between increased neutrophils and sinusitis may be clouded in the individual patient who has allergic rhinitis and/or irritant-exposure rhinitis. It is also clear that many patients with clinical and radiologically confirmed sinusitis do not have bacteria in their nasal mucosal specimen.[63]

In viral nasal infections, ciliated epithelial cells undergo destructive changes termed "ciliocytophthoria". The features of the cytopathic effects of the viruses include clumping of the nuclear chromatin material, margination of the pyknotic chromatin mass attached to inclusion material within the nucleus, halo formation around the nucleus, increased granulation of the cytoplasm, constriction of the ciliated cell, and finally separation of the nucleus-containing basal portion from the ciliated apical portion.[64] After the considerable fall in the number of ciliated cells due to the viral infection, regeneration is usually slow.[65] This may produce long-lasting impairment of nasal mucociliary clearance function.

Nasal polyps

Nasal polyps have been studied histologically. In comparison to healthy nasal and sinus mucosa and mucosa of patients with chronic sinusitis, polyps show a statistically significant increase in the number of eosinophils. Patients with nasal polyps had up to 10 times more eosinophils per surface unit than patients with sinusitis or healthy mucosa.[66] In patients with nasal polyps, basophilic cells were also more numerous. They were found in 65% of these patients as compared with 5% of normal controls, 14% of patients with chronic sinusitis and 91% of patients with nasal allergy.[67]

Atrophic rhinitis

Atrophic rhinitis on cytologic examination reveals epithelial squamous metaplasia and a chronic inflammatory cell infiltrate.[68]

Table 8.5 summarizes the current data on nasal cytology findings in various clinical conditions.

Cytology findings consequent to therapeutic agents

Saline and distilled water

Cause no change in the number or types of cells in nasal lavage fluid.[56]

Propylene and polyethylene-glycol

Cause a trend toward a decrease in eosinophils seen on nasal smear.[69]

Antihistamines

Oral antihistamines, such as terfenadine and cetirizine given prior to an allergen challenge, have no significant effect on the increase in the number and percentage of eosinophils which are noted after allergen challenge.[70] In one clinical trial, cetirizine showed no effect in preventing an increased percentage (10%) and number (67 cells/mm^2) of eosinophils in smears and biopsies of patients with seasonal allergic rhinitis compared with placebo (8%, 12 cells/mm^2).[71] In another clinical trial, following terfenadine 60 mg BID for 4 weeks, there was no significant change in the presence of eosinophils, basophilic cells or neutrophils.[72]

There are no data available on topical antihistamines.

Decongestants

No data are available on oral and intermittent topical use. Rhinitis medicamentosa due to intranasal

Table 8.5. *Nasal cytology in various clinical conditions.*

	Eosinophils	Basophilic cells	Neutrophils	Bacteria	Ciliated cells	Comments
Normal	0	0	0-1+	0	NL	
Allergic rhinitis	1-4+	1-4+	1-4+	0	NL	May occur with others
Vasomotor rhinitis	0	0	0-1+	0	NL	
NARES	1-4+	1-4+	?	0	NL	
Pregnancy	0	0	0-1+	0	NL	
Rhinitis medicamentosa	0	0	0-1+	0	NL	
Irritants	0	0	1-4+	0	NL	May see dysplasia, metaplasia
Bacterial rhinosinusitis	0	0	1-4+	1-4+	NL	Bacteria may be intracellular; may not see bacteria
Viral rhinitis	0	0	1-4+	0	Decreased	Ciliocytophthoria
Polyps	1-4+	0-4+	?	?	Decreased	
Atrophic rhinitis	0	0	1-4+	0	Decreased	Metaplasia

alpha adrenergic agents appears to cause no significant change in nasal cytology.

Anticholinergic agents

Ipratropium bromide has been studied extensively as treatment for both allergic rhinitis and perennial nonallergic rhinitis.[73] No significant change in the percentages of eosinophils, basophilic cells, neutrophils or bacteria found in nasal scrapings has been noted following ipratropium therapy for either of these rhinopathies.

Cromolyn sodium

It has been noted that patients with allergic rhinitis have increased inflammatory cells in blown secretions. In preliminary reports by Pelikan,[74, 75] the response to allergen challenge was examined in 12 patients with and without pretreatment with intranasal cromolyn sodium (sodium cromoglycate). He found that the immediate nasal response without pretreatment was accompanied by changes in the count of eosinophils in 66%, basophilic cells in 8% and neutrophils in 42% of challenges. No significant changes in the counts of these cells were recorded during the immediate nasal response after pretreatment with cromolyn sodium. In the late nasal response, the non-pretreated patients developed changes of eosinophils in 58%, basophilic cells in 8% and neutrophils in 75% of challenges. The changes in those pretreated with cromolyn sodium were less pronounced for the eosinophils and neutrophils and were not statistically significant.

In a clinical study by Orgel et al,[72] there was a statistically significant decrease in eosinophils, but not basophilic cells or neutrophils, in patients treated with intranasal cromolyn 4%, 4 times a day for 4 weeks. In Okuda's study,[76] nasal basophilic cells did not decrease after 2 weeks of intranasal cromolyn.

Topical corticosteroids

Intranasal corticosteroids are known to be highly effective in reducing allergic symptomatology. Their effect on nasal cytology has been evaluated in a number of studies. With allergen challenges, the immediate nasal response in the number of eosinophils and neutrophils in nasal secretions was not affected by pretreatment with the topical glucocorticoid budesonide.[74] In the late nasal response to allergen challenge[75] budesonide, however, did lower the number of eosinophils and neutrophils in secretions. Topical steroid pretreatment with flunisolide for 1 week before allergen challenge blocked the influx of eosinophils, neutrophils and basophilic cells (68% identified as basophils) in the late-phase response examined in nasal washings.[48]

In clinical studies, nasal secretion eosinophilia has been decreased after beclomethasone dipropionate in both seasonal and perennial rhinitis patients as compared with the effect of placebo.[77] A decrease in eosinophils after treatment by beclomethasone dipropionate has also been observed in nasal scrapings. This occurred with both the aerosol and the aqueous formulations in patients with allergic rhinitis in doses as low as 42 μg per nostril twice a day.[78] Another topical corticosteroid, flunisolide, has, like beclomethasone, been shown after 4 weeks of twice-a-day treatment to decrease the number of allergic rhinitis patients with nasal eosinophilia.[79]

Beclomethasone has been shown to inhibit the increase in density of basophilic cells that occurs in the nasal mucosa during the pollen season. Gomez et al[80] studied allergic rhinitis patients by biopsy at the start and after 3 months of a pollen season. Significantly fewer basophilic cells were seen in the corticosteroid-treated group than in those receiving placebo.

Okuda and coworkers[76] studied nasal surface basophilic metachromatic cells in epithelial scrapings from symptomatic allergic rhinitis patients before and after 2 weeks of treatment with beclomethasone. The number of basophilic cells was significantly reduced in the beclomethasone group (64%) as compared with the controls (20%). The mean number was 647 cells/mm^2 before and 205 cells/mm^2 after beclomethasone; it was 708 cells/mm^2 before and 718 cells/mm^2 after treatment with placebo. Otsuka[81] reported that the basophils and formalin-sensitive mast cells found in the superficial epithelial layers were more susceptible to the effects of corticosteroids than formalin-resistant mast cells. Pipkorn[82, 83] also saw no quantitative effect of budesonide on subepithelial mast cells in biopsy specimens taken either out-of-season or in-season from patients with allergic rhinitis.

Examination of nasal scraping specimens of allergic rhinitis patients treated with fluticasone propionate, a new glucocorticosteroid, revealed a striking decrease in eosinophils. In a study in which symptomatic patients received one of three doses of fluticasone (25, 100 or 400 µg twice daily) or placebo, over 80% had nasal eosinophilia before treatment. The graded eosinophil score decreased in 50-70% of patients treated with fluticasone propionate for 2 weeks and in only 20% of placebo-treated patients. Forty-two percent of the patients had basophils present before treatment. After treatment with fluticasone propionate, basophil numbers decreased in a significantly greater number of patients than after treatment with placebo. Neutrophils were demonstrated in the cytograms of 64% of patients. A decrease in these inflammatory cells occurred in a smaller but still significant number of patients following treatment with the two larger doses of fluticasone propionate compared with placebo[39] (Fig. 8.3).

The response to topical steroids of nasal mucosal cells obtained by biopsy has confirmed the absence of atrophy or other possible steroid damage.[84, 85]

In a study in which biopsy specimens were examined by light microscopy after 1 year of intranasal treatment with fluocortin butyl, special attention was paid to the surface epithelium. The results showed that long-term topical therapy with this glucocorticoid led to a change from squamous metaplasia to normal columnar epithelium in some patients. Nasal biopsies also revealed decreases in mucosal eosinophils, basophilic cells and neutrophils as has been shown to occur in nasal secretions and mucosal scrapings after treatment with topical corticosteroids. A number of patients had an increase in intact mast cells, suggesting that long-term therapy may inhibit degranulation.[86] In summary, the effects of topical corticosteroids in allergic rhinitis include: improvement of the epithelial barrier, inhibition of eosinophil influx and reduction of numbers present, inhibition of basophilic cell influx and reduction of numbers present, inhibition of neutrophil influx and modest reduction of numbers present, no change in numbers of submucosal mast cells and reduction in secondary monocyte influx.

Oral corticosteroids

Oral prednisone has been studied for its effect on the late nasal response to allergen challenge. Studies by Bascom and colleagues[87, 88] demonstrated that pretreatment for 2 days with pred-

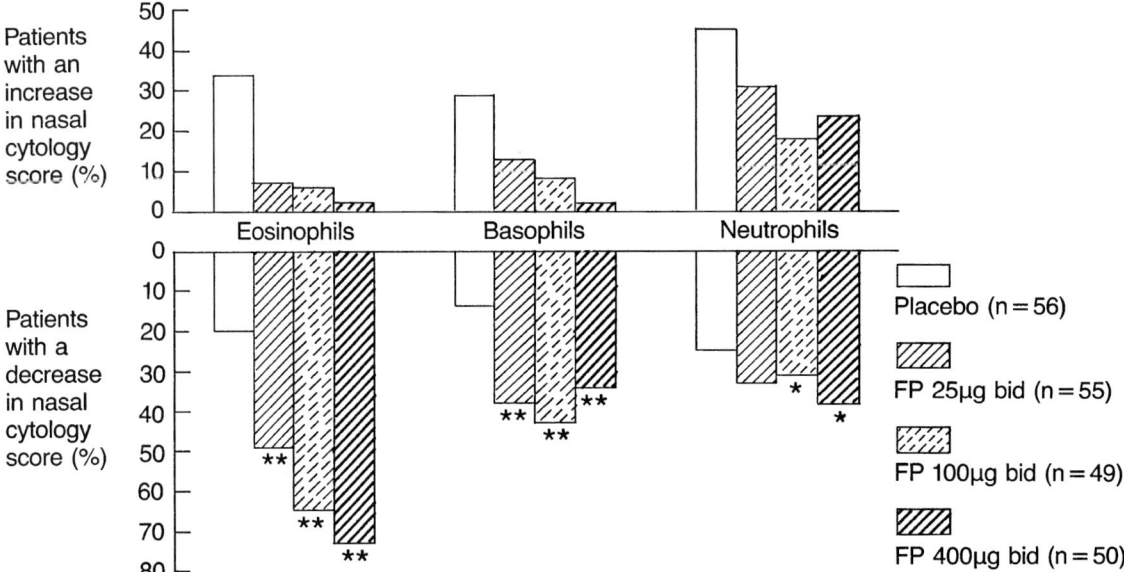

Fig. 8.3. Percent of patients demonstrating increases or decreases in eosinophils, basophils, and neutrophils among patients with evaluable nasal mucosal specimens on both days 1 and 15; * $p < 0.05$ and ** $p \leq 0.003$: fluticasone propionate aqueous nasal spray-treated patients by comparison with placebo. From Meltzer EO, Orgel HA, Bronsky EA, et al. A dose-ranging study of fluticasone propionate aqueous nasal spray for seasonal allergic rhinitis assessed by symptoms, rhinomanometry and nasal cytology. *J Allergy Clin Immunol* 1990; *86*: 221-30.

nisone will block influx of eosinophils but not of neutrophils or mononuclear cells.

Immunotherapy

Nasal allergen challenges will induce influx of eosinophils, basophilic cells and neutrophils in sensitive subjects. The effects of immunotherapy on this influx have been evaluated. In a study by Iliopoulos and colleagues,[89] there was no significant difference in the number of eosinophils, basophilic cells, neutrophils and mononuclear cells prior to a ragweed allergen challenge in two groups of ragweed-sensitive hayfever patients. One of the groups (n = 20) was treated for 8 months with placebo and the other (n = 21) with a moderate dose of ragweed antigen extract. Following challenge, the increase in eosinophils, basophilic cells and neutrophils was not significantly different between the groups. Further work from this Johns Hopkins group has determined that higher immunotherapy doses can decrease eosinophil influx.[90]

In Otsuka's clinical study[91] evaluating the nasal cytologic changes due to immunotherapy, 25 patients with perennial allergic rhinitis were divided into two groups. Eleven served as controls and 14 underwent allergen injection treatments. At the initiation of the study, the number of basophilic cells in nasal mucosal scrapings was not significantly different between groups. Following 3 and 6 months of immunotherapy, nasal symptom scores, nasal provocation sensitivity and the number of basophilic cells were significantly reduced ($p < 0.05$) in the antigen immunotherapy group, but unchanged in the control group compared to pretreatment values.

Antibiotics

In a recently completed study of 51 patients with documented sinusitis, 46 (90%) had neutrophils noted on the initial scraped nasal mucosal specimen. Forty-four had adequate specimens for evaluation both prior to and following a course of amoxicillin/clavulanate potassium (Augmentin®) 500 mg, given 3 times a day for 3 weeks. Of these 44 patients, 39 (89%) had neutrophils present at the first visit and 37 (84%) has neutrophils noted after the Augmentin®. Following the antibiotic treatment, 11 of 44 (25%) had an increase in the neutrophil grade, 18 of 44 (41%) had a decrease in the neutrophil grade and 15 of 44 showed no change. Thus antibiotic intervention in documented sinusitis will not have a predictable effect on the numbers of neutrophils in the nasal cytogram.

Twelve of the 51 sinusitis patients (24%) had bacteria observed in the initial nasal scrapings. After the course of Augmentin®, 1 patient specimen was inadequate for interpretation. For the 11 patients with evaluable samples both before and after antibiotic therapy, 4 had bacteria still present (36%), and 7 of the 11 had no bacteria observed (64%). Thus the trend with antibiotic treatment was to reduce the bacteria seen in the nasal cytograms.[63]

Conclusion

While interest in nasal cytology as a method for evaluating disease and treatment has progressed, several factors have, in the past, diminished its usefulness. Some of these have been the inability to procure adequate samples consistently and with minimal discomfort, the limited use of Hansel's stain, the variety of methods for grading results, the fact that eosinophils are not pathognomonic for allergy, the lack of available data on how to interpret findings, and the assumption that the procedure was not cost-effective. This review has attempted to demonstrate that techniques for obtaining, staining and interpreting nasal cytology specimens are improving. These have contributed to the ability to differentiate the chronic rhinopathies, monitor their course and develop meaningful therapies. The prospect of greater satisfaction for both clinicians and the patients they serve is advanced by this scientific understanding.

References

1. Meltzer EO. Evaluating rhinitis: Clinical rhinomanometric and cytologic assessments. *J Allergy Clin Immunol* 1988; *82:* 900-8.
2. Meltzer EO, Schatz M, Zeiger RS. Allergic and non-allergic rhinitis. In: Middleton E Jr, Reed CE, Ellis EF, eds. *Allergy: Principles and Practice*, 3rd edn. St. Louis: The C. V. Mosby Company, 1988. 1253-89.
3. Hansel FK. Observation on the cytology of the secretions in allergy of the nose and paranasal sinuses. *J Allergy* 1934; *5:* 357-66.
4. Hastie R, Heroy JH, Levy DA. Basophil leukocytes and mast cells in human nasal secretions and scrapings studied by light microscopy. *Lab Invest* 1979; *49:* 541-54.
5. Bryan WTK, Bryan MT. Cytologic diagnosis in otolaryngology. *Trans Am Acad Ophthalmol Otolaryngol* 1959; *63:* 597-611.
6. Pipkorn U, Karlsson G. Methods for obtaining specimens from the nasal mucosa for morphological and biochemical analysis. *Eur Respir J* 1988; *1:* 856-62.
7. Pipkorn U, Karlsson G, Enerback L. A brush method to harvest cells from the nasal mucosa for microscopic and biochemical analysis. *J Immunological Methods* 1988; *112:* 37-42.
8. Jalowayski AA, Zeiger RS. Examination of nasal or conjunctival epithelial specimens. In: Lawlor GJ Jr, Fischer TJ, eds. *Manual of Allergy and Immunology*, 2nd edn. Boston: Little, Brown and Company, 1988: 432-4.
9. Meltzer EO, Jalowayski AA. Nasal cytology in clinical practice. *Am J Rhinol* 1988; *2:* 47-54.
10. Jalowayski AA, Meltzer EO, Orgel HA, et al. Nasal histamine levels in young children with allergic and non allergic rhinitis and chronic otitis. *J Allergy Clin Immunol* 1991; *87:* 146.
11. Welch MJ, Meltzer EO, Kemp JP, et al. Comparison of two different techniques for obtaining specimens for nasal cytology: Nose-blowing vs. nasal mucosal scraping. *J Allergy Clin Immunol* 1991; *87:* 144.
12. Galindo G, Jalowayski A, Meltzer E. Correlation between nasal cytogram and blown technique for the diagnosis of allergic rhinitis. *Ann Allergy* 1991; *66:* 86.
13. Angel-Solano G, Shturman R. Comparative cytology of nasal secretions and nasal mucosa in allergic rhinitis. *Ann Allergy* 1986; *56:* 521.
14. Naclerio RM, Meier HL, Kagey-Sobotka A, et al. Mediator release after nasal airway challenge with allergen. *Am Rev Respir Dis* 1983; *128:* 597-602.
15. Piancentini GL, Kaulbach HC, Scott T, et al. Correlation between inflammatory cell responses in nasal mucosal scrapings and lavages after allergen challenge. *J Allergy Clin Immunol* 1991; *87:* 145.
16. Brown M, Lim M, Furin M, et al. A comparison between antigen-induced leukocyte populations in the nasal mucosa and nasal secretions. *J Allergy Clin Immunol* 1991; *87:* 145.
17. Cohen GA, MacPherson GA, Golembesky HE, et al. Normal nasal cytology in infancy. *Ann Allergy* 1985; *54:* 112-24.
18. Bryan MP, Bryan WTK. Cytologic diagnosis in allergic disorders. *Otolaryngol Clin N Am* 1974; *7:* 637-66.
19. Bickmore JT. Nasal cytology in allergy and infection. *ORL Allergy* 1978; *40:* 39-46.
20. Ohtsuka H, Okuda M. Important factors in the nasal manifestations of allergy. *Arch Otorhinolaryngol* 1981; *233:* 227–35.
21. Miller RE, Paradise JL, Friday GA, et al. The nasal smear for eosinophils. *Am J Dis Child* 1982; *136:* 1009-11.
22. Lans DM, Alfano N, Rocklin R. Nasal eosinophilia in allergic and non-allergic rhinitis: Usefulness of the nasal smear in the diagnosis of allergic rhinitis. *Allergy Proc* 1989; *10:* 275-80.
23. Pelikan Z, Pelikan-Filipek M. Cytologic changes in the nasal secretions during the immediate nasal response. *J Allergy Clin Immunol* 1988; *82:* 1103-12.
24. Klementsson H, Andersson M, Baumgarten CR, et al. Changes in non-specific nasal reactivity and eosinophil influx and activation after allergen challenge. *Clin Exp Allergy* 1990; *20:* 539-47.
25. Pipkorn U, Karlsson G, Enerback L. Nasal mucosal response to repeated challenges with pollen allergen. *Am Rev Respir Dis* 1989; *140:* 729-36.
26. Pelikan Z, Pelikan-Filipek M. Cytologic changes in the nasal secretions during the late nasal response. *J Allergy Clin Immunol* 1989; *83:* 1068-79.
27. Togias A, Naclerio RM, Proud D, et al. Studies on the allergic and non-allergic inflammation. *J Allergy Clin Immunol* 1988; *81:* 782-90.
28. Pipkorn U, Karlsson G, Enerback L. The cellular response of the human allergic mucosa to natural allergen exposure. *J Allergy Clin Immunol* 1988; *82:* 1046-54.
29. Karlsson G, Pipkorn U. Natural allergen exposure does not influence the density of goblet cells in the nasal mucosa of patients with seasonal allergic rhinitis. *J Otorhinolaryngol* 1989; *51:* 171-4.
30. Malmberg H. Symptoms of chronic and allergic rhinitis and occurrence of nasal secretion granulocytes in university students, school children and infants. *Allergy* 1979; *34:* 389-94.
31. Murray AB, Anderson DO. The epidemiologic relationship of clinical nasal allergy to eosinophils and to goblet cells in the nasal smear. *J Allergy* 1969; *43:* 1.
32. Hansel FK. Cytologic diagnosis in respiratory allergy and infection. *Ann Allergy* 1966; *24:* 564-9.
33. Orgel HA, Kemp JP, Meltzer EO, et al. Atopy and IgE in a pediatric allergy practice. *Ann Allergy* 1977; *39:* 161-8.
34. Salas A, Wilson N, Hamburger RN. Relation of serum IgE level to the cells observed in the nasal cytograms. *Ann Allergy* 1988; *60:* 175.
35. Gristwood RE. Observations on the histopathology of allergic rhinitis: regional differences in mucosal eosinophilia. *J Laryng Otol* 1982; *49:* 270.
36. Vaheri E. Nasal allergy with special reference to eosinophilia and histopathology. *Acta Allergol* 1956; *10:* 203–11.
37. Kaufman HS, Rosen I, Shaposhnikov N, et al. Nasal eosinophilia. *Ann Allergy* 1982; *49:* 270–1.
38. Meltzer EO. Unpublished data.
39. Meltzer EO, Orgel HA, Bronsky EA, et al. A dose-ranging study of fluticasone propionate aqueous nasal spray for seasonal allergic rhinitis assessed by symptoms, rhinomanometry and nasal cytology. *J Allergy Clin Immunol* 1990; *86:* 221-30.
40. Connell JT. Nasal disease: Mechanisms and classification. *Ann Allergy* 1983; *50:* 227-35.
41. Connell JT. Nasal Mastocytosis. *J Allergy* 1969; *43:* 182.
42. Borres MP, Irander K, Bjorksten B. Metachromatic cells in nasal mucosa after allergen challenge. *Allergy* 1990; *45:* 98-103.
43. Wihl J-A, Brofeldt S, Gronborg H, et al. Blind study of basophilic cells in nasal smears from patients with grass pollen hayfever. *Eur J Respir Dis* 1983; *64 (suppl):* 383.
44. Okuda M, Otsuka H. Basophilic cells in allergic nasal secretions. *Arch Otorhinolaryngol* 1977; *214:* 283-9.
45. Lang DM, Howland WC, Stevenson DD. Sensitivity and features of nasal cytology in diagnosis of allergic (IgE mediated) rhinitis. *Ann Allergy* 1988; *60:* 176.
46. Otsuka H, Denburg J, Dolovich J, et al. Heterogeneity of metachromatic cells in human nose: Significance of mucosal mast cells. *J Allergy Clin Immunol* 1985; *76:* 695-702.
47. Jalowayski AA, Maes TW, Wasserman SI, et al. Histochemical differentiation of the human nasal mucosa mast cells from basophil leukocytes. *J Allergy Clin Immunol* 1983; *71:* 89.
48. Bascom R, Waschs M, Naclerio RM, et al. Basophil influx occurs after nasal antigen challenge: Effects of topical corticosteroid pretreatment. *J Allergy Clin Immunol* 1988; *81:* 580-9.
49. Viegas M, Gomez E, Brooks J, et al. Changes in nasal mast cell numbers in and out of pollen season. *Int Arch Allergy Appl Immunol* 1987; *82:* 275-6.

50. Mullarkey MF, Hill JS, Webb DR. Allergic and non-allergic rhinitis: Their characterization with attention to the meaning of nasal eosinophilia. *J Allergy Clin Immunol* 1980; 65: 122-6.
51. Elwany S, Bumsted R. Ultrastructural observations on vasomotor rhinitis. *J Oto-Rhino-Laryngol* 1987; 49: 199-205.
52. Jacobs RL, Freedman PM, Boswell RN. Nonallergic rhinitis with eosinophils (NARES syndrome). *J Allergy Clin Immunol* 1981; 67: 253-62.
53. Davidson AE, Miller SD, Settipane RJ, et al. Delayed nasal mucociliary clearance in patients with nonallergic rhinitis and nasal eosinophilia. *Allergy Proc* 1992; 13: 81–4.
54. Settipane GA, Klein DE. Non-allergic rhinitis: Demography of eosinophils in nasal smear, blood total eosinophil counts and IgE levels. *NER Allergy Proc* 1985; 6: 363-6.
55. Schatz M, Zeiger RS. Diagnosis and management of rhinitis during pregnancy. *Allergy Proc* 1988; 9: 545-54.
56. Meslier N, Braunstein G, Lacronique J, et al. Local cellular and humoral responses to antigenic and distilled water challenge in subjects with allergic rhinitis. *Am Rev Respir Dis* 1988; 137: 617-24.
57. Boysen M, Zadig E, Digernes V, et al. Nasal mucosa in workers exposed to formaldehyde: A pilot study. *Br J Industr Med* 1990; 47: 116-21.
58. Togias A. Unpublished data.
59. Petruson B, Hansson HA. Nasal mucosal changes in children with frequent infections. *Arch Otolaryngol Head Neck Surg* 1987; 113: 1294-300.
60. Wilson NW, Jalowayski AA, Hamburger RN. A comparison of nasal cytology with sinus x-rays for the diagnosis of sinusitis. *Am J Rhinol* 1988; 2: 55-9.
61. Gill FF, Neiburger JB. The role of nasal cytology in the diagnosis of chronic sinusitis. *Am J rhinol* 1989; 3: 13-5.
62. Melen I, Pipkorn S, Pipkorn U. Mast cells on the surface of the mucous membrane – a general feature of inflammatory reactions in the nose? *Rhinology* 1985; 23: 187-90.
63. Meltzer EO. Unpublished data.
64. Bryan WTK, Bryan MP, Smith CA. Human ciliated epithelial cells in nasal secretions. Morphologic and histochemical aspects. *Ann Otol Rhinol Laryngol* 1964; 73: 474.
65. Pedersen M, Sakakura Y, Winther B, et al. Nasal mucociliary transport, number of ciliated cells, and beating pattern in naturally acquired common colds. *Eur J Resp Dis* 1983; 128 (suppl, part 1): 355-65.
66. Jankowski R, Bene MC, Moneret-Vautrin AD, et al. Immunohistological characteristics of nasal polyps. A comparison with healthy mucosa and chronic sinusitis. *Rhinology* 1989; 8: 51-8.
67. Sakaguchi K, Okuda M, Ushijima K, et al. Study of nasal surface basophilic cells in patients with nasal polyp. *Acta Oto-Laryngol (Stockh)* 1986; 430: 28-33.
68. Abdel-Latif SM, Baheeg SS, Aglan YI, et al. Chronic atrophic rhinitis with fetor (ozena): a histopathologic treatise. *Rhinology* 1987; 25: 117-20.
69. Spector SL, Toshener D, Gay I, et al. Beneficial effects of propylene and polyethylene glycol and saline in the treatment of perennial rhinitis. *Clin Allergy* 1982; 12: 187-96.
70. Klementsson H, Andersson M, Pipkorn U. Allergen-induced increase in nonspecific nasal reactivity is blocked by antihistamines without a clear-cut relationship to eosinophil influx. *J Allergy Clin Immunol* 1990; 86: 466-72.
71. Howarth PH, Wilson SJ, Brewster H. The influence of cetirizine on symptom generation and nasal eosinophilia in seasonal allergic rhinitis. *J Allergy Clin Immunol* 1991; 87: 151.
72. Orgel HA, Meltzer EO, Kemp JP, et al. Comparison of intranasal cromolyn sodium, 4%, and oral terfenadine for allergic rhinitis: Symptoms, nasal cytology, nasal clearance, and rhinomanometry. *Ann Allergy* 1991; 66: 237-44.
73. Meltzer EO, Bronsky, EA, Findlay SR, et al. Dose response study of ipratropium bromide nasal spray in perennial allergic rhinitis. *J Allergy Clin Immunol* 1991; 87: 150.
74. Pelikan-Filipek M, Pelikan Z. Nasal secretions cytology during the immediate nasal response pretreated with disodium cromoglycate and budesonide. *J Allergy Clin Immunol* 1991; 87: 144.
75. Pelikan Z, Pelikan-Filipek M. Cytologic changes in nasal secretions during the late nasal response pretreated with disodium cromoglycate and beclomethasone dipropionate or budesonide. *J Allergy Clin Immunol* 1991; 87: 281.
76. Okuda M, Otsuka H, Sakaguchi K, et al. Effect of anti-allergic treatment on nasal surface basophilic metachromatic cells in allergic rhinitis. *Allergy Proc* 1989; 10: 23-6.
77. Holopainen E, Malmberg H, Tarkiainen E. Experiences of treating allergic rhinitis with intra-nasal beclomethasone dipropionate. *Acta Allergol* 1977; 32: 263-77.
78. Orgel HA, Meltzer EO, Kemp JP, et al. Clinical, rhinomanometric, and cytologic evaluation of seasonal allergic rhinitis treated with beclomethasone dipropionate as aqueous nasal spray or pressurized aerosol. *J Allergy Clin Immunol* 1986; 77: 858-64.
79. Meltzer EO, Orgel HA, Bush RK, et al. Evaluation of symptom relief, nasal airflow, nasal cytology, and acceptability of two formulations of flunisolide nasal spray in patients with perennial allergic rhinitis. *Ann Allergy* 1990; 64: 536-40.
80. Gomez E, Claque JE, Gatland D, et al. Effect of topical corticosteroids on seasonally induced increases in nasal mast cells. *Br Med J* 1988; 296: 1572-73.
81. Otsuka H, Denburg JA, Befus AD, et al. Effect of beclomethasone dipropionate on nasal metachromatic cell subpopulations. *Clin Allergy* 1986; 16: 589-95.
82. Pipkorn U. Effect of topical glucocorticoid treatment on nasal mucosal mast cells in allergic rhinitis. *Allergy* 1983; 38: 125-9.
83. Pipkorn U, Enerback L. Nasal mucosal mast cells and histamine in hayfever. *Int Arch Allergy Appl Immunol* 1987; 84: 123-8.
84. Holopainen E, Malmberg H, Binder E. Longterm follow-up of intranasal beclomethasone treatment. A clinical and histologic study. *Acta Otolaryngol (Stockh)* 1982; 386: 270-5.
85. Pipkorn U, Pukander J, Suonpaa J, et al. Long-term safety of budesonide nasal aerosol: a 5.5 year follow-up study. *Clin Allergy* 1988; 18: 253-9.
86. Orgel HA, Meltzer EO, Bierman CW, et al. Intranasal fluocortin butyl in patients with perennial rhinitis: A twelve-month efficacy and safety study including nasal biopsy. *J Allergy Clin Immunol* 1991; 88: 257-64.
87. Bascom R, Pipkorn U, Gleich G, et al. Effect of systemic steroids on eosinophils and major basic protein during nasal antigen challenge. *J Allergy Clin Immunol* 1986; 77: 246.
88. Bascom R, Pipkorn U, Lichtenstein LM, et al. The influx of inflammatory cells into nasal washings during the late response to antigen challenge. Effect of systemic steroid pretreatment. *Am Rev Respir Dis* 1988; 138: 406-12.
89. Iliopoulos O, Proud D, Adkinson NF Jr, et al. Effects of immunotherapy on the early, late, and rechallenge nasal reaction to provocation with allergen: Changes in inflammatory mediators and cells. *J Allergy Clin Immunol* 1991; 87: 855-66.
90. Furin MJ, Norman PS, Creticos PS, et al. Immunotherapy decreases antigen-induced eosinophil cell migration into the nasal cavity. *J Allergy Clin Immunol* 1991; 88: 27-32.
91. Otsuka H, Mezawa A, Ohnishi M, et al. Changes in nasal metachromatic cells during allergen immunotherapy. *Clin Exp Allergy* 1991; 21: 115-9.

CHAPTER 9

Allergy diagnosis

STEN DREBORG

Introduction

Allergic diseases include many states of illnesses, caused by several mechanisms. This paper is restricted to the diagnosis of IgE-mediated or atopic rhinitis, *i.e.* rhinitis caused by interaction between allergen and specific IgE on the surface of mast cells and other effector cells.

The diagnosis of allergic rhinitis is based upon a thorough clinical history, *i.e.* the history of exposure to allergens and symptoms related to this exposure, and it might be supported by diagnostic tests.

Allergists

It is necessary for the allergist to know not only the allergic diseases, but also the distribution of allergens in the environment, and the methods used for investigation of allergen exposure.

Much is known about the seasonal variation in the number of pollen grains and mold spores in the air and also about the conditions favoring accumulation of indoor allergens. However, the local distribution of allergens must be investigated in each region separately. Local pollen counts vary between years. The prevalence of mold spores also varies between years and, in addition, it varies indoors in the same house due to changes in the indoor climate or ventilation systems. Only by continuous detailed study of these and other relevant parameters can the allergist give the specialized advice he or she is obliged to provide to patients.

A special problem which will be discussed further below is the amount of indoor allergens present in homes and office buildings. This exposure is not obvious to the patient and most often results in non-specific nasal hyperreactivity.

Clinical history

Questionnaires are used in most countries, and they are very helpful when taking a history. However, answers to questions must be carefully interpreted by the allergist, especially in perennial rhinitis.

Only 10% of children without allergy amongst close relatives will develop allergic symptoms during childhood, whereas no less than 75% of children whose parents both suffer from the same allergic disease, e.g. allergic rhinitis, become allergic before school age.[26] Thus, heredity is of importance for predicting whether rhinitis symptoms are of allergic origin or not. Another important predictor of allergy, as a cause of rhinitis, is a history of other allergic diseases. This is especially true in the case of children and young adults.

A truism that is important to mention is that no sensitization occurs without repeated exposure to the allergen in question, or to allergens cross reacting with this allergen, and that there are no symptoms without exposure to the allergen. Therefore, it is important to consider present and previous exposure to allergens. It is easy to find out, for example, whether there has been a cat at home. Cat allergen will be present for years in that home, provided the house is not thoroughly cleaned by washing clothing and wet-cleaning floors and furniture.[47] However, cat dander might also be present in the dust of homes without known contact with a cat,[41,44] in the dust of day-care centers and schools,[35] and probably also in the dust of trains and other public places.[44] This exposure is not obvious to the patient (see below).

There will probably be a rapid accumulation of data on the distribution of environmental allergens, which must be considered in clinical practice. Investigation of the allergen content of the dust and air in homes of patients with allergic perennial rhinitis should be part of the normal diagnostic procedure.

The clinical history is obvious in most cases of pollinosis when there is a short, well-defined season. In Northern Europe, birch pollinosis is an example of such a pollinosis with well-characterized features. The diagnosis is not only founded on the seasonal appearance of nasal symptoms, but also on the occurrence of oral itching upon eating apples, nuts, etc. These symptoms are present in all children with severe birch pollinosis, but in only 50% of adults with birch pollinosis.[9]

The diagnosis of animal dander allergy is easy when symptoms appear upon direct contact with cats or dogs.[14] However, only a minor proportion of patients who have found themselves to be allergic to pets get such immediate symptoms: most react after a prolonged visit to homes keeping pets, or find that they experience alleviation of symptoms of rhinitis after leaving homes where pets are kept.

Allergic patients exposed to animal dander and mite-sensitized patients most often show more or less continuous symptoms of nasal hyperresponsiveness at exposure to non-specific stimuli such as cigarette smoke, pollutants and cold air. There is a risk that these patients will be considered non-allergic, since the relation between exposure and symptoms is not obvious. If they are not given any advice to remove the offending animal, clean the house and avoid all contact with pets, their symptoms will continue for long periods of time.

A common history in children sensitized to dog and cat is that their symptoms are less pronounced during the summer vacations, but reappear when school starts again. This has been ascribed to indirect contact, *i.e.* contact with other pupils who keep pets at home. Recently, we found that the content of cat allergen I or *Fel d* I in schoolrooms, was nearly as high (1 µg/g fine dust) as that present in cat-inhabited homes, and that in the dust from school chairs the concentration of the major dog allergen, *Can f* I, was 10 to 100 times higher than that of cat allergen.[35] In fact, the concentration on Swedish school chairs was the same as found in American homes with dogs.[40] These results indicate that, until it has been proven that no allergen can be found in the environment of the patient, so-called non-specific symptoms should be considered to be of allergic origin in individuals sensitized to environmental allergens present in the dust of schools or office buildings. This stresses the necessity to actively investigate allergen contamination of the environment, both in homes and work places such as schools and offices. Methods for determination of the major allergen content in dusts are now available and should be used not only in scientific investigations but also in daily practice. A special case is the patient with a cat or a dog at home who does not show obvious symptoms upon direct contact. This is not unusual in pet-keeping allergics. If the pet is removed, symptoms most often become obvious when the patient is later exposed to the same pet elsewhere.

Both the doctor and the patient can become falsely convinced that the pet has no causative relation to the rhinitis symptoms since, when the pet is removed, symptoms often continue. This can, as mentioned earlier, be ascribed to the fact that cat dander allergen is present for years in the dust of the home in almost the same concentration as before removal of the cat (pet).[44, 47]

Diagnostic tests

Diagnostic *in vivo* and *in vitro* tests can support the clinical history but can never replace it. A history without supporting tests can be questioned. Positive tests without plausibly positive clinical history indicate sensitization but not necessarily clinical disease (latent allergy, see below).

In vivo diagnostic tests

A specific allergy can be demonstrated by skin testing and by allergen challenge tests. However, the relevance of test results depends on the composition and potency of the allergenic extract used. All allergen sources are composed of a number of allergenic proteins. All relevant allergens must be present in the extract in relevant concentrations to make the diagnostic material reliable. The total allergenic potency must be well-defined because, the higher the potency, the more patients with true clinical symptoms due to the allergen in question will be diagnosed by the test, *i.e.* the sensitivity of the test increases. In parallel with increasing sensitivity, the specificity decreases, *i.e.* more and more patients without symptoms related to the allergen produce positive tests. For most kinds of diagnostic tests, sensitivity and specificity is not a great problem, since there is often a gap between normal values and values found in patients with disease. In allergy diagnosis, however, the problem is of great importance. In Fig. 9.1 the relation between potency, sensitivity and specificity is illustrated according to Gerhardt & Keller,[21] with an example from a recent diagnostic allergy study.[14] Both the varying degree of sensitivity to the many allergenic molecules present in allergen source materials, such as pollen grains, and the difference in amount of allergenic components in the raw materials contributes to the less distinct limit between values obtained in allergics and non-allergics. It is like a mosaic. The ratio of IgE molecules to allergenic molecules varies between patients in an unpredictable way.

All diagnostic procedures should be performed using either fresh material, e.g. pollen grains[1, 2] or fresh fruits,[17] powdered allergen[34] or standardized allergenic extracts.[22]

The presence of a specific IgE-mediated allergy is most easily demonstrated by skin prick (puncture) test (SPT), which should be performed according to established methods.[10] In the range of weal reactions, 3-8 mm in diameter, the diameters of weals must not vary more than ±1 mm at repeated testing.[8, 10, 11]

The size of the weal reaction is often taken as a direct measure of skin sensitivity to the allergen. However, it is not a good measure since the mean weal diameter only increases by a factor of 1.5 (the area by 2.5)[5, 10] when the allergen concentration is increased 10-fold. This is illustrated in Fig. 9.2. It is now understandable why even a difference of 2 mm between duplicate tests means poor precision, especially at low response levels. In routine clinical work, the coefficient of variation if often high, even more than 100%.[11, 18] It can be improved by training and by using standardized techniques. The technique can be checked by always using duplicate tests or by now and then repeating 20 tests with the same substance in the same patient.[8, 10, 11] Then, the coefficient of variation can be kept at low values, *i.e.* less than 10% when based on weal diameter and less than 20% when based on weal area.[11]

The presence of IgE on skin mast cells does not necessarily prove the presence of clinically relevant IgE also in the nose. Some patients with positive SPT have only conjunctivitis, and others have

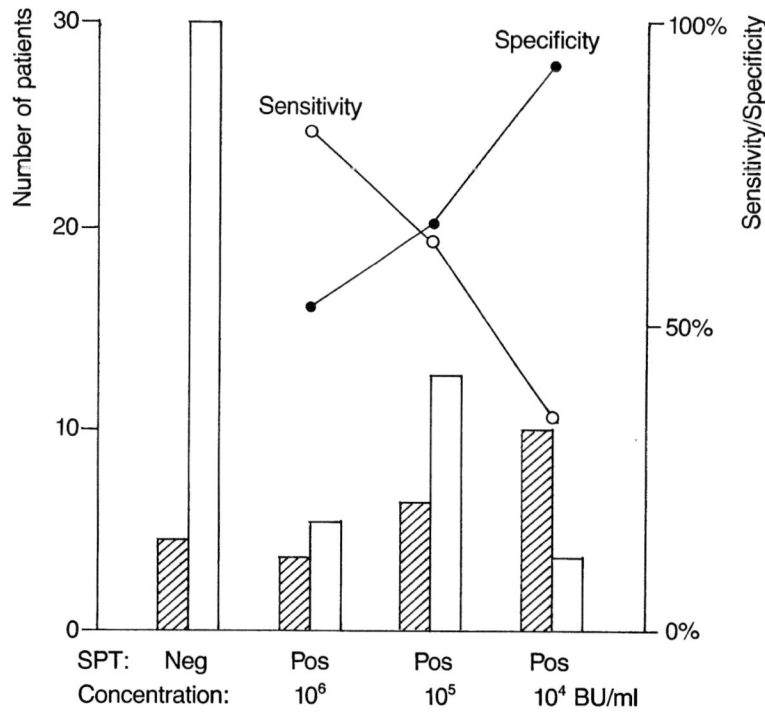

Fig. 9.1. Results of skin prick testing (SPT) with three concentrations of allergen extract in individuals with a positive history of allergy to dog (N=27; hatched bars), and in control individuals with a negative history (N=54; open bars). The sensitivity and specificity of the test is expressed in per cent. The results depend on the strength of the allergen extract used.[14, 20, 21]

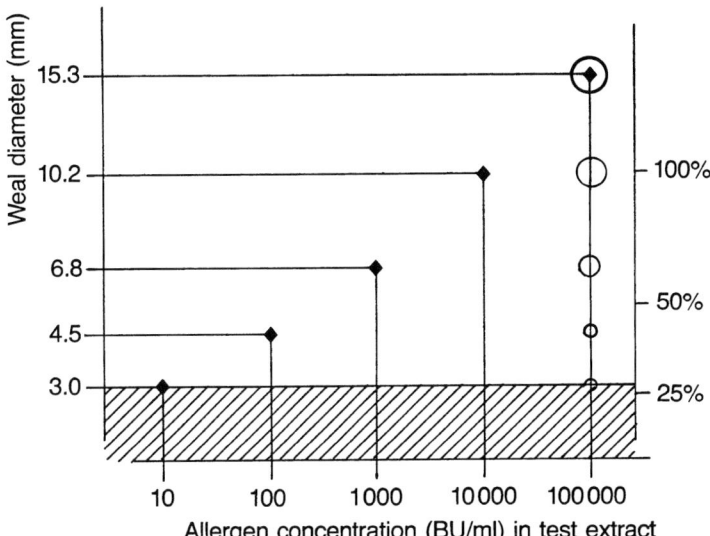

Fig. 9.2. An example of the allergen dose-response relationship for skin prick testing. The open circles illustrate that 5 patients, having 10-fold differences in skin sensitivity, only show relatively small differences in weal size. The filled squares show the weal response in the most sensitive patient when tested with 10-fold dilutions of the highest concentration. Absolute changes in weal diameter or area or percentage changes in these parameters, are often presented in papers. These measures of changes are not appropriate. Instead, the change or difference in skin sensitivity (open circles) or potency of allergen extracts (filled squares) should be used as illustrated on the right y-axis.[5]

asthma caused by the allergen in question. Therefore, a positive SPT, like a positive *in vitro* test, must be considered a sign of sensitization, not necessarily of clinical allergy. However, since young people sensitized to an allergen often show symptoms after continued exposure of the nasal mucosa,[4] the question of sensitization *vs* clinical allergy is more or less of purely academic interest. When the history is unclear and tests do not explain the history, then a nasal allergen provocation test might be useful. As a rule there is sensitization of both the eye and nose,[14, 38] and the simple and rapid procedure for conjunctival provocation test proposed by Möller & Dreborg[7] can replace the more complicated nasal provocation test.

A provocation test mimics the natural situation of sudden direct contact with an allergen. Whether a certain amount of allergen will induce immediate symptoms or not depends on the sensitivity to the allergen of the individual patient. Lower doses, however, may be needed to induce signs of chronic inflammation, which is a typical clinical feature of chronic rhinitis.

The sensitivity to all types of common inhalant allergens varies by 4 powers of ten between patients referred to a university clinic.[11] This is true for the skin[11] as well as shock organs.[6, 19] When the variation between patients in the general population is considered, then another 2 powers of ten must be added.[14]

The most sensitive cat-allergic patients will react with symptoms after 1 minute in a home with a cat. The amount of major allergen (*Fel d* I) inhaled during this period is about 0.2 ng.[29, 42] When challenged in the eye, these patients will react with symptoms to 1 ng/ml, *i.e.* an allergen dose of the same order of magnitude as during natural exposure.

The variation in allergen sensitivity between individuals with a positive history has been estimated to be 1 million-fold,[14] and the dose necessary to cause immediate symptoms in the least sensitive persons is about 200 µg, and this is roughly what is needed for a positive conjunctival test. Theoretically, symptoms would take 1 million minutes, or nearly 2 years, to appear in such patients exposed to the amount of allergen present in the air of homes with cats, but symptoms may present earlier or at lower allergen doses because the IgE-mediated immediate reaction is followed by allergic inflammation and hyperreactivity.

The possible importance of these late-occurring allergic responses can be illustrated by a recent study of patients with a positive history of allergy to dog.[14] As much as 1 million BU/ml, equal to about 1 mg of the major allergen *Can f* I (1 drop = 50 µg),[15] was needed to induce a positive conjunctival test in all patients. It will take about 20 weeks to inhale 50 µg of major allergen in a home with a dog (Fig. 9.3a).

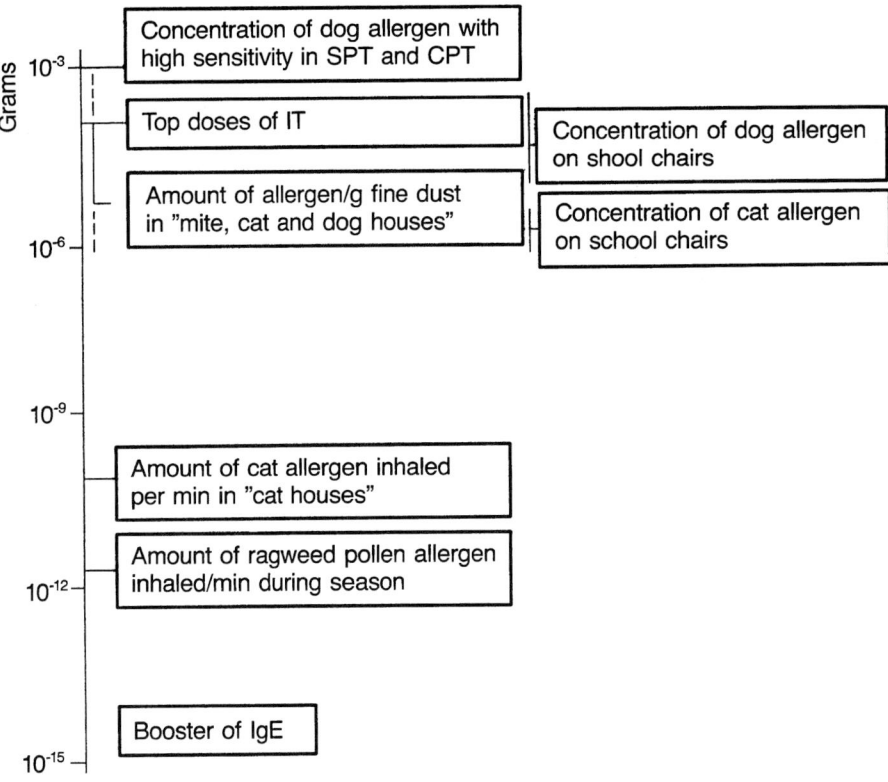

Fig. 9.3a. The different concentrations (from top to bottom) and doses of allergen used for diagnostic procedures with a high sensitivity,[20, 25] high-dose immunotherapy,[35] amount of allergen per gram fine dust,[35, 39-42, 44] concentration of animal allergen on school chairs (to the right), amount of allergen inhaled during natural exposure, as well as the amount of allergen believed to be sufficient to boost the production of IgE.

There are no well-documented data in the literature on the allergen dose necessary to cause chronic low-grade nasal symptoms at continuous contact. As the least sensitive patients, in theory, need 1 million minutes to inhale the dose that would cause immediate symptoms in the most sensitive patients, it is theoretically possible that as little as 10^{-6} of the dose causing immediate symptoms can induce inflammation, hyperreactivity and chronic symptoms.

Based on this type of clinical observation and theoretical thinking, it can be calculated that there may be a difference as high as 10^{12} between the tiny amount of allergen necessary to induce inflammation, hyperreactivity and chronic symptoms in highly sensitive patients, and the huge dose needed to provoke immediate symptoms in the least sensitive persons (Fig. 9.3b–c).

The hypothesis that very low doses of allergen are of clinical importance in patients with rhinitis needs further experimental documentation. In asthmatics, Ihre & Zetterström[24] have recently shown that 1% of the dose causing immediate symptoms induced chronic hyperreactivity when inhaled every morning for 7 days.

The late inflammatory reaction and non-specific hyperreactivity following the immediate allergic reaction last for a few weeks after a single allergen contact. The late reaction with mucosal swelling and increased mucosal reactivity represents an experimental model for the study of chronic rhinitis, which can be triggered by repeated low-dose allergen challenge, as demonstrated by Connell.[4]

Patients with birch pollinosis are influenced for at least 1 week by a single pollen peak in the season according to Broström & Möller,[3] who developed a time-series model for the investigation of this influence. Thus, allergic symptoms are more easily induced by allergens and non-allergic triggering factors after a previous allergen exposure that induced allergic inflammation and hyperreactivity.

The non-specific reactivity of the nose can be investigated by methacholine and histamine provocation tests and the late reaction can be studied by determination of nasal air flow and mediator release.[36] However, these methods are not of practical clinical value at present.

It should also be added that panels of SPT's can be used as a screening test to diagnose the atopic trait, i.e. to establish whether a person has an in-

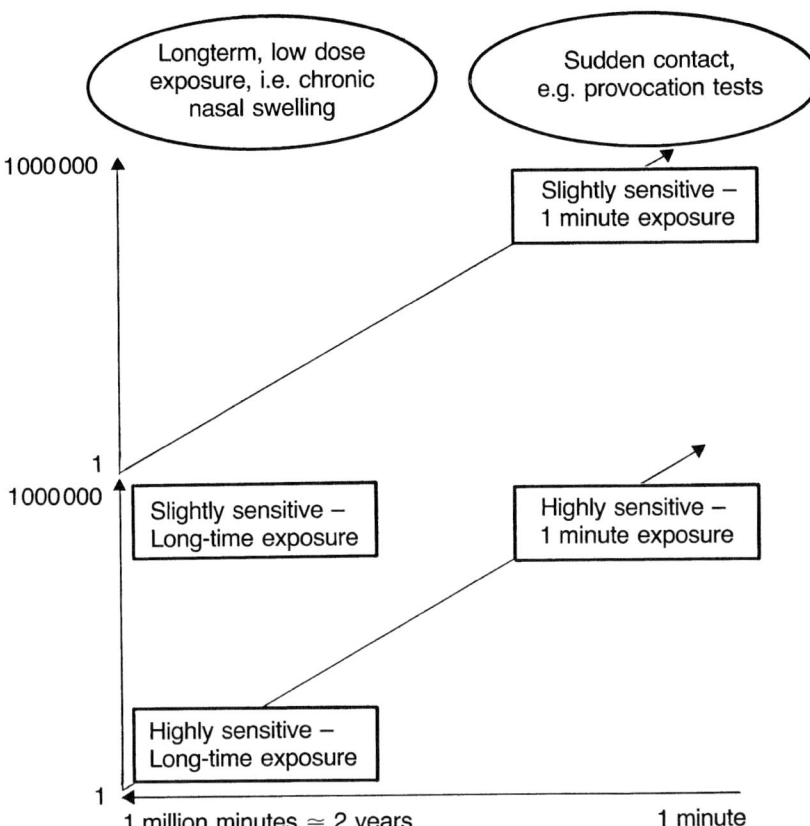

Fig. 9.3b. Theoretical model illustrating the possible relationship between allergen doses and periods of exposure necessary to produce nasal symptoms in patients with a very high degree of allergy and in patients with a very low degree of allergy. The figure indicates that there may be a maximum of a 1 million-fold difference between the allergen doses causing immediate symptoms in the two groups of patients, and the same difference between the allergen doses causing immediate symptoms from short-term exposure and those causing chronic symptoms from long-term exposure.

creased tendency to respond with high-level and long-standing IgE production upon contact with common environmental allergens. Any positive reaction to a panel of common allergens in SPT is taken as an indication that the individual is prone to respond with significant and persisting IgE production after contact with allergens, *i.e.* the subject is an atopic individual. This is an indicator that an allergic origin of symptoms should be considered.

In vitro diagnostic tests

In vitro diagnostic tests based on determination of IgE can be used both for screening of atopy, as just mentioned for SPT, and for confirmation of allergy to defined allergens.

For 20 years, the amount of total IgE in serum has been used for the diagnosis of atopy, *i.e.* the inherited tendency to produce a more pronounced and/or prolonged IgE antibody response upon contact with new proteins of suitable size and configuration. Unfortunately, total IgE does not discriminate very well between atopic and non-atopic individuals.[49] Therefore, tests have been developed based on the fact that atopic individuals show an increased and prolonged IgE response after contact with common allergens. In screening tests of this type, several allergens are coupled to the solid phase. The sum of IgE-antibodies attaching to these allergens on the solid phase is determined. The tests are most often designed to give a yes or no answer, atopy or not. An example is given in Fig. 9.4, which clearly shows that such tests are to be preferred for screening purposes.

An example of the more pronounced and long-lasting IgE response to common allergens is the high and often prolonged IgE response towards hen's egg white found in children at the age of about 8 months, *i.e.* after the introduction of hen's egg to the diet. Increased levels of hen's egg IgE can predict allergic symptoms before the age of 7 years as shown in a study of Swedish children.[22]

Specific allergy diagnosis can be supported by a variety of commercial tests, with the original RAST test as an example. Provided the test is specific, *i.e.* measures only antibodies specific for the allergen under investigation, then positive tests

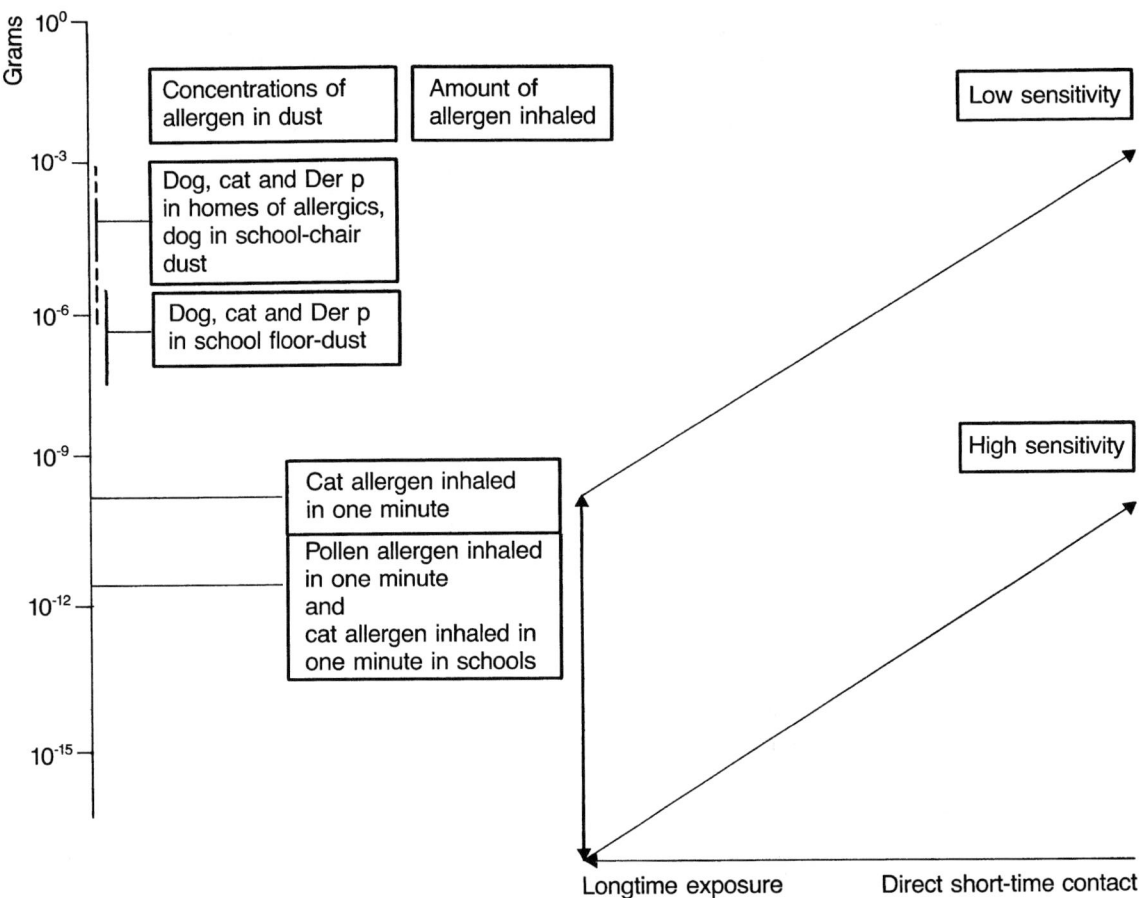

Fig. 9.3c. This figure combines Fig. 9.3a and Fig. 9.3b. Since the allergen concentration necessary for diagnosing all patients with clinical allergy has been estimated to be about 1 mg of major allergen/ml, i.e. about 50 μg (50×10^{-6}) instilled in one drop of test solution in the eye, it is the author's hypothesis that natural exposure of doses about 10^{-12} g may cause immediate symptoms in the most sensitive patients within 1 minute, and that still lower doses, maybe 10^{-15} to 10^{-18} g inhaled during long periods of time might induce inflammation, hyperreactivity and chronic symptoms in highly sensitive individuals.

prove the presence in serum (or other body fluids) of allergen-specific (epitope-specific) IgE-antibodies directed against the allergenic material coupled to the solid phase. However, thorough documentation of the diagnostic capacity of commercially available tests, *i.e.* their sensitivity and specificity, in relation to clinical allergy is most often lacking. The same problems exist with composition and potency of allergenic extracts used for *in vitro* tests as for those discussed for *in vivo* tests. Furthermore, proteins bind to a different degree to the solid phase to which they are passively or actively coupled. Therefore, the proportion between allergenic components on the solid phase is not always the same as in the natural source material, which further complicates the situation. Although the sensitivity of *in vivo* allergy tests is good for pollen allergens, these tests are still not sufficiently sensitive for other allergens such as dog[14] and molds.[37] On the other hand, the specificity of *in vitro* tests is high, *i.e.* patients with a positive test are definitively sensitized.

Use of *in vitro* tests should be considered in small children, in whom it is difficult to perform many SPT's. *In vitro* tests should also be preferred in patients with ongoing allergic symptoms, in order to avoid allergic reactions. Medication that might interfere with SPT results[10] and dermatitis in the test region are other indications. Furthermore, in general practice it might be of value to screen some patients with unclear symtpoms for specific IgE by using a series of panel RAST tests. These tests can diagnose, e.g., the presence of tree-specific IgE or animal dander-specific IgE.

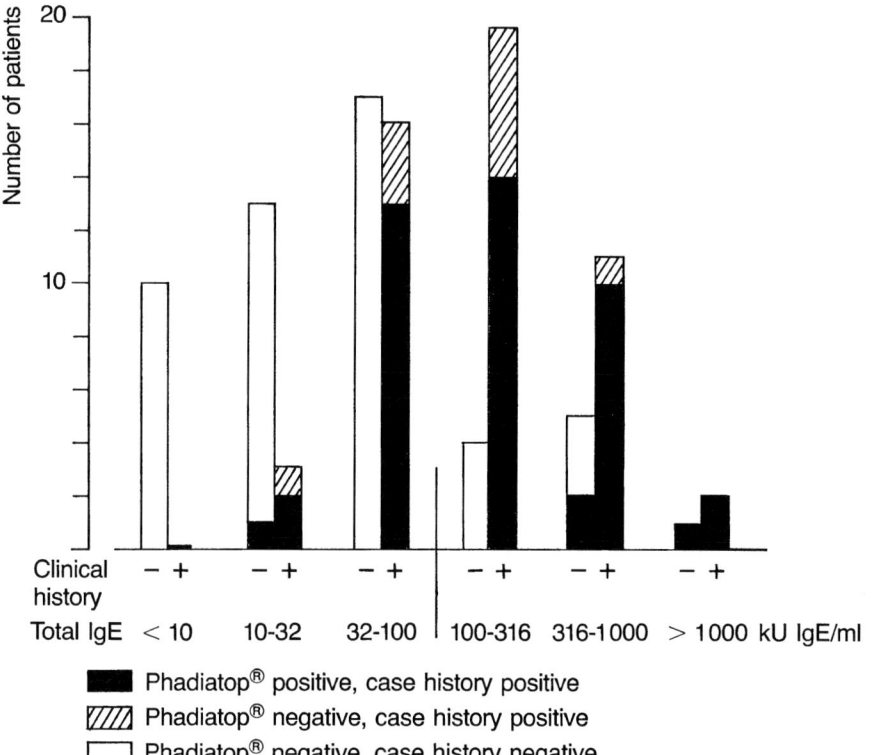

Fig. 9.4. Serum from patients with a positive and a negative history of allergy, tested for total IgE and with Phadiatop®. As shown, the Phadiatop® test better discriminates between those regarded as atopic and those regarded as non-atopic, based on the case history by an experienced allergist, than does total IgE using a discriminating level of 100 kU/l between atopics and non-atopics.[49]

Latent allergy

Latent allergy means a positive test in the absence of clinical symptoms (Fig. 9.5). This term was first suggested by Carl Juhlin-Dannfeldt,[25] who noticed positive intradermal tests to allergens not known to be of clinical relevance to the patient. He found such reactions in patients with previous clinical allergy to the allergen in question, but also in patients who developed symptoms upon contact with the same allergen later in life. Especially atopic children are prone to develop new allergies. Horak[23] followed a group of children with positive tests against inhalant allergens. Within a few years, more than 30% of asymptomatic children with positive SPT developed rhinitis from exposure to the allergens positive in SPT.

Significance of study and test population

It is well known that diagnostic tests differ in their diagnostic characteristics between populations with different disease prevalence.[8] Thus, the number of false positives increases in populations with low prevalence of disease. There will, for example, be many false positive tests to flour in children, if the test has been originally documented in bakers who have a high prevalence of clinical allergy due to pronounced exposure. Similarly, the proportion of false negatives increases in populations with a high prevalence of disease, e.g., when the same test is first documented in children not heavily exposed to flour and is then applied to a group of bakers. The situation is further complicated by the fact that sensitivity to a certain allergen differs between populations, e.g. there are many more individuals

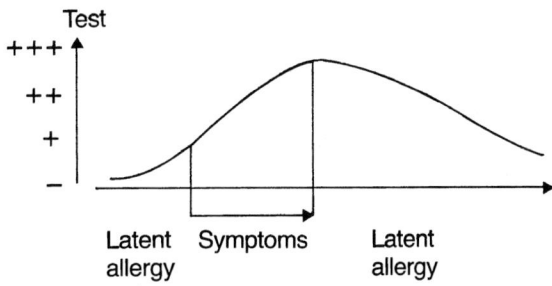

Fig. 9.5. Latent allergy is defined as signs of sensitization without allergic symptoms. The number of individuals with latent allergy in a sample varies with the sensitivity of the *in vitro* or *in vivo* test. In the case of *in vivo* tests the concentration of allergen in the test solution as well as the technique applied influences the sensitivity of the test.[10]

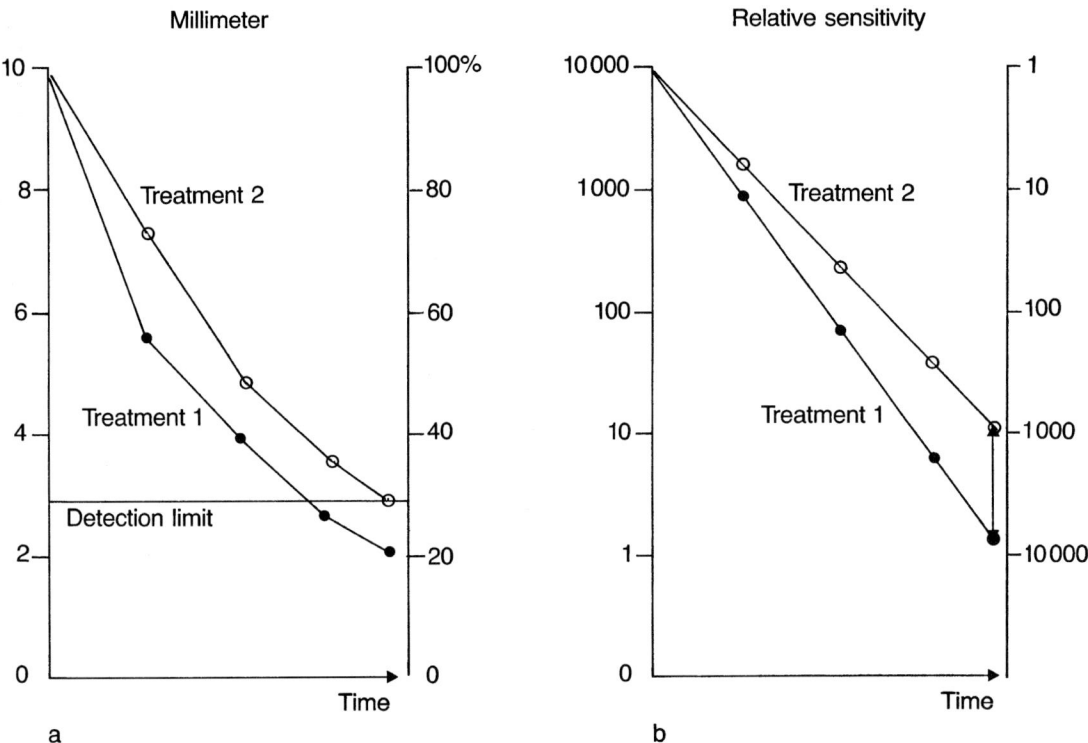

Fig. 9.6. This theoretical example illustrates two ways of presenting the change in skin sensitivity during, e.g., treatment with two dosages of an antihistamine.

Fig. 9.6a shows the ordinary method[28] for giving changes in sensitivity, *i.e.* the change in weal diameter obtained by SPT. The reduction in skin reaction after administration of the antihistamine is shown to the left and the reduction in per cent of the initial skin response to the right. A decrease from 3 to 2 mm in diameter corresponds to a change of 10%.

Fig. 9.6b shows the same data transformed into changes in concentration inducing the same weal response, as estimated by parallel line bio-assay. To the left is the relative decrease in skin response and to the right the decrease in skin reactivity. Thus there is a 10-fold difference in reduced skin response after the two dosages of antihistamine, as indicated by the arrow at the right.[8, 10] When the weal diameter is reduced by a factor of 1.5, then the skin sensitivity is reduced by a factor of 10. More valuable information is obtained by using the method presented in Fig. 9.6b than that in Fig. 9.6a. However, as yet there are no publications using this method of evaluating the effect of antihistamines on the skin reaction.

with low sensitivity in the general population than amongst patients referred to allergy clinics.[14] There are few publications on this important subject and no commercial tests available at present have been thoroughly documented regarding their diagnostic characteristics in specialized clinics or in general practice.

Interpretation of test results

In vivo tests

The sensitivity of a test is high when most clinically sensitive individuals are diagnosed (Fig. 9.1). However, at the same time, many healthy individuals are also found positive (low specificity), *i.e.* the number of negative tests is low amongst healthy individuals. The predictive value of a positive and a negative test, *i.e.* the information provided by the test result, is largely independent of allergen concentration used for SPT, and the information obtained is not impressive. However, the aim of SPT should be to detect allergens of possible pathogenetic importance for the patient. Therefore, diagnostic tests should have high sensitivity, and when SPT is used for diagnostic screening, then high concentrations of allergen should be used.

Some years ago most allergists used end-point titration by the intradermal test method, *i.e.* they used the lowest concentration eliciting a positive result as a measure of skin sensitivity; but this

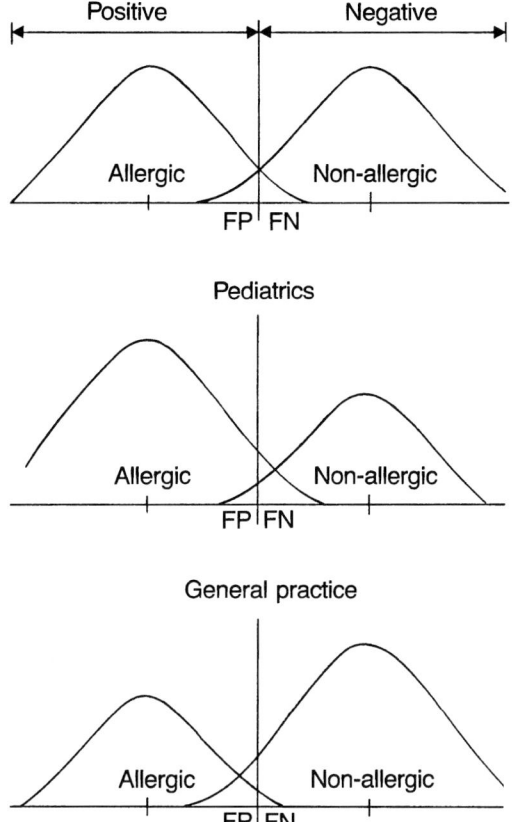

Fig. 9.7. The diagnostic capacity of allergy tests, both *in vivo* and *in vitro* tests, varies with the prevalence of allergic disease in the population being investigated. This figure illustrates the differences in false positives (FP) and false negatives (FN), using a test initially documented in a chest clinic (upper part of figure), with moderate disease prevalence, in a pediatric allergy clinic (middle part of the figure) with high prevalence of disease, and in general practice (lower part of the figure) with low prevalence of disease among the patients tested. In this figure,[8] the skin sensitivity to allergen in patients with disease is assumed to be the same. However, we found patients in the general population to be much less sensitive than patients referred to a university clinic.[26] This clearly complicates the picture and indicates that more research is needed to document the diagnostic capacity of the diagnostic tests in different populations.

method does not give reproducible results.[31] In the last decade, there has been an increase in the use of SPT with standardized allergens, standardized needles with 1 mm tip and standardized technique.[10]

Most allergists use changes in the size of the weal reaction as a measure of changes in skin sensitivity.[28] The change is often expressed as change in diameter or given as percentage of the initial reaction. However, due to the flat dose-response curve of the skin sensitivity to allergen,[11, 18] a small change in diameter corresponds to a large change in sensitivity (Fig. 9.6).[5] Patients are often tested with the same material several times, e.g. during trials evaluating antihistamines or immunotherapy, or with different materials at the same time, evaluating differences in total allergenic activity. In that case a change in weal diameter does not give as good information as the change in concentration inducing the same response before and after therapy. Such information can be obtained by using parallel line bioassay,[8, 12] regression analysis,[30] or simple one-point methods as described by Dreborg et al.[12]

Fig. 9.2, to the right, indicates the change in percent and to the left the change in potency using a log log model. It is obvious that a decrease in skin sensitivity from, e.g., 10.2 to 6.8 mm in diameter, i.e. by 35%, that seems to be a pronounced decrease, corresponds to a decrease of 10-fold, and that a decrease from 3 to 2 mm in diameter, *i.e.* by 10%, that seems to be a limited decrease, also corresponds to a 10-fold decrease in skin sensitivity. To understand this relation, and use it in practice, is of great importance. Fig. 9.7 shows two curves, both illustrating the decrease in skin sensitivity during antihistamine therapy, with the same scale on the x-axis, but weal size to the left and, to the right, change in allergen concentration giving the same response. Until now there have been no reports evaluating SPT results from trials with antihistamines using the decrease in skin sensitivity, as expressed in -fold change in skin sensitivity. There are a few reports on such evaluations of the effect of immunotherapy, either by parallel line assay, by regression analysis or, most easily, by using one concentration of allergen and estimating the change using the common slope of the allergen dose-response relationship.[12, 30]

In vitro tests

Laboratory results are most often well-documented regarding normal values, sensitivity/specificity, and results from clinical chemistry tests are highly reproducible. Furthermore, the clinical importance of changes form normal to pathological values is most often well-documented. However, *in vitro* allergy tests have a low sensitivity when related to clinical disease. The sensitivity of the test depends on the amount of allergenic molecules attached to the solid phase. There are obvious difficulties in binding all types of proteins to the type of solid phases used. Also high titers of other idiotypes than IgE, especially IgG, might decrease binding to allergenic epitopes by competition.

In general, *in vitro* tests are less sensitive than *in vivo* tests with high concentrations of allergen.[14] Therefore, positive *in vitro* tests should be taken as a sign of sensitization, whereas negative tests must be interpreted with caution. Negative tests cannot be taken as an indicator that sensitization has not taken place. It must also be stressed that the documentation available on the diagnostic capacity of most *in vitro* as well as *in vivo* tests in relation to clinical disease is scarce.

Furthermore, there are several commercial tests on the market, the results of which are not directly comparable to the standard RAST test. Results of *in vitro* allergy tests must therefore be interpreted with caution. Provided the test has been shown to give negative results with non-specific IgE, e.g. myeloma IgE at high concentrations, then a positive result indicates presence of specific IgE in the body fluid investigated. However, many commercial tests are not documented regarding the influence of non-specific IgE on test results.

Positive test results clearly show the presence of IgE antibodies. However, it has recently been claimed that not all IgE antibodies release histamine and other mediators from basophils and mast cells.[27, 32, 43] Provided these results are further clinically documented, then the clinical value of *in vitro* IgE testing must be reconsidered.

Future development

At the moment, it is important further to document the clinical features of diagnostic *in vivo* and *in vitro* tests as their sensitivity and specificity in different diagnostic situations is often poorly documented.

During the next decade, genetic probes for screening of IgE responders and other genetic entities will probably be introduced. Estimation of levels and changes in interleukines and mediators may soon be of clinical importance.

The most astonishing trend will probably be development of intelligent computer programs for the diagnosis of allergic diseases including allergic rhinitis. Probably, the clinical history will be too complex and variable to be correctly interpreted by computers. On the other hand, diagnostic tests are often difficult for clinicians to interpret. Therefore, the first step would probably be the development of programs combining the clinical history as interpreted by doctors with results of objectively evaluated allergy results.

Conclusion

Diagnosis of immediate-type, IgE-mediated allergy is based on the case history supplemented by *in vivo* and *in vitro* allergy tests. Allergens present in the environment are potential sensitizers and exposure can induce symptoms in sensitized individuals. Continuous exposure to small amounts of allergen might induce chronic allergic symptoms, although there may be no obvious contact between the patient and the allergen, and there is a need for further studies of the significance of 'invisible' allergen sources. The results of both *in vivo* and *in vitro* diagnostic tests depend on the potency and the composition of the allergen extract and of the technique used. These factors determine the diagnostic characteristics of a test, *i.e.* its ability to detect sensitized individuals (sensitivity) and exclude healthy subjects (specificity). A diagnosis of clinical allergy is based on the case history together with a positive allergy test, but the history can be negative ('invisible' allergen source), and a test with a low sensitivity cannot exclude a cause-relationship. Evaluation of a skin test result is preferably based on the allergen dose-response relationship. It may be possible to further improve the clinical value of the allergy tests by investigating their sensitivity and specificity, using standardized allergen extract, in various well-defined study populations, e.g., patients attending a university department and patients visiting their general practitioner.

References

1. Blumstein GI. The dry pollen nasal test. Its technique, interpretation, and indications. *J Allergy* 1937; *8:* 321-6.
2. Bousquet J, Lebel B, Dhivert H, Bataille Y, Martinot B, Michel FB. Nasal challenge with pollen grains, skin prick tests and specific IgE in patients with grass pollen allergy. *Clin Allergy* 1987; *17:* 529-36.
3. Broström G, Möller C. A new method to relate system scores with pollen counts. A dynamic model for comparison of treatments of allergy. *Grana* 1990; *28:* 123-8.
4. Connell JT. Quantitative intranasal pollen challenge III. The priming effect in allergic rhinitis. *J Allergy* 1969; *43:* 33-8.
5. Dreborg S. The skin prick test in diagnosis of atopic allergy. In: LaRosa M, ed. Proceedings of the "50 Congresso dell Associazione per la prevenzione delle allergopattie infantili". Sciacca, 1988: 1-19.
6. Dreborg S. *Bronchial provocation tests with biologically standardized allergenic preparations.* Toronto & Philadelphia: Decker Inc, 1990: 185-93.
7. Dreborg S. Conjunctival provocation test. *Allergy* 1985; *40 (suppl 4):* 66-7.
8. Dreborg S. The skin prick test. Methodological studies and clinical applications, Linköping University, Medical Dissertations No 239, 1987: 1-148.
9. Dreborg S. Food allergy in pollen sensitive patients. *Ann Allergy* 1988; *61:* 41-6.
10. Dreborg S, Backman A, Basomba A, Bousquet J, Dieges P, Malling H-J. Skin tests used in type 1 allergy testing. Position paper prepared by the Sub-Committee on Skin Tests of the European Academy of Allergology and Clinical Immunology. *Allergy* 1989; *44 (suppl. 10):* 1-59.
11. Dreborg S, Basomba A, Belin L, et al. Biological equilibration of allergenic preparations. Methodological aspects and reproducibility. *Clin Allergy* 1987; *17:* 537-50.
12. Dreborg S, Basomba A, Löfkvist T, Möller C, Holgersson M. Suppression of immediate skin reactions by immunotherapy with birch, D. farinae and Wall Pellitory allergen preparations. In: Dreborg S, ed. The skin prick test. Methodological studies and clinical applications, Linköping University Medical Dissertation No 239, Linköping, 1987: 133-48.
13. Dreborg S, Björkstén B, Kjellman N-I M, Rimås M. How to define allergy to dog and what's the optimal concentration for diagnosis of allergy to dog by skin prick test? *Allergy* (submitted).
14. Dreborg S, Einarsson R. The major allergen content of allergenic preparations reflects their biological activity. *Allergy* (in press).
15. Dreborg S, Einarsson R, Longbottom J. The chemistry and standardization of allergens. In: Weir DM, ed. *Handbook of experimental immunology.* Oxford: Blackwell, 1986; vol. 1: 1-28.
16. Dreborg S, Foucard T. Allergy to apple, carrot and potato in children with birch pollen allergy. *Allergy* 1983; *38:* 167-71.
17. Dreborg S, Holgersson M, Nilsson G, Zetterström O. Dose response relationship of allergen, histamine, and histamine releasers in skin prick test and the precision of the method. *Allergy* 1987; *42:* 117-25.
18. Dreborg S, Rosendahl A, Einarsson R. The activity of biologically equilibrated allergen preparations in conjunctival provocation test and leucocyte histamine release. In: Dreborg S, ed. The skin prick test. Methodological aspects and clinical applications. Linköping University Medical Dissertation No 239, Linköping, 1987: 123-32.
19. Galen RS, Gambino SR. *Beyond normality. The predictive value and efficiency of medical diagnoses.* New York: John Wiley & Sons, 1975; 115-6.
20. Gerhardt W, Keller H. Evaluation of test data from clinical studies. I. Terminology, graphic interpretation, diagnostic strategies and selection of sample groups. *Scand J Clin Lab Invest* 1986; *46 (suppl 181):* 5-42.
21. Hattevig G, Johansson SGO, Björkstén B. Clinical symptoms and IgE responses to common food proteins in atopic and healthy children. *Clin Allergy* 1984; *14:* 551-9.
22. Horak F. Manifestation of allergic rhinitis in latent-sensitized patients. A prospective study. *Arch Otorhinolaryngol* 1985; *242:* 242-9.
23. Ihre E, Axelsson IGK, Zetterström O. Late asthmatic reactions and bronchial variability after challenge with low doses of allergen. *Clin Allergy* 1988; *18:* 557-68.
24. Ihre E, Zetterström O. Increase in bronchial reactivity after inhalation of low doses of allergen. Abstracts from XIV ICAIC, Kyoto 13-18 October, 1991. *Allergy Clin Immunol News* 1991; *3 (suppl 1):* 227.
25. Juhlin-Dannfeldt C. About the occurrence of various forms of pollen allergy in Sweden. *Acta Med Scand* 1948; *26:* 563-77.
26. Kjellman NIM. Atopic disease in seven-year-old children. *Acta Pæd Scand* 1977; *22:* 465-71.
27. Lichtenstein LM. Histamine-releasing factors and IgE heterogeneity. *J Allergy Clin Immunol* 1988; *81:* 814-20.
28. Lindgren BR, Brundin A, Andersson GG. Inhibitory effects of clonidine on the allergen-induced wheal and flare reactions in patients with extrinsic asthma. *J Allergy Clin Immunol* 1987; *79:* 941-6.
29. Luczynska CM, Li Y, Chapman M, Platts-Mills TAE. Airborne concentrations and particle size distribution of allergen derived from domestic cats (Felix domesticus). *Am Rev Respir Dis* 1990; *141:* 361-7.
30. Löfqvist T, Svensson G, Agrell B, Dreborg S. Immunotherapy with a purified, standardized mite (*D. farinae*) allergen preparation in patients with mite rhinitis. *Allergy* (submitted).
31. Malling H-J. Diagnosis and immunotherapy of mould allergy. II. Reproducibility and relationship between skin sensitivity estimated by end point titration and histamine equivalent reaction using skin prick test and intradermal test. *Allergy* 1985; *40:* 354-62.
32. Malling HJ, Stahl Skov P. Diagnosis and immunotherapy of mould allergy. VIII. Quantitative and qualitative estimation of IgE in Cladosporium immunotherapy. *Allergy* 1988; *43:* 228-35.
33. Marsh DG. Allergens and the genetics of allergy. In: Sela M, ed. *The antigens.* New York: Academic Press, 1975; *3:* 271-359.
34. Melillo G. Allergen inhalation challenge with a micronized freeze-dried extract administered by a powder inhaler. In: Mellillo G, Norman PS, Marone G, eds. *Respiratory allergy.* Toronto, Philadelphia: Decker, 1990: 207-15.
35. Munir AKM, Einarsson R, Schou C, Dreborg S. Allergens in school dust. I the amount of major cat (Fel d 1) and dog (Can f 1) allergens in dust from Swedish schools is high enough to probably cause perennial symptoms in most asthmatic children sensitized to cat and dog. *J Allergy Clin Immunol* (submitted).
36. Naclerio RM, Meier HL, Kagey-Sobotka A, Lichtenstein LM. Mediator release after nasal airway challenge with allergen. *Am Rev Respir Dis* 1983; *128:* 597-602.
37. Nordvall L, Agrell B, Malling H-J, Dreborg S. Diagnosis of mold allergy by RAST and skin prick testing. *Ann Allergy* 1990; *65:* 418-22.
38. Petersson G, Dreborg S, Ingestad R. Clinical history, skin prick test and RAST in the diagnosis of birch and timothy pollinosis. *Allergy* 1986; *41:* 398-407.
39. Platts-Mills TAE, de Weck AL. Dust mite allergens and asthma. *J Allergy Clin Immunol* 1989; *83:* 4176-27.
40. Schou C, Hansen JN, Lintner T, Løwenstein H. Assay for the major dog allergen, *Can f* 1. Investigation of house dust samples and commercial dog extracts. *J Allergy Clin Immunol* (in press).
41. Shamie S, Enberg R, Terry L, Ownby D. The consistent presence of cat allergen (*Fel d* 1) in various types of public places. *J Allergy Clin Immunol* 1990; *85:* 226-30.

42 Swanson MC, Campbell AR, Klauck MJ, Reed CE. Correlations between levels of mite and cat allergens in settled and airborne dust. *J Allergy Clin Immunol* 1989; *83:* 776-83.
43 Urbanek R, Kuhn W, Holgersson M, Dreborg S. Changes in conjunctival provocation test (CPT) and skin prick test (SPT), specific IgE and specific IgG during immunotherapy (IT) with grass pollen preparations (PP). *Ann Allergy* 1985; *55:* 259.
44 van der Brumpt X, Charpin D, Haddi E, da Mata P, Vervloet D. Cat removal and Fel d 1 levels in mattresses. *J Allergy Clin Immunol* 1991; *87:* 595-6.
45 Van Metre TE, Marsh DG, Adkinson NF Jr, et al. Dose of cat (Felix domesticus) allergen (Fel d 1) that induces asthma. *J Allergy Clin Immunol* 1986; *78:* 62-75.
46 Warner JA, Little SA, Warner JO. Comparison of two IgE antibody tests with skin test and clinical history in asthmatic patients. *Ped Allergy Immunol* 1990; *1:* 34-40.
47 Weeke B, Davies RJ, Okuda M. Allergy diagnosis in vivo. In: Mygind N, Weeke B, eds. *Allergic and vasomotor rhinitis: Clinical aspects*. Copenhagen: Munksgaard, 1985: 97-107.
48 Wood RA, Chapman MD, Adkinson NF Jr, Eggleston PA. The effect of cat removal on allergen content in household-dust samples. *J Allergy Clin Immunol* 1989; *83:* 730-4.
49 Zetterström O, Osterman K, Axelsson G. Differential diagnosis of atopic allergy in asthma and rhinitis with an improved technology applying the Phadiatop principle. In: Johansson SGO, ed. Clinical workshop, IgE-antibodies and the Pharmacia CAP system in allergy diagnosis. A report of an international workshop, June 23, 1988. Pharmacia, Uppsala, Sweden.

CHAPTER 10

Vasoconstrictors

LARS MALM
ANDERS ÄNGGÅRD

Introduction

The use of vasoconstrictors is rooted in antiquity. Ephedrine is the active constituent of Ma Huang, a Chinese herbal medicine which has been used for more than 5,000 years.[22] This compound was studied by Chen & Schmidt[10] in 1924, and introduced for clinical use in 1927. Subsequently, other sympathomimetic agents, including phenylephrine, pseudoephedrine and phenylpropanolamine became available in the 1940's. Cocaine, which is well-known for its vasoconstrictive properties, has been widely used in some countries prior to surgical procedures to provide mucosal vasoconstriction and analgesia. The total amount used by ENT departments in England is about 960 kg per year at a cost of over 100,000 pounds.[26] In Sweden, where topical vasoconstrictors previously only could be obtained following a doctor's prescription, the market for topical vasoconstrictors has markedly increased since nose drops were freed for purchase by the public (Fig. 10.1). Whether this increase in the use of vasoconstrictors is of benefit for the patient or represents an overconsumption is unknown. Nose drop abuse was first pointed out by Hünerman in 1942[15] and Gollum in 1944[13] described a group of 30 patients who had become "addicted to the use of Privine®" (naphazoline). Privine® belongs to the same group of imidazoline derivatives as the "modern nose drops" (Table 10.1). Even if presently available nose drops have been said to possess less tendency to produce rebound vasodilatation[23] this potential complication remains. This chapter aims to provide guidance for the rational use of nasal vasoconstricting drugs in clinical practice.

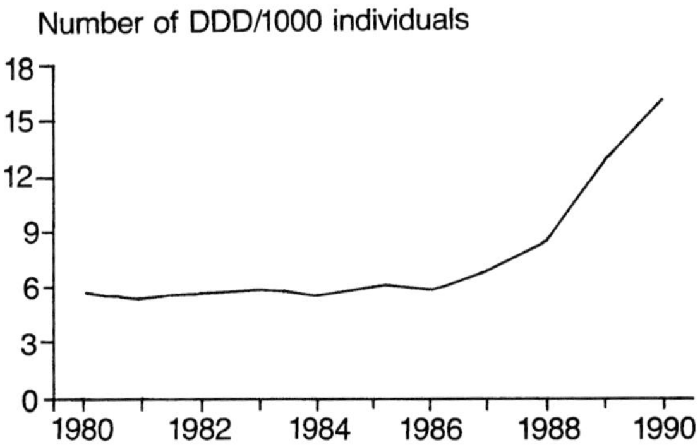

Fig. 10.1. Swedish sale of vasoconstrictor sprays which in 1987 became available over-the-counter.

Pharmacology of nasal vasoconstrictors

The blood vessels of the nasal mucosa have a rich sympathetic innervation. In experimental studies the amount of noradrenaline (NA) has been found to be around 14 nmol/g nasal mucosa[18] which is comparable to other organs particularly rich in NA such as the heart, spleen and vas deferens which have levels around 5-50 nmol/g tissue. It has been demonstrated that under physiological conditions changes in nasal patency are modulated by changes in sympathetic nervous activity and during normal conditions sympathetic nervous activity maintains the venous sinusoids contracted at about half of the maximal contractile state. At exercise sympathetic activity is further increased, resulting in further decongestion and increase in nasal patency.[27] A similar effect is obtained by topical administration of nasal vasoconstrictors.

Table 10.1. *Different types of vasoconstrictors.*

	Adrenergic receptor activity	Attributes	Usual route of administration
β-*phenylethylamine derivatives*			
Ephedrine sulphate	$\alpha_1, \alpha_2, \beta_1, \beta_2$	Significant CNS stimulation	Oral and topical
Pseudoephedrine hydrochloride	$\alpha_1, \alpha_2, \beta_1, \beta_2$	Less CNS stimulation than ephedrine; less potent vasoconstrictor	Oral
Phenylephrine hydrochloride	α_1	Less CNS stimulation than ephedrine; more potent vasoconstrictor	Topical
Phenylpropanolamine hydrochloride	α_1, α_2	Rapid GI tract metabolism	Oral
Imidazoline derivatives			
Oxymetazoline hydrochloride	α_2	Long-acting	Topical
Xylometazoline hydrochloride	α_2	Long-acting	Topical
Naphazoline hydrochloride	α_2	Significant CNS depression in excess: mucosal irritation	Topical

All the commercially available nasal vasoconstrictors for use in rhinitis possess α-adrenergic agonist properties thus interfering with sympathetic adrenergic transmission (Fig. 10.2). The

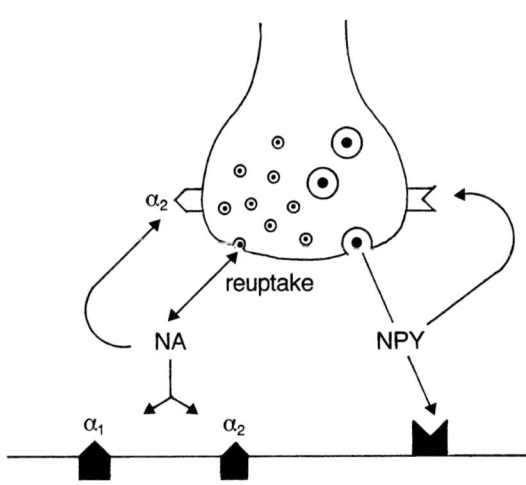

Fig. 10.2. Schematic drawing of some pre- and postjunctional adrenergic and non-adrenergic mechanisms regulating nasal vascular control. Co-release of NA and NPY from sympathetic nerve varicosities presumably occurs via exocytosis. The release seems to be regulated via prejunctional α_2-adrenoceptor mechanisms. Furthermore, the release of NA and NPY seems to be inhibited via prejunctional NPY receptors. Filled receptor symbols on the vascular smooth muscle mediates vasoconstriction.

characteristics of adrenergic transmission in the nasal mucosa is of major importance for understanding the pharmacology of nasal vasoconstrictors and will be briefly reviewed. The autonomic sympathetic innervation of the nasal vascular bed has been extensively studied and the adrenoceptor mechanisms influencing the total blood flow, blood volume and superficial blood flow in the nasal mucosa have been characterized.[18]

In the sympathetic adrenergic nerve terminal NA, the classical transmitter is biosynthesized, stored in small and large dense-cored vesicles and released by exocytosis (Fig. 10.2). However, in the last decade many reports have suggested the occurrence of a component of the sympathetic nerve-mediated contractile response in a number of tissues and blood vessels, including the nasal mucosa, that is resistant to α-adrenoceptor antagonists. One candidate for these non-adrenergic vasoconstrictor mechanisms is neuropeptide Y (NPY). NPY seems to be stored mainly in the large dense-cored vesicles and released simultaneously with NA at sympathetic activation.[18] The presently used nasal vasoconstrictors interact with classical adrenergic mechanisms and do not interact with NPY.

The classification of adrenergic receptors in α_1- and α_2-receptor subtypes has been a result of the development of selective agonists and antagonists.

In the nasal vascular bed it is likely that postsynaptic α_1- and α_2-adrenoceptor mechanisms are present both in resistance vessels, regulating blood flow, as well as in capacitance vessels, regulating blood volume changes. In the capacitance vessels, α_2-receptors dominate over α_1-responses. Of particular interest is the evidence suggesting that noradrenaline, by acting on presynaptic receptors, can regulate its own release and these inhibitory feedback mechanisms operate through α_2-receptors.[18] Beta-receptors of β_2-type have been demonstrated in the nasal mucosa but they are of minor importance in nasal vascular function. Reuptake of NA by adrenergic nerve terminals and by other cells is the main mechanism by which the released transmitter is inactivated. Circulating adrenaline and noradrenaline are degraded enzymatically but much more slowly than e.g. acetylcholine. The two main enzymes, monoamine oxidase (MAO) and cathecol-O-methyl transferase (COMT) are both located intracellularly, so uptake into cells is necessary for metabolic degradation. Sympathomimetic nose drops act through similar mechanisms and the principal ways in which nasal vasoconstrictors stimulate the adrenoceptors of the nasal blood vessels are listed in Table 10.2.

The potency of vasoconstrictors depends on the affinity and efficacy for adrenoceptors, interaction with neuronal uptake systems or interaction with degrading enzymes. The effect of various adrenergic agonists on the nasal vascular bed has been studied in the pig nasal mucosa[18] and their relative potency is shown in Table 10.3.

Table 10.2. *Nasal vasoconstrictors: mode of action.*

Direct action (α-adrenoceptor stimulation)
  noradrenaline
  adrenaline
  metaoxedrine
  tetrahydrozoline
  xylometazoline
  oxymetazoline

Direct and indirect action (stimulates release of NA)
  ephedrine
  pseudoephedrine
  phenylpropanolamine

Indirect action (prevents reuptake or degradation of NA)
  tricyclic antidepressants
  cocaine
  MAO-inhibitors

Drugs available and their effect on nasal obstruction

The most common α-adrenergic vasoconstrictors available for clinical use are listed in Table 10.1. The clinical pharmacology of these and other related preparations are detailed in standard pharmacology and allergy textbooks.[30, 32]

Most studies suggest that vasoconstrictors reduce nasal blockage and are therefore indicated for this symptom. The pathophysiological mechanisms leading to nasal vascular congestion, whether related to allergic or non-allergic factors, do not appear to be relevant to the efficacy of vasoconstrictors, since they have been useful in all disease categories.[2] Though α-adrenergic vasoconstrictors are highly effective in alleviating nasal obstruction, it should be noticed that these drugs have no effect in reducing sneezing or nasal secretion; at least in animal models they actually increased nasal secretion.[20]

On theoretical grounds stimulation of either α_1- or α_2-receptors would be expected to reverse vascular congestion. However, it has been reported that the resistance vessels which determine the blood flow through the nasal mucosa are less affected by α_1-agonist[1] whereas a reduction in blood flow of about 30-40% was recorded when studying the effects of oxymetazoline – an α_2 agonist.[6] Thus, in order to decongest the nasal mucosa but not reduce blood flow, adrenergic agonists with α_1 specificity might be preferable to those with α_2 specificity. Using a 2.5% solution topically applied onto the nasal mucosa a 40% decongestant effect was observed which was comparable to that induced by physical exercise.[4] However, the decongestion only lasted for about 3 hours[5] which may be too short for clinical use and much shorter than that of oxymetazoline or xylometazoline which lasts for about 6 hours.[6]

Oral vasoconstrictors – efficacy in rhinitis

There have been very few well-controlled clinical trials on the efficacy of oral vasoconstrictors in allergic rhinitis. Pseudoephedrine as a sustained release preparation has been shown to decrease

Table 10.3. α-agonist potency studied in pig nasal vasculature. Blood flow (BF). Volume changes (V). LDF denotes the superficial mucosal blood flow as recorded with a laser Doppler flowmeter probe.[18]

BF	UK 14304 > Oxymetazoline > NA > Phenylephrine > Adrenaline
V	UK 14304 > Oxymetazoline = NA = Adrenaline > Phenylephrine
LDF	UK 14304 = NA = Adrenaline > Oxymetazoline > Phenylephrine
BF	Relative potency $\alpha_1/\alpha_2 = 1/10$

both the nasal obstruction and nasal airway resistance in patients with symptoms of hay fever.[11, 33] However, in principle, the mixing of drugs in a single preparation is undesirable and limits the way in which the drugs can be individually tailored to the patient's needs.

Nasal obstruction is a particularly prominent symptom of vasomotor rhinitis, indicating vasoconstrictor therapy. Both pseudoephedrine and phenylpropranolamine reduce nasal obstruction and nasal airway resistance but only at doses where there is a high risk of systemic side-effects.[7, 9] In allergic rhinitis there have been many more investigations with combined antihistamine and vasoconstrictor preparations[19] and, although there is little doubt that they are highly beneficial in reducing clinical symptoms, there have been no convincing demonstrations that they reduce nasal airway resistance.[9]

Local side-effects

Vasoconstrictor agents may be administered either locally in the nose or orally. Local treatment with vasoconstrictors administered as nasal drops or sprays reduces mucosal congestion very effectively. However, their continued use can only be recommended for a maximum of 10 days in any single course of treatment since, for periods longer than this, there is a distinct risk of developing rhinitis medicamentosa (nose drop abuse). This condition is characterized by nasal obstruction which is less responsive to vasoconstrictor drugs. Furthermore, when fully established it may not always respond to withdrawal of the offending vasoconstrictor agent and under these conditions a short course of topical intranasal steroids or systemic steroids may help reverse the process.

The pathophysiology of rhinitis medicamentosa is unknown. The occurrence of the condition in the presence of high local concentrations of α-adrenergic agonists suggests that the sensitivity of the α-adrenergic receptors in the mucosal blood vessels of the nose is reduced and that tolerance has developed. In the normal nose, adrenergic tone is important in adjusting nasal blood flow in response to changing ambient conditions. It is possible that during prolonged and frequent exposure to an α-adrenergic agonist the nasal vasculature will be desensitized or tachyphylactic, not only to the vasoconstrictor drug locally administered but also to endogenous NA released from adrenergic nerve terminals in the nasal mucosa. It might also be speculated whether long-term use of an α_2-agonist may reduce the endogenous release of NA by stimulation of presynaptic α_2-receptors. This is substantiated by the findings that in the dog nasal mucosa pretreatment with an α_2-agonist reduced the response to sympathetic nerve activation.[8] Thus, loss of α-adrenergic tone would be expected to persist as long as the patient continues to use vasoconstrictor drugs, despite resolution of the original cause of the nasal obstruction.[25]

Systemic side-effects

Cocaine

Cocaine is widely used in some countries prior to or during surgical procedures to provide mucosal vasoconstriction and analgesia. Resorption is quite high and causes CNS side-effects and other systemic side-effects in doses which are commonly used for nasal surgery. These systemic effects can be markedly reduced if another vasoconstricting drug, e.g. oxymetazoline, is administered locally before or at application of the cocaine.[24] This will induce vasoconstriction and subsequently reduced absorption.

Oral vasoconstrictors

Since allergic and vasomotor rhinitis are diseases whose symptoms usually extend beyond a 10-day period, vasoconstrictor agents administered orally have found wide acceptance, especially since there is no evidence that rhinitis medicamentosa occurs with this route of administration. However, in oral doses necessary to decongest the nasal mucosa, systemic drug levels are achieved which may cause disturbing side-effects. Because of these adrenergic side-effects, a number of studies have been undertaken to more clearly define the clinical indication for oral vasoconstrictors and the optimal therapeutic doses which cause minimal side-effects.[2,12] However, on account of their sympathomimetic effects, oral α-adrenergic agonists are contraindicated in hypertension, coronary artery disease, hyperthyroidism, diabetes mellitus, narrow angle glaucoma and in patients who are taking monoamine oxidase inhibitors. Since cardiac effects have not been reported when vasoconstrictors are administered locally into the nose this is clearly an advantage for this form of treatment.[21,31]

Non-vascular effects in the nose

In the nose, α-adrenergic agonists may also exert pharmacological activities on other tissues such as the epithelium, nerves, glands and basophil leokocytes, all of which are located in the nasal mucosa. Sackner[28] has found an increased mucociliary transport of teflon discs after local α-adrenergic administration. This effect is unlikely to be due to increased ciliary beat frequency, as α-adrenergic agonists reduce the ciliary wave frequency in vivo.[16] A more likely explanation is that α-agonists increase fluid secretion onto the nasal mucosa.[20]

Conclusion

Basic mechanisms regarding regulation of the nasal vasculature are well known. Pharmacological studies regarding nasal vasoconstrictors with preferential α_2 activity have demonstrated clear-cut effects with about 40% improvements in nasal patency lasting for around 6 hours. However, simultaneously a 30% reduction in blood flow occurs which may be deleterious to the nasal mucosa. It may be speculated that this, apart from intervention with adrenergic mechanisms, may be a pathophysiological factor in the development of nose drop abuse. Oral vasoconstrictors have been shown to improve nasal patency but only in doses where side-effects become apparent. Topical vasoconstrictors should therefore preferably be used when symptomatic vascular decongestion is indicated for alleviation of nasal obstruction. However, therapy should not be prolonged for an extended time in order to diminish the risk of development of nose drop abuse.

References

1. Andersson KE, Bende M. Adrenoceptors in the control of human nasal mucosal blood flow. *Ann Otol Rhinol Laryngol* 1984; *93:* 179-82.
2. Änggård A, Malm L. Orally administered decongestant drugs in disorders of the upper respiratory passages: A survey of clinical results. *Clin Otolaryngol* 1984; *9:* 43-9.
3. Bende M. The effect of topical decongestant on blood flow in normal and infected nasal mucosa. *Acta Otolaryngol (Stockh)* 1983; *96:* 523-7.
4. Bende M, Andersson KE, Johansson CJ, Sjögren C, Svensson G. Dose-response relationship of a topical nasal decongestant phenylpropanolamine. *Acta Otolaryngol (Stockh)* 1987; *98:* 543-7.
5. Bende M, Andersson KE, Johansson CJ, Sjögren C, Svensson G. Vascular effects of phenylpropanolamine on human nasal mucosa. *Rhinology* 1985; *23:* 43-8.
6. Bende M, Loth S. Vascular effects of topical oxymetazoline on human nasal mucosa. *J Laryngol Otol* 1986; *100:* 285-8.
7. Benson MK. Maximal nasal inspiratory flow rate: Its use in assessing the effect of pseudoephedrine in vasomotor rhintis. *Eur J Clin Pharmacol* 1971; *3:* 182-4.
8. Berridge TL, Roach AG. Characterization of alpha-adrenoceptors in the vasculature of the canine nasal mucosa. *Br J Pharmacol* 1986; *88:* 345-54.
9. Broms P, Malm L. Oral vasoconstrictors in perennial non-allergic rhinitis. *Allergy* 1982; *37:* 67-74.
10. Chen KK, Schmidt CF. The action of ephedrine, the active principle of the Chinese drug Ma Huang. *J Pharmacol Exp Ther* 1924; *24:* 192.
11. Empey DW, Bye C, Hodder M, Hughes DTD. A double-blind crossover trial of pseudoephedrine and triprolidine, alone and in combination, for the treatment of allergic rhinitis. *Ann Allergy* 1973; *34:* 41-6.
12. Empey DW, Young GA, Letley E, et al. Dose-response study of the nasal decongestant and cardiovascular effects of pseudoephedrine. *Br J Clin Pharmacol* 1980; *9:* 351-8.
13. Gollum J. The problem of nasal medication with particular reference to Privine HCL 0,1%. *Can Med Assoc J* 1944; *51:* 123-6.

14 Hamilton LH, Chobanian SL, Cato A, Perkins JG. A study of sustained action pseudoephedrine in allergic rhinitis. *Ann Allergy* 1982; *48:* 87-9.
15 Hünerman T. Kritisches zur Schnupfentherapie. *Deutsche Medizinische Wochenschrift* 1942; *68:* 580-1.
16 Hybinette JC, Mercke U. Effects of sympathomimetic agonists and antagonists on mucociliary activity. *Acta Otolaryngol (Stockh)* 1982; *94:* 121-30.
17 Ishibe T, Yamashita T, Kumazawa T, Tanaka C. Adrenergic and cholinergic receptors in human nasal mucosa in cases of nasal allergy. *Arch Otorhinolaryngol* 1983; *238:* 167-73.
18 Lacroix JS. Adrenergic and non-adrenergic mechanisms in sympathetic vascular control of the nasal mucosa. *Acta Physiol Scand* 1989; *136:* 1-63.
19 Löfkvist T, Svensson G. A comparative evaluation of oral decongestants in the treatment of vasomotor rhinitis. *J Int Med Res* 1978; *6:* 56-60.
20 Malm L, Mc Caffrey TV, Kern EB. Alpha-adrenoceptor-mediated secretion from the anterior nasal glands of the dog. *Acta Otolaryngol (Stockh)* 1983; *96:* 149-55.
21 Myers MG, Iazetta JJ. Intranasally administered phenylephrine and blood pressure. *Can Med Assoc J* 1982; *127:* 365-8.
22 NIAID Task Force Report: Asthma and the other allergic diseases. U.S. Department of Health, Education and Welfare. NIH Publication 1979; No. 79: 387.
23 Petruson B, Hansson H. Function and structure of the nasal mucosa after 6 weeks use of nose-drops. *Acta Otolaryngol (Stockh)* 1982; *94:* 563-9.
24 Pfleiderer AG, Brockbank M. Cocaine and adrenaline: a safe or necessary combination in the nose? A study to determine the effect of adrenaline on the absorption and adverse side effects of cocaine. *Clin Otolaryngol* 1988; *13:* 421-6.
25 Proctor DF, Adams GK III. Physiology and pharmacology of nasal function and mucus secretion. *Pharmacol Ther Bull* 1976; *2:* 493-509.
26 Quiney RE. Intranasal topical cocaine: Moffet's method or topical paste? *J Laryngol Otol* 1986; *100:* 279-93.
27 Richerson HB, Seebohm PM. Nasal airway response to exercise. *J Allergy* 1968; *41:* 269-84.
28 Sackner MA. Mucociliary transport. *Ann Otol Rhinol Laryngol* 1978; *87:* 474-83.
29 Spector SL, Toshener D, Gay I, Rosenmann E. Beneficial effects of propylene and polyethylene glycol and saline in the treatment of perennial rhinitis. *Clin Allergy* 1982; *12:* 187-96.
30 Tennenbaum JI. Allergic rhinitis. In: Patterson R, ed. *Allergic diseases: diagnosis and management.* 2nd edn. Philadelphia: Lippincott, 1980: 179-203.
31 van Alyea OE, Donnelly WA. Systemic effects of intranasal medication. *Eye, Ear, Nose and Throat Monthly* 1952; *31:* 1-8.
32 Wade A, ed. Martindale. *The Extra Pharmacopoeia,* 27th edn. London: Pharmaceutical Press, 1977.
33 Weippl G, Mauracher EH. The use of azatadine maleate and pseudoephedrine sulfate in relieving symptoms in allergic rhinitis. *Curr Ther Res* 1982; *32:* 678-85.

CHAPTER 11

Cromoglycate

PETER HOWARTH

Introduction

Sodium cromoglycate was synthesized in 1965 as part of a program investigating the smooth muscle relaxant properties of Khellin, a chromone derivative from the seeds of an Eastern Mediterranean plant, *Ammi Visnaga*. In humans, this bis-chromone was found to have a protective effect on the immediate airway response to allergen, in the absence of any bronchodilator effect.[1] Subsequent studies established that sodium cromoglycate exerted this protective effect without any discernible anti-histaminic, anti-cholinergic, anti-leukotriene, anti-bradykinin, anti-serotonin, corticosteroid-like or adrenergic agonist activity.[2] Further evaluation identified an inhibitory action against immunological degranulation of rat peritoneal mast cells.[3] This led to the concept that sodium cromoglycate acted through mast cell "stabilization" and to its classification as an "anti-allergic" compound. Subsequent development led to the synthesis of nedocromil sodium, a disodium pyranoquinoline dicarboxylic acid, which is more potent than sodium cromoglycate in inhibiting immunologically stimulated mediator release from dispersed lung and airway mast cells.[4] Although both these compounds have a clinical effect in allergic rhinitis, it is uncertain whether their beneficial effect in this condition relates primarily to an action on nasal mast cells or to an action on other cellular components.

Mechanism of action

The mechanism of action of both sodium cromoglycate and nedocromil sodium within the nose in rhinitis is incompletely defined. While both these drugs have been demonstrated to influence immunologic mast cell degranulation, in *in vitro* studies on dispersed human lung mast cell and mast cells recovered by bronchoalveolar lavage,[4] no inhibitory effect has been demonstrated on histamine release from cells recovered by nasal scrapings in rhinits.[5] One explanation for this is that these nasal mast cells represent a population distinct from those recovered from the lower airways and exhibit pharmacological heterogeneity. Consistent with this, ultrastructural investigations have suggested that nasal metachromatic cells, recovered by epithelial scraping, have greater resemblance to blood basophils than tissue mast cells.[6] As sodium cromoglycate does not influence basophils degranulation, other modes of action may be pertinent and several have now been described with both sodium cromoglycate and nedocromil sodium that are of relevance to rhinitis. Both these compounds have been shown to influence granulocyte chemotaxis and cell activation *in vitro* and clinical studies have demonstrated a reduction in mucusal surface eosinophils in both the upper and lower airways with sodium cromoglycate.[7-10] By contrast, nasal biopsy studies with nedocromil sodium have not identified any effect on eosinophil numbers but have suggested that this drug modulates seasonal increments in nasal mast cells in rhinitis.[11] This action on cell recruitment may be secondary to modulation of cytokine release locally within the nasal musoca. Although this has not been defined in direct relation to rhinitis, studies on cultured skin have demonstrated that immunologic upregulation of endothelial adhesion molecule expression, which is mediated by TNFα, is inhibited by prior exposure to sodium cromoglycate.[12]

In addition to these cellular actions, both sodium cromoglycate and nedocromil sodium have been shown to inhibit non-IgE mediated airway responses within the lower airways.[13] This action has been attributed to an inhibitory effect on sensory neural stimulation and is supported by animal studies investigating this mode of action.[14]

Clinical Effect

Laboratory challenge

Under controlled conditions in the laboratory, pretreatment with either sodium cromoglycate or nedocromil sodium inhibits the immediate sneezing, rhinorrhea and blockage following nasal allergen insufflation.[15, 16] Thus both these drugs exert prophylactic effects if administered prior to allergen exposure.

Seasonal rhinitis

Placebo-controlled studies have demonstrated the superiority of sodium cromoglycate to placebo in therapeutic trials in seasonal allergic rhinitis[10, 17, 18] (Fig. 11.1). Not all trials have, however, identified clear benefit[19] and the greatest effect appears to be in those patients with a) the highest IgE levels, b) with the greatest allergen exposure. This suggests that in clinical disease the predominant effect of cromoglycate may be on secondary cell recruitment and cell activation rather than on mast cell degranulation, in contrast to the demonstration of effect in the immediate response in allergen challenge models. Consistent with this, sodium cromoglycate has been shown to reduce mucosal eosinophil numbers in allergic rhinitis.[10]

A number of placebo-controlled studies have now been undertaken with nedocromil sodium in seasonal allergic rhinitis (Table 11.1). These demonstrate clinical benefit. A comparative study of nedocromil sodium 1% with sodium cromoglycate 4% nasal sprays, each used four times per day, in the treatment of ragweed seasonal rhinitis identified no difference between treatments.[23]

Perennial rhinitis

Sodium cromoglycate has been shown in placebo controlled studies to provide significant symptom relief in perennial allergic rhinitis (Fig. 11.2). These studies identify a 20-30% improvement with the least benefit on nasal blockage.[24, 25] Similar to the findings in seasonal rhinitis, there is a variability in response and, based on clinical experience, it has been proposed that the best clinical benefit is seen in patients who fulfill the following criteria: a) an obvious allergic etiology, b) nasal eosinophilia, c) predominance of sneezing and watery rhinorrhea, d) absence of nasal polyps, e) young age and f) short duration of disease.[26]

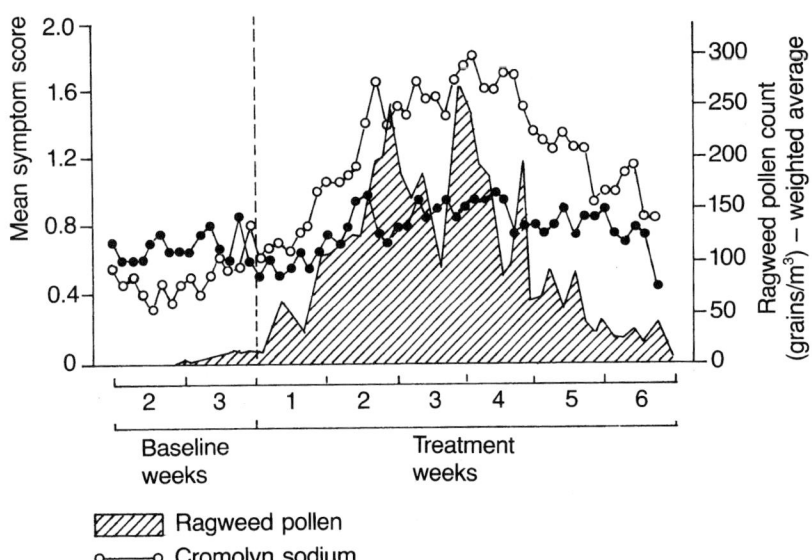

Fig. 11.1. Daily symptom scores for rhinorrhea in ragweed-allergic patients treated with 4% cromoglycate (cromolyn sodium) nasal solution or placebo. From Handelman NI, Friday GA, Schwartz, et al. Cromolyn sodium nasal solution in the prophylactic treatment of pollen-induced seasonal allergic rhinitis. *J Allergy Clin Immunol* 1977; *59:* 237-42.

Table 11.1. *Nedocromil sodium 1%: placebo controlled trials in seasonal allergic rhinitis.*

Trial	Subject numbers	Escape medication use N < P	Clinical symptom improvement N > P ($p \leq 0.05$)
Sipila et al[20]	54	$p < 0.01$	I
Ruhno et al[21]	36	$p < 0.004$	R, B
Bellioni et al[22]	38	NA	I, S, R, B
Lozewicz et al[11]	22	$p < 0.025$	NA
Schuller et al[23]	233	NS	I, S, R, B
Druce et al[24]	177	NS	I, S, R, B

N = nedocromil sodium, P = placebo, NA = not available, NS = not significant, I = nasal itching, R = rhinorrhea, S = sneezing, B = nasal blockage.

Drug administration

Sodium cromoglycate is available for nasal insufflation as a powder preparation (10 mg per capsule), as a 2% metered dose pump spray (2.6 mg per metered dose), and in the U.S.A. as a 4% metered dose spray (5.2 mg per metered dose), as well as in the form of 2% nasal drops. Due to its relatively short duration of action, the drug should be administered every 3-4 hours and the prophylactic nature of the treatment explained to the patient. In symptomatic patients no immediate symptom relief will be evident. If the nasal cavity is too obstructed to permit easy administration, the use of a vasoconstrictor spray 10 minutes prior to cromoglycate administration may be beneficial. In addition, a compound preparation of sodium cromoglycate (2% w/v) and the vasoconstrictor xylometazoline hydrochloride (0.025% w/v) is available, delivering approximately 2.6 mg sodium cromoglycate and 0.0325 mg of xylometazoline per metered dose. Sodium cromoglycate may be co-administered with other treatments, such as H_1-antihistamines, corticosteroids and immunotherapy with no adverse interaction.

Nedocromil sodium is available as a 1% w/v nasal spray delivering 1.3 mg per metered dose. Treatment recommended is one to two applications per nostril four times per day. Similar to sodium cromoglycate, its therapeutic application is as a prophylactic medication requiring regular administration.

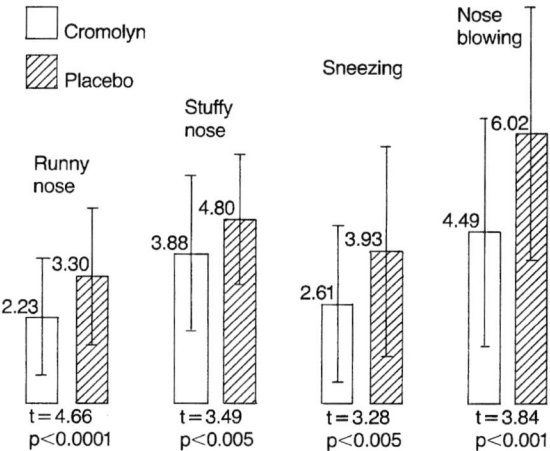

Fig. 11.2. Daily symptom scores (mean, SD) in 34 adult patients with perennial allergic rhinitis, receiving either 4% sodium cromoglycate or placebo 6 times daily. From Cohan RH, Bloom FL, Rhoades RB, Wittig HJ, Haugh LD. Treatment of perennial allergic rhinitis with cromolyn sodium. *J Allergy Clin Immunol* 1976; *58:* 121-8.

Adverse effects

Both sodium cromoglycate and nedocromil sodium are safe therapies with a limited adverse effect profile. Nedocromil sodium has been reported to have an unpleasant taste and sodium cromoglycate occasionally to induce a burning sensation in the nasal mucosa immediately following administration. Both these effects are transient and occur in approximately 10% of patients.[23]

Comparison with other medications

Other than the comparison with sodium cromoglycate, no comparative studies with other agents have been reported with nedocromil sodium.[23] Regular therapy with sodium cromoglycate compares favorably with H_1-antihistamines[10, 27] and immunotherapy[28] whereas topical corticosteroid therapy provides superior control in seasonal allergic rhinitis.[29] The choice of therapy will depend upon the patients' informed preference for the differing therapeutic modes and their clinical experience with these differing modalities. The guidelines detailed in the section on perennial rhinitis identify those patients in whom the greatest benefit with sodium cromoglycate would be anticipated.

References

1. Altounyan REG. Inhibition of experimental asthma by a new compound disodium cromoglycate "Intal". *Acta Allergol* 1967; *22:* 487.
2. Brogden RN, Speicht TM, Avery GS. Sodium cromoglycate (cromolyn sodium): A review of its mode of action, pharmacology, therapeutic efficacy and use. *Drugs* 1974; *7:* 164-282.
3. Cos JSG. Disodium cromoglycate (FPL 670 "Intal"): a specific inhibitor of reaginic antigen-antibody mechanisms. *Nature (London)* 1967; *216:* 1328-9.
4. Pearce FL, Al-Laith M, Bosman L, et al. Effects of sodium cromoglycate and nedocromil sodium on histamine secretion from mast cells from various locations. *Drugs* 1989; *37 (suppl):* 37-43.
5. Okuda M, Ohnishi M, Ohtsuka H. The effect of cromolyn sodium on the nasal mast cells. *Ann Allergy* 1985; *55:* 721-3.
6. Kawabori S, Unno T, Okuda M, Otsuka H. Electron microscopic study of basophilic cells in allergic nasal secretions and mucous membranes. *Rhinology* 1981; *(suppl 1):* 115-23.
7. Kay AB, Walsh GM, Moqbel R, et al. Disodium cromoglycate inhibits activation of human inflammatory cells *in vitro*. *J Allergy Clin Immunol* 1987; *80:* 1-8.
8. Moqbel R, Crommell O, Walsh GM, Wardlaw KJ, Kurlak L, Kay AB. The effects of nedocromil sodium (Tilade) on activation of human eosinophils, neutrophils and histamine release from mast cells. *Allergy* 1988; *43:* 268-76.
9. Diaz P, Galleguillas FR, Gonzalez MC, Pantin CFA, Kay AB. Bronchoalveolar lavage in asthma. The effect of disodium cromoglycate (cromolyn) on leucocyte counts, immunoglobulins and complement. *J Allergy Clin Immunol* 1984; *74:* 41-8.
10. Orgel HA, Meltzer EO, Kemp JP, Osborn NK, Welch MJ. Comparison of intranasal cromolyn sodium, 4%, and oral terfenadine for allergic rhinitis: symptoms, nasal cytology, nasal ciliary clearance and rhinomanometry. *Ann Allergy* 1991; *66:* 237-44.
11. Lozewicz S, Gomez E, Clague J, Gatland D, Davies RJ. Allergen-induced changes in the nasal mucous membrane is seasonal allergic rhinitis. Effect on nedocromil sodium. *J Allergy Clin Immunol* 1990; *85:* 125-1.
12. Klein LM, Larker RM, Matis WL, Murphy GF. Degranulation of human mast cells induces an endothelial antigen central to leucocyte adhesion. *Proc Natl Acad Sci* 1989; *86:* 8972-6.
13. Sheppard D, Nadel JA, Bonshey HA. Inhibition of sulphur dioxide-induced bronchoconstriction by disodium cromoglycate in asthmatic subjects. *Am Rev Respir Dis* 1981; *124:* 257-9.
14. Dixon M, Jackson DM, Richards IM. The action of sodium cromoglycate on "c-fibre" endings in the dog lung. *Br J Pharmacol* 1980; *70:* 11-3.
15. Orie NGM, Booij-Nord H, Pelikan Z, et al. Protective effect of disodium cromoglycate on nasal and bronchial reactions after allergen challenge. In: Pepys J, Frankland AW, eds. *Disodium cromolycate in allergic airways disease.* London: Butterworth, 1970: 33-41.
16. Corrado OJ, Gomez E, Baldwin DL, Clague JF, Davies RJ. The effect of nedocromil sodium on nasal provocation with allergen. *J Allergy Clin Immunol* 1987; *80:* 218-22.
17. Holopainen E, Backman A, Salo OP. Effect of disodium cromoglycate on seasonal allergic rhinitis. *Lancet* 1971; *1:* 55-7.
18. Handelman NI, Friday GA, Schwartz HJ, et al. Cromolyn sodium nasal solution in the prophylactic treatment of pollen-induced seasonal allergic rhinitis. *J Allergy Clin Immunol* 1977; *59:* 237-42.
19. Leiferman KM, Younginger JW, Larson JB, Gleich GJ. The effect of cromolyn sodium powder as a treatment for ragweed pollinosis. *J Allergy Clin Immunol* 1975; *56:* 481-90.
20. Sipila P, Sorri M, Pukander J. Double-blind comparison of nedocomil sodium (1% nasal spray) and placebo in rhinitis caused by birch pollen. *Clin Otolaryngol* 1987; *12:* 365-70.
21. Ruhno J, Denburg J, Dolovitch J. Intranasal nedocromil sodium in the treatment of ragweed allergic rhinitis. *J Allergy Clin Immunol* 1988; *81:* 570-4.
22. Bellioni P, Savinelli, Patalano F, Ruggieri F. A double-blind group comparative study of nedocromil sodium in the treatment of seasonal allergic rhinitis. *Rhinology* 1988; *26:* 281-7.
23. Schuller De, Selcow JE, Joos TH, et al. A multicentre trial of nedocromil sodium, 1% nasal solution, compared with cromolyn sodium and placebo in ragweed seasonal allergic rhinitis. *J Allergy Clin Immunol* 1990; *86:* 554-61.
24. Druce HM, Goldstein S, Melamed J, Grossman J, Moss BA, Townley RG. Multicentre placebo-controlled study of nedocromil sodium 1% nasal solution in ragweed seasonal allergic rhinitis. *Ann Allergy* 1990; *65:* 212-6.
25. Cohan RH, Bloom FL, Rhwades RB, Wittig HJ, Haugh LD. Treatments of perennial allergic rhinitis with cromolyn sodium. *J Allergy Clin Immunol* 1976; *58:* 121-8.
26. Resta O, Foschino Barbaro MP, Carnimeo N. A comparison of sodium cromoglycate nasal solution and powder in the treatment of allergic rhinitis. *Br J Clin Pract* 1982; *36:* 94-8.
26a. Mygind N. *Nasal allergy*, 2nd edn. Oxford: Blackwell, 1979.
27. Lindsay-Miller ACM, Chambers A. Group comparative trial of cromolyn sodium and terfenadine in the treatment of seasonal allergic rhinitis. *Ann Allergy* 1987; *58:* 23-32.
28. Anderson NH, Jeppesen F, Schiøler T, Østerballe O. Treatment of hay fever with sodium cromoglycate, hyposensitisation, or a combination. *Allergy* 1987; *42:* 343-51.
29. Welsh PW, Sticker WE, Chu-Pin Chu MS, et al. Efficacy of beclomethasone nasal solution, flunisolide and cromolyn in relieving symptoms of ragweed allergy. *Mayo Clin Proc* 1987; *62:* 125-34.

CHAPTER 12

Anticholinergic medication

JERRY DOLOVICH
NIELS MYGIND

Introduction

Topical respiratory anticholinergic treatment dates back to the use of preparations containing atropine, stramonium and related compounds in ancient medicine.[1] The recognition that anticholinergic compounds with quaternary amine structure are poorly absorbed following topical application to mucosal surfaces and are relatively slow to cross the blood-brain barrier led to the commercial development of ipratropium bromide for inhalational use. Inhaled ipratropium bromide in doses sufficient to elicit bronchodilatation had no demonstrable systemic effect and 5-fold greater doses did not inhibit ciliary beat frequency or muco-ciliary transport in the lungs.[2] Borum and coworkers then found that topical nasal treatment with ipratropium bromide is effective for the paroxysmal rhinorrhea of perennial rhinitis.[3] Intranasal ipratropium bromide, 400 μg, 5 times the usual dose, had little or only marginal systemic effects.[4] The observed relatively low plasma level of ipratropium bromide after 240 μg intranasally supports these findings.[5]

Stimulation of parasympathetic nerves to the nasal mucosa is known to lead to watery nasal secretion. Section of the vidian nerve, which deprives the nasal mucosa of parasympathetic stimulation, provides temporary relief from the rhinorrhea of vasomotor rhinitis. Borum showed that in patients with perennial rhinitis with nasal hypersecretion there is a hyperresponsiveness of the nasal mucosa to cholinergic stimulation; the volume of secretion stimulated by intranasal methacholine was considerably larger than in normal subjects,[6] indicating that the rhinorrhea in these patients is probably due to an abnormality in a nasal mucosal hyperresponsiveness to methacholine in perennial rhinitis. These findings indicate that usual nasal mucosal reflexes, initiated by various common stimuli including temperature changes and irritants, possibly mediated in part through the action of neuropeptides,[7,8] could produce nasal hypersecretion in affected people.

The nasal discharge stimulated by topical nasal methacholine or the ingestion of hot spicy foods is rich in secretory IgA, lysosyme and lactoferrin which are secretory products of the serous components of submucous glands.[8] The increased secretion of this protein-rich fluid is blocked by topical atropine, indicating cholinergic control of the secretion of these protective substances by the nasal mucosa. There is a theoretical possibility that treatment which produces a chronic inhibition of secretion of these protective molecules could reduce mucosal defenses against infection. The demonstration of muscarinic acetylcholine receptors on glandular cells in studies of tissue sections with a selective receptor radioligand combined with autoradiography[9] is consistent with the observed responsiveness of the acinar cells of the submucous glands to cholinergic stimulation.

In vasomotor rhinitis with rhinorrhea, there is frequent and often prolonged nasal secretion of clear watery fluid but an absence of inflammatory cells. Histamine can elicit nasal discharge through stimulation of reflex secretory mechanisms as well as direct vascular effects leading to plasma exudation. The latter leads to the presence of albumin, IgG and serum-type IgA in the nasal discharge (Table 12.1).

Histamine as well as other active molecules such as TAME esterase are present in the nasal discharge fluid stimulated by inhaled cold dry air. The observation that steroid treatment reduces the histamine

Table 12.1. *Increases in the concentration of proteins in nasal cavity fluid after intranasal challenge. Adapted from Raphael et al.[8]*

Challenge with:	Large increase	Small increase
Methacholine*	lactoferrin	albumin
	lysozyme	IgG
	secretory IgA	IgA (serum type)
Histamine	albumin	lactoferrin
	IgG	lysozyme
	IgA (serum type)	secretory IgA

* Responses are inhibited by prior treatment with intranasal atropine.

release but does not reduce the clinical response to cold dry air indicates a limited relevance of histamine in the generation of the nasal discharge.[10] This is supported by the apparent low level of efficacy of H_1 antihistamine in the treatment of perennial rhinitis with watery rhinorrhea.

Terminology

Topical nasal anticholinergic treatment has found its main application in people in whom profuse watery rhinorrhea is the main symptom. The condition has variously been termed vasomotor rhinitis, paroxysmal rhinorrhea, profuse rhinorrhea, watery rhinorrhea or secretory rhinitis. Since this condition is now well-characterized as a disorder of hypersecretion and since there is no major component of inflammation, perhaps a preferable term would be secretory rhinopathy. Nevertheless, this brief review generally adheres to the terminology as used in the articles quoted.

Clinical trials of ipratropium bromide

In 1979, Borum et al reported in 20 adults, with perennial rhinitis and severe watery rhinorrhea as the main symptom, that ipratropium bromide 40 µg in each nasal cavity 4 times daily reduced the volume of rhinorrhea.[3] In this placebo-controlled, cross-over trial, 14 out of 20 subjects showed preference for the active treatment. There was no reduction in sneezing or nasal blockade. Most of the patients had not previously had satisfactory relief from other forms of treatment. Rhinorrhea returned when the ipratropium bromide was stopped. There was no decrease in the sense of smell. This study design including the total dose of 320 µg/day has been reproduced in many clinical trials with nasal ipratropium bromide since that time. The anticholinergic treatment of watery rhinorrhea has recently been reviewed by Mygind & Borum.[11]

In 1983, Jokinen and Sipila similarly showed marked efficacy in the reduction of hypersecretion and the number of nasal tissues used by affected subjects.[12] There was no effect on nasal obstruction or sneezing. Nasal smears for cytology did not change with the treatment. Nasal irritation and dryness were more common in the ipratropium bromide group than in the placebo group. Nasal bleeding and headache were also reported in single cases.

In 1983, Borum et al reported an open follow-up study lasting 10 months or more in 20 patients with perennial rhinitis with severe watery rhinorrhea. In long-term follow-up, the patients selected their own doses. Eight continued to use a total of 320 µg/day but 6 chose a reduced dosage and 6 stopped the treatment. The appearance of the mucosa at rhinoscopy and the sense of smell did not change and the secretory hyperresponsiveness to methacholine had decreased by the end of the study.[13]

In 1983 Malmberg et al reported effects of topical nasal ipratropium bromide, 320 µg/day in 34 patients, 60 years of age or older with watery vasomotor rhinorrhea.[14] The authors remarked that this is often an irritating condition in elderly people. The reduction of the rhinorrhea was marked ($p < 0.001$) and the nasal discharge in reponse to methacholine was decreased.

Kirkegaard et al, in 36 adults with perennial non-allergic rhinitis, found that ipratropium bromide, 320 µg/day, markedly reduced nasal hypersecretion by comparison with placebo ($p < 0.001$).[15] For comparison, a much higher dosage, 400 µg four times daily was used. The higher dosage had only a marginal advantage in reducing the hypersecretion

Table 12.2. *Efficacy of ipratropium bromide in a 3-week trial in 25 patients with vasomotor rhinitis.*[17]

Daytime symptoms	p-value*
Severity of nasal discharge	<0.00005
Duration of nasal discharge	<0.00005
Number of nasal tissues per day	0.002
Severity of nasal stuffiness	0.48 NS
Duration of nasal stuffiness	0.60 NS

* In each case, the symptom level was lower in the treatment than the placebo group.

Table 12.3. *Self-selected doses of ipratropium bromide (20 μg/spray) at the end of 1 year in two long-term trials.*

Number of sprays each side per day	Trial 1 (ref 17) Percent of subjects	Trial 2 (ref 20) Percent of days
<1	35	14
1	18	11
2	11	16
3	18	8
4	6	23
6	6	21
8	6	5

($p<0.05$) but local side-effects were more marked and some systemic side-effects were noted.

Using a protocol similar to that used by Knight et al,[16] we compared ipratropium bromide, 250 μg/day, with placebo in a cross-over trial in 25 patients with vasomotor rhinitis (Table 12.2).[17] The criteria for selection were: (1) clear watery nasal discharge more than 1 hour each day; (2) absent or mild nasal obstruction; (3) no known allergic cause, and (4) no satisfactory response to previous alternative medication. The difference between active treatment and placebo was marked ($p<00005$) for both daytime severity and duration of nasal discharge and there was the usual greater reduction in nasal tissue use and a preference for the active treatment. There were no systemic side-effects. Local side-effects occurred in 84% of subjects during active treatment and 32% with placebo ($p=0.0004$). The local side-effects, more numerous with ipratropium bromide, included stuffy nose, and blood spotting of nasal discharge. Twenty-one of the patients enrolled in a follow-up trial of at least 1 year. Over that time, the dose selected by most patients was lower than the initial 320 μg/day (Table 12.3). During the year, there were several dropouts due to insufficient efficacy or due to side-effects. Of the 17 that continued in the open trial for at least 1 year, all claimed good therapeutic results and no side-effects. Subsequently, in 26 subjects, ipratropium bromide, 160 μg/day and 320 μg/day, were found to have equal efficacy. Local nasal side-effects were equally prevalent in the two groups, except that less stuffiness was reported at the lower dosage.

In clinical trials such as those cited above, reduction of rhinorrhea has been uniformly demonstrated. The magnitude of improvement probably is a function of patient selection. Rigorous criteria such as those outlined above may be optimal to demonstrate efficacy in clinical trials but do not necessarily allow for the range of patients in whom topical nasal anticholinergic treatment may be useful. Bende & Rundcrantz compared topical nasal ipratropium bromide with budesonide in a group of non-allergic patients who had additional symptoms including nasal blockage, sneezing and itching.[18] They found no significant reduction in rhinorrhea with ipratropium bromide while budesonide significantly reduced symptoms of secretion and sneezing. Jessen & Bylander[19] compared topical nasal ipratropium bromide with topical nasal beclomethasone in 24 patients with non-allergic watery nasal hypersecretion. The variability among the subjects is indicated by the fact that many had nasal discharge less than an hour at a time and 3 did not have daily symptoms. Eight of the patients turned out to have eosinophilia in the nasal smear. In general, those with eosinophilia were more likely to prefer beclomethasone and those without eosinophilia were more likely to prefer ipratropium. Overall, there was equal efficacy with the two types of treatment.

Nasal mucosal effects of ipratropium bromide

Short-term clinical trials have typically been conducted with one or two specified doses of ipratropium bromide compared with placebo. As has been mentioned above, local mucosal side-effects,

Table 12.4. *Lack of tissue effects of topical nasal ipratropium bromide administered for more than 12 months for rhinorrhea (n = 12).*

Associated with treatment there were no significant changes in:

1 Gross rhinoscopic appearance
2 Sense of smell threshold (pyridine scale)
3 Ciliary beat frequency
4 Electron microscopic assessment of ciliary morphology
5 Light microscopic semi-quantitative assessment of: epithelium, cell type, leukocytes, submucosa, edema, inflammatory cells, submucous glands and numbers

particularly drying of the mucosa, are common. Open studies have demonstrated that different patients choose widely different doses for control of symptoms and patient-initiated doses elicit fewer side-effects.[17]

In a study of the tissue effects of long-term ipratropium bromide, it was decided to have the 20 patients use a self-selected dose (Table 12.4).[20] Thirty-four percent elected to use one spray per dose on each side, and the rest elected to use two sprays per dose on each side. Fifty-eight percent used a total of eight puffs per day or less of the spray which delivered 20 μg/puff (Table 12.3). Twelve of the 20 subjects who entered this onerous study, involving nasal brushings and nasal biopsies at the beginning, at 6 months and at 1 year, completed the study. The 8 who failed to complete it gave a variety of reasons but none of the drop-outs stated that it was due to side-effects. One withdrawal was due to lack of efficacy. The 12 subjects who completed the study had continuing control of the nasal discharge. Clinical examination of the nasal cavity at 0, 3, 6, 9 and 12 months revealed no changes in the gross appearance of the nasal mucosa. Any changes noticed at individual visits such as "pale" or "inflamed" mucosa were not persistent throughout the course of the study during which there was continued use of the ipratropium bromide.

The sense of smell was tested with the pyridine scale for measurement of olfactory threshold.[21] There was no significant change with time. Generally, there were more people with an improved threshold rather than decreased threshold during the course of treatment but changes were not significant. Nasal scrapings taken at the beginning, at 6 and at 12 months were studied by transmission electron microscopy to examine ciliary ultrastructure. The percentage of abnormal cilia did not change. Ciliary beat frequency in nasal mucosal brushings was analyzed by a system involving a video motion analyzer attached to a phase contrast microscope.[22] The mean beat frequency at the time of entry for the 12 patients who completed the study was 13.8 ± 1.0 Hz. At 6 months it was 13.7 ± 1.0 and after 12 months it was 13.3 ± 0.6 Hz. There was no change during the course of treatment and no significant difference from normal (12.9 ± 0.4 Hz). By light microscopy, there was no change in the percentage of epithelial cells which were ciliated. Biopsies were examined for additional changes including edema, vascular dilatation, basement membrane thickness and infiltration by vari-

Table 12.5. *Anticholinergic inhibition of rhinorrhea.*

Condition	Inhibition of:	Agent	Reference
Vasomotor rhinitis	chronic nasal discharge	IB	11
Methacholine challenge	nasal discharge	IB	6
	protein secretion	A	8
Ambient cold air	nasal discharge	IB	23
	nasal discharge	A	24
Ingested spicy food	nasal discharge	IB	23
	protein secretion	A	8
Common cold	nasal discharge	IB	25
Experimental rhinovirus infection	nasal discharge	A	26
Perennial allergic rhinitis	nasal discharge	IB	27

IB: ipratropium bromide. A: atropine.

ous inflammatory cells (Table 12.4). Slides were read blind at the end of the study. There was a trend towards a small decrease in the density of inflammatory cells, but the changes were not significant. Minimum thickness of the basement membrane did not change but between the time of entry and the final samples at least 12 months later, there was a significant decrease into the normal range in maximum basement membrane thickness.

Range of conditions in which topical nasal anticholinergic treatment is effective

Østberg et al selected 14 healthy volunteers to receive ipratropium bromide in a single high dose of 200 μg in each nasal cavity.[23] In this placebo-controlled, cross-over study the subjects were evaluated prior to enduring a 40-minute walk outdoors in freezing weather. As a separate challenge, they ingested hot Indian currie soup over a 10-minute period. With ipratropium bromide, there was significantly less discharge ($p < 0.01$) in response to the cold air and in response to ingestion of the hot soup. Similarly, Silver showed that cold-induced rhinorrhea in skiers, which was termed "the skier's nose", was inhibited by topical nasal atropine[24] (Table 12.5).

Raphael et al showed that the increase in the secretion of proteins of glandular origin, lactoferrin, lysosyme and secretory IgA, stimulated by topical nasal methacholine or by ingested hot spicy foods could be prevented by topical nasal atropine.[8]

Borum et al examined the efficacy of topical nasal ipratropium bromide, 40 μg, four times daily, for 1 week in 40 adults with common colds.[25] Ipratropium bromide produced significant reduction in nasal discharge by comparison with placebo ($p < 0.001$), especially in the first 3 days when watery secretion was prominent. Gaffey et al studied intranasal atropine methonitrate in experimental rhinovirus colds.[26] The subjects received 250 or 500 μg/treatment, four times daily, 24 hours after intranasal innoculation of the virus. The nasal mucous production assayed by weight was lower for the higher dose of atropine methonitrate than for placebo, but atropine treatment was associated with mild nasal adverse signs and symptoms.

Since histamine or allergen nasal provocation on one side stimulates nasal hypersecretion in the contralateral nasal mucosa, it can be concluded that a reflex mechanism is involved. Moreover, after topical nasal mucosal challenge with antigen, the components of the resulting nasal cavity fluid indicate that the rhinorrhea is largely due to glandular secretion. H_1 antihistamine can reduce the nasal hypersecretion of allergic rhinitis due to involvement of histamine as a mediator. An effective anticholinergic agent would be expected to interrupt reflex effects and thereby produce a beneficial reduction in the rhinorrhea of allergic rhinitis, but there are surprisingly few studies. Meltzer et al in a dose-response study did find that ipratropium bromide reduced the nasal secretion over a period of 4 weeks in patients with perennial allergic rhinitis.[27]

Conclusions

The enhanced secretory response to topical nasal methacholine in patients with persistent watery rhinorrhea or with allergic rhinitis indicates that there is a hyperresponsiveness of the mucosal glands to cholinergic stimulation. The prevention of rhinorrhea by anticholinergic treatment in patients with chronic rhinitis with rhinorrhea, allergic rhinitis, or nasal discharge after inhaling cold air or ingesting hot spicy foods illustrates the relevance of the anticholinergic agent, ipratropium bromide. The selection, by appropriate patients, of the lowest dose needed is likely to be effective in the control of rhinorrhea without the occurrence of local nasal side-effects.

References

1. Simons FER. Anticholinergic drugs and the airways. "Time future contained in time past". *J Allergy Clin Immunol* 1987; *80:* 239-42.
2. Ruffin RE, Wolff RK, Dolovich MB, Rossman CM, Fitzgerald JD, Newhouse MT. Aerosol therapy with Sch 1000: short-term mucociliary clearance in normal and bronchitic subjects and toxicology in normal subjects. *Chest* 1978; *73:* 501-600.
3. Borum P, Mygind N, Schultz Larsen F. Intranasal ipratropium: a new treatment for perennial rhinitis. *Clin Otolaryngol* 1979; *4:* 407-11.
4. Groth S, Dirksen H, Mygind N. The absence of systemic side-effects from high doses of ipratropium in the nose. *Eur J Respir Dis* 1983; *64 (suppl 128):* 490-3.
5. Laurikainen E, Koulu M, Kaila T, Scheinin M, Isalo E. Evaluation of the systemic anticholinergic activity of nasally administered ipratropium bromide. *Rhinology* 1988; *26:* 133-8.
6. Borum P. Intranasal ipratropium: inhibition of methacholine induced hypersecretion. *Rhinology* 1978; *16:* 225-33.
7. Stjärne P, Lundblad L, Lundberg JM, Änggård A. Capsaicin and nicotine-sensitive afferent neurones and nasal secretion in healthy human volunteers and in patients with vasomotor rhinitis. *Br J Pharmacol* 1989; *96:* 693-701.
8. Raphael GD, Baraniuk JN, Kaliner MA. How and why the nose runs. *J Allergy Clin Immunol* 1991; *87:* 457-67.
9. van Megen YJB, Klaassen ABM, de Miranda JFR, van Ginneken CAM, Wentges BTR. Alterations of muscarinic acetylcholine receptors in the nasal mucosa of allergic patients in comparison with nonallergic individuals. *J Allergy Clin Immunol* 1991; *87:* 521-9.
10. Cruz AA, Togias AG, Lichtenstein LM, Kagey-Sobotka A, Proud D, Naclerio RM. Steroid-induced reduction of histamine release does not alter the clinical nasal response to cold, dry air. *Am Rev Respir Dis* 1991; *143:* 761-5.
11. Mygind N, Borum P. Anticholinergic treatment of watery rhinorrhea. *Am J Rhinology* 1990; *4:* 1-5.
12. Jokinen K, Sipila P. Intranasal ipratropium in the treatment of vasomotor rhinitis. *Rhinology* 1983; *21:* 341-5.
13. Borum P, Mygind N, Schultz Larsen F. Ipratropium treatment for rhinorrhoea in patients with perennial rhinitis. An open follow-up study of efficacy and safety. *Clin Otolaryngol* 1983; *8:* 267-72.
14. Malmberg H, Grahne B, Holopainen E, Binder E. Ipratropium (Atrovent) in the treatment of vasomotor rhinitis of elderly patients. *Clin Otolaryngol* 1983; *8:* 273-6.
15. Kirkegaard J, Mygind N, Mølgaard F, et al. Ordinary and high-dose ipratropium in perennial nonallergic rhinitis. *J Allergy Clin Immunol* 1987; *79:* 585-90.
16. Knight A, Kazim F, Salvatori VA. A trial of intranasal Atrovent versus placebo in the treatment of vasomotor rhinitis. *Ann Allergy* 1986; *57:* 348-54.
17. Dolovich J, Kennedy L, Vickerson F, Kazim F. Control of the hypersecretion of vasomotor rhinitis by topical ipratropium bromide. *J Allergy Clin Immunol* 1987; *80:* 274-8.
18. Bende M, Rundcrantz H. Treatment of perennial secretory rhinitis. *ORL* 1985; *47:* 303-6.
19. Jessen M, Bylander A. Treatment of non-allergic nasal hypersecretion with ipratropium and beclomethasone. *Rhinology* 1990: *28:* 77-81.
20. Dolovich J. Unpublished data.
21. Sherman AH, Amoore JE. The pyridine scale for clinical measurement of olfactory threshold: A quantitative reevaluation. *Otolaryngol Head Neck Surg* 1979; *87:* 717-33.
22. Rossman CM, Lee MKW, Forrest JB, Newhouse MT. Nasal ciliary ultrastructure and function in patients with primary ciliary dyskinesia compared with that in normal subjects and in subjects with various respiratory diseases. *Am Rev Respir Dis* 1984; *129:* 161-7.
23. Østberg B, Winther B, Mygind N. Cold air-induced rhinorrhea treated with ipratropium. *Arch Otolaryngol Head Neck Surg* 1987; *113:* 160-2.
24. Silvers WS. The skier's nose: a model of cold-induced rhinorrhea. *Ann Allergy* 1991; *67:* 32-6.
25. Borum P, Olsen L, Winther B, Mygind N. Ipratropium nasal spray: A new treatment of rhinorrhea in the common cold. *Am Rev Respir Dis* 1981; *123:* 418-20.
26. Gaffey MJ, Gwaltney JM, Dressler WE, Sorrentino JV, Hayden FG. Intranasally administered atropine methonitrate treatment of experimental rhinovirus colds. *Am Rev Respir Dis* 1987; *135:* 241-4.
27. Meltzer EO, Bronsky EA, Findlay SR, et al. Dose-response study of ipratropium bromide nasal spray in perennial allergic rhinitis. (abst) *J Allergy Clin Immunol* 1991; *87:* 150.

CHAPTER 13

Systemic steroids

ELLIOTT MIDDLETON JR

Three forms of rhinopathy may require systemic corticosteroid therapy: 1) severe, intractable allergic rhinoconjunctivitis, 2) rhinitis medicamentosa and 3) obstructing nasal polyps. A suggested regimen of corticosteroid administration for each of these conditions is provided in a separate section below.

Intractable allergic rhinoconjunctivitis

The range of severity of symptoms in patients with allergic rhinitis or rhinoconjunctivitis can run from mild, episodic and marginally distressing to severe, persistent and refractory to therapy.[1-3] When the latter situation occurs, the patient's quality of life can be markedly affected with disabling sneezing, itching, rhinorrhea, congestion and itchy red, tearing eyes (occasionally with worrisome chemosis). Under these circumstances patients may develop insomnia, easy fatiguability, irritability and inability to work. In addition, patients may develop extranasal and extraocular symptoms such as cough and wheezing and occasionally erythema and urticaria, substantiating the systemic nature of the IgE-dependent sensitivity. Individuals with this degree of hypersensitivity often respond poorly or not at all to oral antihistamines and decongestant therapy or to topical corticosteroids because the drug cannot be introduced sufficiently deeply into the nose to reach the target mucous membranes and exert an anti-inflammatory effect.

Patients with symptoms of allergic rhinoconjunctivitis of this order of magnitude generally are exquisitely allergic to a particular pollen or animal protein, as in laboratory technicians, for example. Prick skin tests reveal striking wheal and erythema reactions.

Patients with severe allergic rhinitis may also develop the complication of purulent sinusitis, especially in the presence of a deviated nasal septum (with or without polyps). Although infrequently necessary, these patients may benefit from a brief course (5-10 days) of oral corticosteroids.

Rhinitis medicamentosa

Since individuals with the degree of severity of allergic rhinoconjunctivitis described above often fail to gain relief with oral antihistamine and oral decongestant therapy and even topical corticosteroids, they may resort to topical decongestants. These agents provide temporary help but can, with prolonged use, cause the development of severe rebound congestion, ultimately with difficult-to-reverse habituation and rhinitis medicamentosa. It may be necessary to allow patients with this disorder to continue to use the topical decongestant for 2-3 days during the initial days of systemic corticosteroid therapy. When the corticosteroid effect has set in, then the patient can discontinue the topical decongestant.

Nasal polyposis

Nasal polyposis can be another indication for systemic corticosteroid therapy in selected patients. Nasal polyps develop in patients with chronic sinus disease, aspirin intolerance (often with associated asthma), cystic fibrosis (especially polyps in early childhood), and in the rare disorder, primary ciliary dyskinesia. Polyposis may possibly occur with greater frequency in patients with non-allergic rhinitis with nasal eosinophilia.[1] The role of oral corticosteroid therapy in non-allergic perennial rhinitis without nasal polyps has not been clarified to date. If such patients are symptomatically seriously discomfited and if nasal eosinophilia is present then they might be expected to benefit from oral corticosteroid therapy of brief duration, for example, a 1- to 2-week course.

Corticosteroid administration

Both acute, severe, intractable allergic rhinoconjunctivitis and prolonged use of topical decongestants with associated habituation/rhinitis medicamentosa, as well as large nasal polyps, are indications for the use of systemic corticosteroid therapy. The duration of therapy will be determined in part by the response. A fairly common practice is to administer prednisone 25 mg daily for 7-14 days and then to discontinue the treatment. This approach is generally accompanied by an excellent clinical response. During the period of symptom abatement, therapy with a topical corticosteroid preparation can be started and then continued after the oral corticosteroid has been stopped.

Systemic corticosteroid therapy may be very helpful in reducing nasal congestion due to polyps and in restoring a normal sense of smell, as the nerve endings of the olfactory nerve become unoccluded and free to interact with the ambient environment in a normal fashion. The anti-inflammatory action of systemic corticosteroid treatment causes prompt decrease in both polyp and other nasal mucous membrane swelling, thus improving airflow, promoting normal osteomeatal function with improved sinus drainage, and improving the sense of smell.

Treatment of nasal polyposis with corticosteroids might involve 1 to 2 weeks of therapy with prednisone, 25 mg daily, for example (together with appropriate antibiotic and decongestant therapy as indicated). During this time topical intranasal corticosteroid therapy can be instituted with the ultimate aim of preventing significant polyp regrowth. In some patients it may be desirable nonetheless to perform polypectomies, provide a good airway and hope that the topical corticosteroid treatment will prevent regrowth of the polyps. The response to oral corticosteroids will influence consideration of polypectomy. If oral therapy provides substantial polyp shrinkage and return of a good nasal airway with satisfactory sense of smell, then surgery can be forestalled. On the other hand, if oral therapy is less than satisfactory, then polypectomy may be necessary. In patients about to undergo polypectomy it may be desirable to give a burst of oral corticosteroid therapy preoperatively.

Usually patients tolerate oral corticosteroid dosing regimens such as suggested here without developing any adverse effects. It is prudent, however, to inquire about potentially troublesome conditions that might modify the corticosteroid dosing plan such as diabetes, hypertension, psychic instability, infection, and muscle weakness, for example. Corticosteroid therapy can modify insulin requirements in diabetes mellitus, increase blood pressure, cause fluid retention, aggravate ulcer symptoms, cause mental changes from euphoria to psychosis and can cause a steroid myopathy. With short courses of therapy these problems tend generally not to be of great significance. In the occasional patient with recurrent nasal polyposis it may be necessary to prescribe alternate-day corticosteroid therapy which may be necessary for months. In this situation the patient should be forewarned about long-term complications of corticosteroid therapy such as weight gain, cushingoid features, acne, ecchymoses, striae, osteoporosis, cataract formation and glaucoma. Ophthalmologic examination every 6 months is recommended as well as regular monitoring for blood pressure and periodic blood chemistries.

Some physicians give injections of depot (slowly absorbed) corticosteroid preparations (e.g. triamcinolone, methylprednisolone) before the beginning of a pollen season in order to suppress development

Table 13.1. *Measures to minimize hypothalamic-pituitary-adrenal suppression in patients receiving oral corticosteroid therapy.*

* Use short-acting preparation at lowest effective dose
* Use inhaled formulations if possible
* Give entire daily dose at 8 a.m. except when twice-daily dosing may be required initially
* Switch to alternate-day therapy as soon as clinical condition permits
* Limit duration of therapy if possible

of symptoms of allergic rhinoconjunctivitis. While such therapy may be clinically effective[4-6] it is a practice that cannot be recommended by this author although some authorities would disagree.[2,5] Depot corticosteroid preparations expose the hypothalamic-pituitary-adrenal axis to protracted elevation of plasma corticosteriod concentrations which effectively turns off endogenous cortisol secretion[7,8] in a dose- and time-dependent manner and with considerable interpatient variation. Decreased plasma cortisol concentrations occur in some patients for some weeks, thereby putting the individual at risk in case of illness or accident.[9,10] The adrenal response to tetracosactrin (or corticotrophin) may be suppressed for some weeks in occasional patients. Therefore, it is prudent to use oral prednisone in the management of the rhinopathies discussed here. Table 13.1 shows ways in which HPA suppression can be reduced in patients requiring oral steroids. It is preferable to be able to regulate steroid dosage using the oral route of administration.

Conclusion

Systemic corticosteroid therapy may be required in three forms of rhinopathy: 1) severe, intractable allergic rhinoconjunctivitis, 2) rhinitis medicamentosa, and 3) obstructing nasal polyposis. When a patient afflicted with one of these conditions fails to respond to conventional therapy with antihistamines, decongestants and topical corticosteroid then he/she is a candidate for systemic corticosteroid treatment to reverse the symptom-producing inflammatory pathology. Oral prednisone is the most commonly prescribed corticosteroid and may be administered for variable periods to achieve the desired result. The practice of administering corticosteroids by intramuscular injection is not recommended although some authorities use this approach. It should be emphasized, however, that injected corticosteroid may produce a state of prolonged adrenal cortical hyporesponsiveness. Administration of prednisone orally permits appropriate regulation of dosage.

References

1 Mathews KP. Allergic and nonallergic rhinitis, nasal polyposis and sinusitis. In: Kaplan AP, ed. *Allergy*. New York: Churchill Livingstone, 1985: 323-66.
2 Mygind N. *Nasal allergy*, 2nd edn. Oxford: Blackwell Scientific Publications, 1979: 1-363.
3 Meltzer EO, Schatz M, Zeiger RS. In: Middleton E Jr, Reed CE, Ellis EF, Adkinson NF, Yunginger JCV, eds. *Allergic and nonallergic rhinitis*. St Louis: The CV Mosby Company, 1988: 1253-89.
4 Brown E, Seideman T, Siegelaub AB, Popovitz C. Depot-methylprednisolone in the treatment of ragweed hay fever. *Ann Allergy* 1960; *18:* 1321-30.
5 Borum P, Grønborg H, Mygind N. Seasonal allergic rhinitis and depot injection of a corticosteroid. Evaluation of the efficacy of medication early and late in the season based on detailed symptom recording. *Allergy* 1987; *42:* 26-32.
6 Ohlander BO, Hansson RE, Karlsson KE. A comparison of three injectable corticosteroids for the treatment of patients with seasonal hay fever. *J Int Med Res* 1980; *8:* 63-9.
7 Dujovne A, Azarnoff DL. In: Azarnoff DL, ed. *Clinical implication of corticosteroid therapy. A selected review in steroid therapy*. Philadelphia: WB Saunders, 1975: 27-41.
8 Hedner P, Persson G. Suppression of hypothalamo-pituitary-adrenal axis after a single intramuscular injection of methylprednisolone acetate. *Ann Allergy* 1981; *47:* 176-9.
9 Ganderton MA, James VHT. Clinical and endocrine side-effects of methylprednisolone acetate as used in hay fever. *Br Med J* 1970; *1:* 267-9.
10 Helfer EL, Rose LI. Corticosteroids and adrenal suppression characterizing and avoiding the problem. *Drug* 1989; *38:* 838-45.

CHAPTER 14

Intranasal steroids

ROBERT M NACLERIO
NIELS MYGIND

Glucocorticosteroids (steroids) are currently the most potent medications available for the treatment of allergic rhinitis.[1-4] Intranasal preparations eliminate the systemic side-effects and equal or exceed the efficacy of their oral counterparts.[5] Initially reserved as a second-line agent, the role of intranasal steroids may be changing. Unlike immunotherapy, steroid therapy is nonspecific and has efficacy in some types of nonallergic rhinitis.

Mechanism of action

Hydrocortisone is the parent molecule from which natural and synthetic anti-inflammatory steroids are derived (Fig. 14.1). The structure-activity relationships of the steroid molecule have been intensively investigated.[5] The lipophilic nature of steroids permits rapid absorption across mucosal surfaces. Systemically absorbed steroids bind to

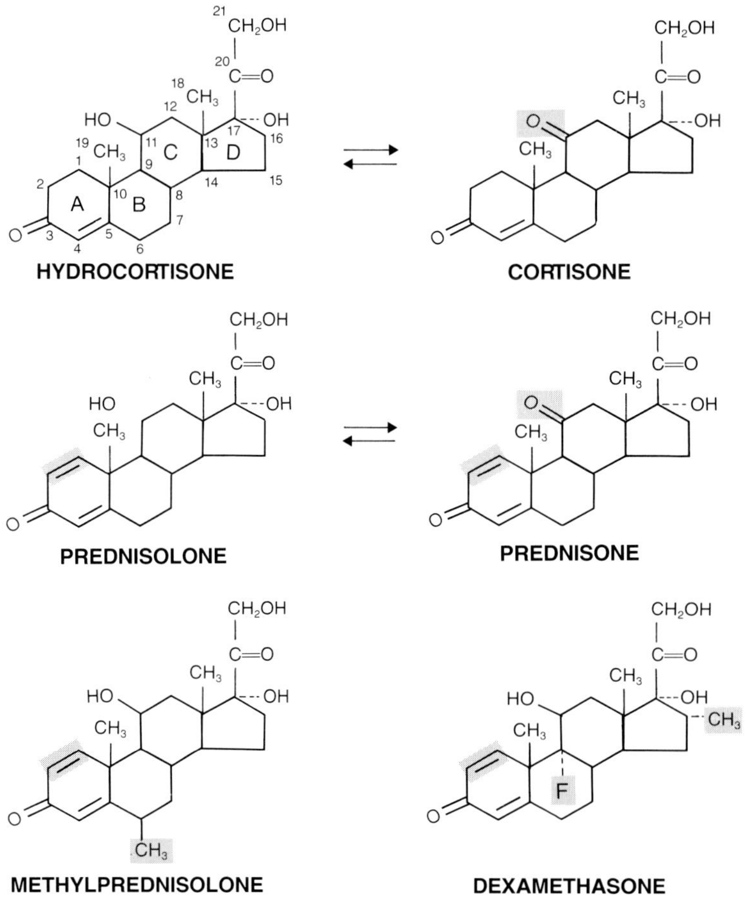

Fig. 14.1. Chemical structure of some important glucocorticoids. Reprinted with permission from CV Mosby, St. Louis. *Allergy: Principles and Practice*, 3rd edn. 1991: 739-65.

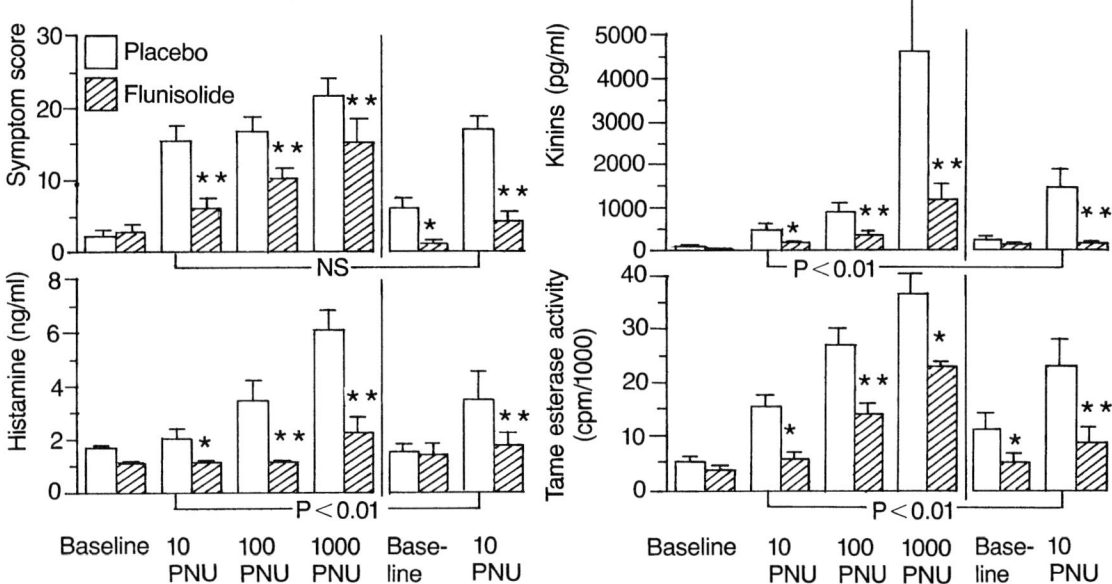

Fig. 14.2. Levels of histamine, TAME-esterase activity and kinins and symptom scores (includes number of sneezes) 10 minutes after each challenge (mean ± SEM). Statistical comparison of results after placebo and topical glucocorticosteroid pretreatment are indicated (* = p<0.05; ** = p<0.01; NS = not significant). The vertical line indicates 11 hours' separation in time between challenges. The connecting line indicates the comparison between the two 10 PNU challenges on the placebo day. The second challenge, 11 hours after the first, is augmented and is not statistically different from the initial 100 PNU challenge. Adapted and reprinted with permission from *N Engl J Med* 1987; *316:* 1506-10.

plasma proteins and undergo metabolism in the liver before being excreted in the urine. Their action on individual cells begins when the free steroid molecule diffuses across the cell membrane and binds to steroid receptors within the cell. The complex interacts with the nucleus to eventually form messenger RNA transcripts. The posttranscriptional proteins then mediate drug effects. The need for transcription and translation account for the time delay between administration and clinical activity.

The accessibility of the nose has permitted an evaluation of some of the myriad effects of these drugs on the pathophysiology of allergic rhinitis. Initial studies using 2-week pretreatment with dexamethasone isonicotinate and using 1-week pretreatment with beclomethasone showed no effect on nasal airway resistance during the early response to antigen provocation.[6,7] More recent studies by Vilsvik[8] and Pipkorn[9] have shown significant inhibition of antigen-provoked increase in nasal airway resistance with 1-week pretreatment with beclomethasone and budesonide, respectively. Okuda & Senba reported inhibitory effects of 2-week pretreatment with beclomethasone on allergen-induced symptoms.[10] The duration of treatment seems to be the important variable in establishing an effect on the early response to antigen challenge, which is dominated by mast cell degranulation.

In trying to further understand the effect of intranasal steroids, Pipkorn showed that 1-week pretreatment with budesonide had no effect on histamine provocation, suggesting that these drugs didn't effect the H_1 receptor.[11] Pipkorn then biopsied normal and allergic subjects before and after 1-week pretreatment with 400 μg of budesonide.[12] The number of mast cells remained constant, while the histamine content declined by a small but significant amount in the allergic individuals. Otsuka, using nasal scrapings, later showed that beclomethasone reduced the number of formalin-sensitive metachromatic cells.[13] Treatment with budesonide in normal persons had no effect on either the capacitance vessels, as determined by measurement of nasal airway resistance, or on the resistance vessels, as determined by the xenon washout technique.[14] One-week pretreatment with flunisolide significantly inhibited the release of histamine, TAME-esterase activity and kinins into nasal secretions during the early response to antigen challenge

(Fig. 14.2).[15] Intranasal beclomethasone had no effect on mucociliary transport in 14 normal subjects.[16]

Since the early reaction represents only one component of the response to nasal challenge with antigen, the effect of intranasal steroids on the late inflammatory events has also been investigated. One-week treatment with flunisolide reduced the cellular infiltration, the late-phase reaction and the augmented response to antigen (Fig. 14.2-3). The latter was shown to be inhibited by treating with intranasal steroids after the early response (Fig. 14.4).[17] Anderson showed that the level of eosinophilic cationic protein and the number of eosinophils were also reduced by intranasal budesonide.[18] In other studies, intranasal steroids reduced the increase in nonspecific reactivity which follows the early response to nasal provocation with antigen.[19] Since inflammation does not end with inflammatory events occurring within 24 hours of exposure, an investigation was made of the effect of continuous intranasal steroid usage on the increase in seasonal specific IgE levels.

Treatment continually with beclomethasone reduced the anticipated rise in ragweed-specific IgE.[20] Intranasal steroids seem to function on all aspects of the nasal inflammatory response in which they have been studied.

Many of the effects of intranasal steroids described above can be reproduced in clinical trials during the allergy season. The number of eosinophils, the presence of eosinophil cationic protein and the number of mast cell progenitors are reduced.[21, 22] It is clear that a single mechanism cannot be proposed to account for the multiple actions of steroids. On the contrary, their multiple sites of action may account for their extreme potency.

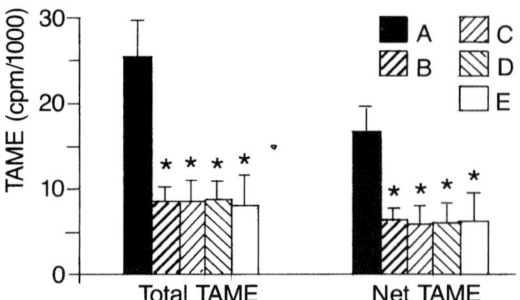

Fig. 14.4. TAME activity levels in nasal lavages at rechallenge (mean ± SEM). Bars on left indicate total values obtained; bars on right indicate net increase (after subtraction of diluent challenge). A, placebo treatment; B, treatment 2 hours after initial challenge; C, 2 hours of pretreatment with topical glucocorticosteroid; D, 12 hours of pretreatment; E, 48 hours of pretreatment with intranasal glucocorticosteroid. *p < 0.05 compared with placebo. Reprinted with permission from *J Allergy Clin Immunol* 1988; *82:* 1019-26.

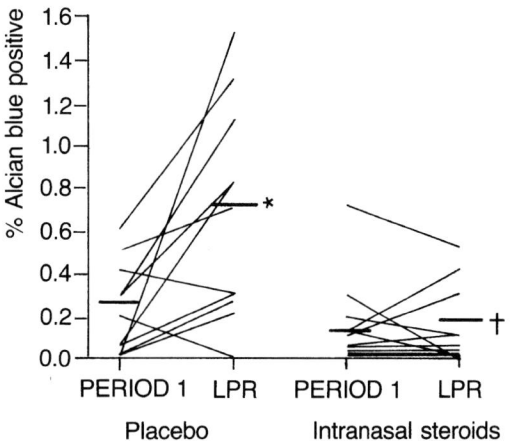

Fig. 14.3. Influx of alcian blue-stained positive cells after nasal antigen challenge in allergic subjects, expressed as the percent of at least 300 cells counted on cytocentrifuge slides. Period 1 represents pooled data from baseline washes and the first 2 hours after antigen challenge. The late phase is 3 to 11 hours after antigen challenge. *Placebo period 1 versus late-phase, p = 0.01. †Placebo treatment late-phase versus intranasal steroid treatment late-phase, p < 0.01. Reprinted with permission from *J Allergy Clin Immunol* 1988; *81:* 580-9.

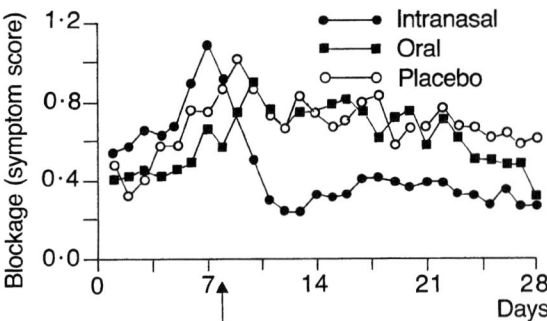

Fig. 14.5. Mean symptom scores for blocked nose for the 4 study weeks. There was no difference between the three treatments in the run-in week. Treatment start is indicated with an arrow. Intranasal topical treatment with budesonide 400 μg/day was significantly more effective than oral budesonide, 500 μg/day (p < 0.01) and placebo (p < 0.01). There were no statistically significant differences between oral budesonide and placebo treatment. Reprinted with permission from *Clin Exp Allergy* 1989; *19:* 71-6.

Clinical usage

The development of intranasal steroids dramatically reduced the need for systemic steroid treatment. Their efficacy for treating allergic rhinitis is indisputable. The effect of topical steroids is based on local activity, since administration of the equivalent amount of drug orally produces no benefit (Fig. 14.5).[23, 24] Their efficacy exceeds that of antihistamines (Fig. 14.6), decongestants and cromolyn (Fig. 14.7).[2-4] Their major limitation lies in the treatment of associated eye symptoms and the relatively slow onset of action. The medications work best on a continual versus an as-needed basis (Fig. 14.8).[25] There is some evidence that intranasal usage during the pollen season reduces symptoms of asthma (Fig. 14.9). We know of only one study comparing intranasal steroids and immunotherapy.[26] This study found intranasal budesonide superior to Pollinex®. The latter treatment is not a standard form of immunotherapy, and further investigations comparing immunotherapy and intranasal steroids are warranted. Intranasal steroids also have efficacy in the treatment of nasal polyps (Fig. 14.10)[27, 28] and in perennial nonallergic rhinitis,[29] particularly if eosinophilia is present.

The first recommendation for treatment of allergic rhinitis is avoidance. If this does not provide significant amelioration or takes a protracted time to accomplish, then pharmacotherapy is introduced. Antihistamines, with or without decongestants, are usually recommended first. If they fail to provide satisfactory relief or if the disease is severe, intranasal steroids should be introduced. This highly effective treatment provides almost complete relief of nasal symptoms. For those with persistent eye complaints, topical eyedrops or oral antihistamines may be necessary to complement intra-

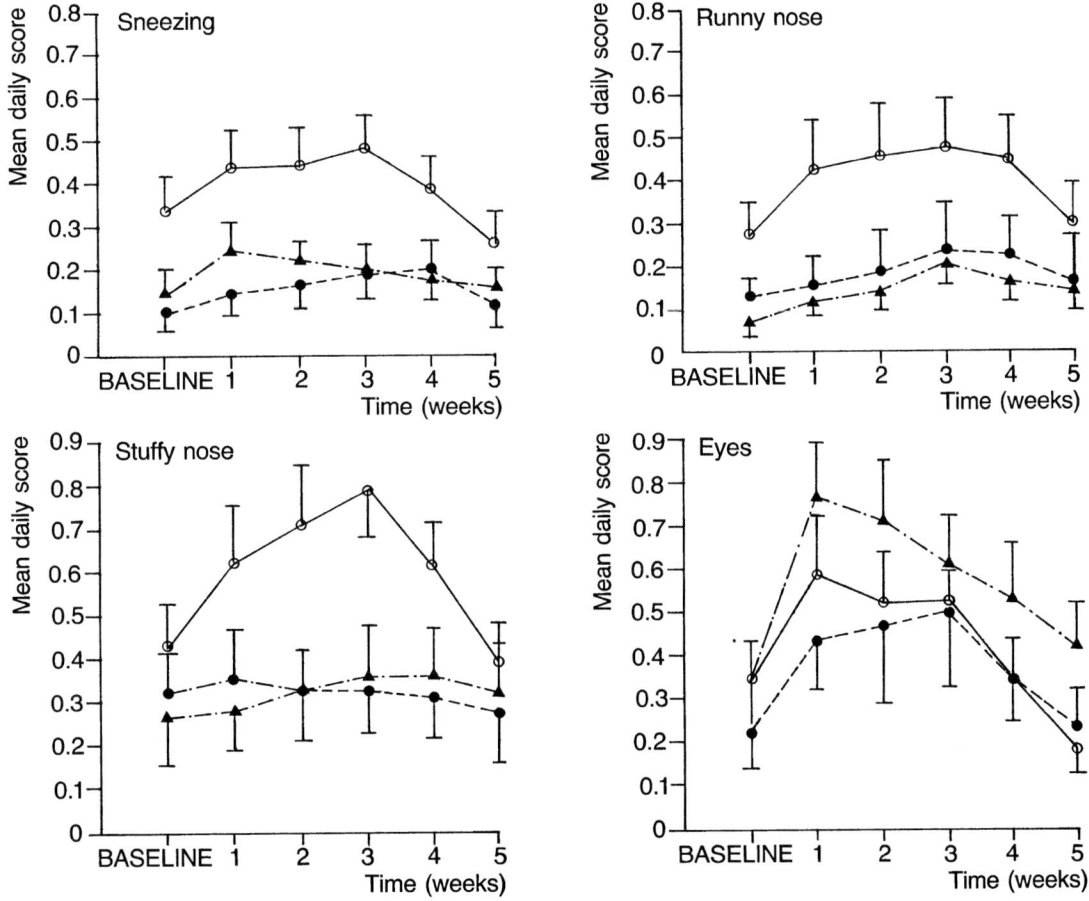

Fig. 14.6. Mean daily nose and eye symptom scores (SEM) before and throughout the ragweed-pollen season; astemizole alone (○); aqueous beclomethasone nasal spray alone (▲); astemizole plus aqueous beclomethasone nasal spray (●). Reprinted with permission from *J Allergy Clin Immunol* 1989; *83*: 627-33.

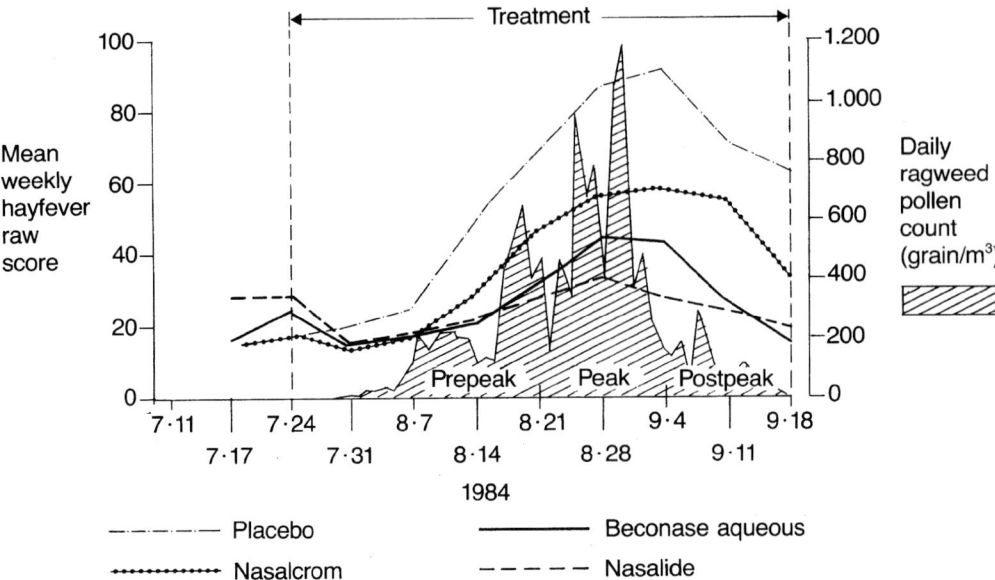

Fig. 14.7. Mean weekly raw scores for symptoms of hay fever among 120 patients in four study groups, based on treatment: placebo, cromolyn sodium (Nasalcrom), flunisolide (Nasalide), and beclomethasone nasal solution (Beconase AQ). Study was conducted during ragweed season in 1984. Daily ragweed pollen count is shown in shaded area. All active treatments were more effective than placebo, and the two glucocorticoids were more effective than cromolyn in preventing symptoms of hay fever. Reprinted with permission from *Mayo Clinic Proc* 1987; *62:* 125-34.

nasal steroids. This is an example of how treatments for allergic rhinitis can be combined to maximize relief.

Pump sprays provide better distribution of drug compared to aerosols.[30, 31] Few studies have directly compared the mode of delivery, but both preparations clearly improve symptoms relative to placebo. The choice of preparation probably depends mostly on patient preference.

Preparations available include beclomethasone, flunisolide, budesonide, triamcinolone and dexamethasone. Fluocortin butylester and fluticasone propionate are in various states of development. The recommended adult starting dose for flunisolide is 50 µg (2 sprays) per nostril twice a day and for beclomethasone is 42 µg (1 spray) per nostril two to four times per day;[32] budesonide, 200 µg BID and triamcinolone, 200 µg QD. After using these doses for 1 to 2 weeks, the patient needs to be reevaluated. First, the nose should be examined for signs of local irritation secondary to the drug or mechanical trauma from the applicator. If no adverse effects are reported or detected at this point, the patient will usually tolerate the mechanism for prolonged periods.

The dose can be adjusted based on clinical response. The goal should be to use the lowest dose which provides efficacy. Once-a-day dosing is often possible with most preparations, a major advantage for compliance. When adjusting the dose, as when initiating therapy, the patient must be informed that the therapeutic effects have a slow onset and offset of activity, unlike the rapid response of decongestants and antihistamines. The physician must also consider whether the environmental allergen load will be increasing or decreasing.

Dexamethasone has minor but detectable systemic effects at clinically recommended doses and should be used with caution.[33] With proper use of intranasal steroids, the physician should expect excellent symptomatic relief in over 90% of properly diagnosed patients.[34]

Patients may present in the middle of a season with total nasal obstruction. This condition not only affects daytime breathing and vocal resonance but can also induce sleep and eustachian tube dysfunction and can predispose to sinus infections.[35, 36] Oral decongestants, with or without antihistamines, will not be effective in such instances, and topical steroids cannot be effectively applied. A short course of oral steroids (e.g., 30 mg of prednisone orally for 3 days, 20 mg orally for 3 days

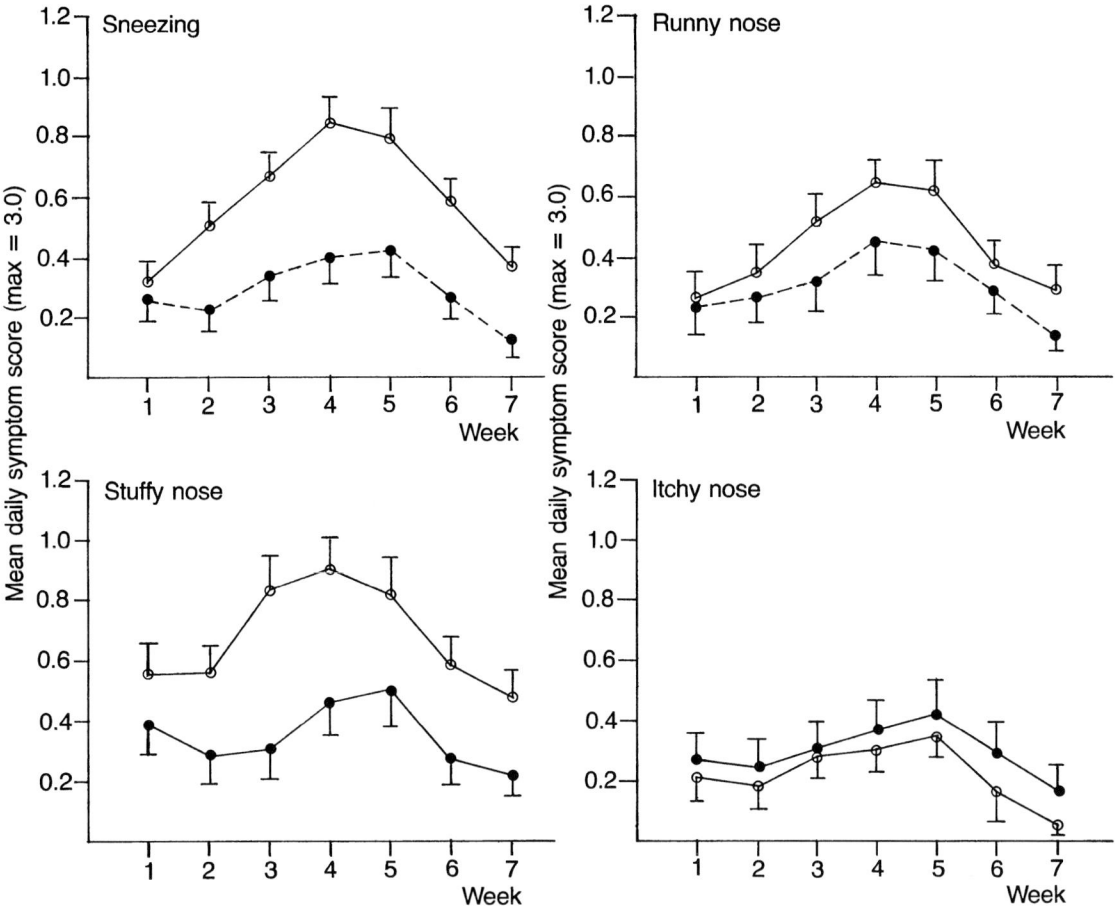

Fig. 14.8. Nasal symptoms during the ragweed-pollen season: beclomethasone as required (○); and regular (●); sneezing, p=0.0002; stuffy nose, p=0.0015; runny nose, p=0.025; itchy nose, p=0.37. Reprinted with permission from *J Allergy Clin Immunol* 1990; *86:* 380-6.

and 10 mg orally for 3 days and then stopping) is an effective approach. Alternatively, a topical decongestant can be used prior to administration of the intranasal steroids. The major reason for the lack of efficacy of intranasal steroids in appropriately diagnosed allergic rhinitis is their inability to gain access to the site of inflammation.

Adverse effects

Local nasal irritation represents the major side-effect of intranasal steroids. About 10% of patients will experience some sensation of irritation, burning or sneezing after administration.[34] About 2% will note a bloody discharge, and rare septal perforations have been detected. Septal perforations may occur more frequently in subjects who have undergone nasal septal reconstructions. The incidence of local irritation has been reduced by the development of aqueous preparations.[32] The reduction in local irritation has increased their use in children. Biopsies of the nasal mucosa obtained from perennial rhinitics who received beclomethasone continuously for 5 years showed no signs of atrophy.[36-38] In a 1-year trial, fluocortin seemed to normalize the mucosa.[29] Candida overgrowth does not occur in the nose.[38]

Systemic side-effects were not detected in clinical trials with beclomethasone, budesonide and flunisolide.[33,38] The fear of systemic side-effects should be discussed with the patient at the time the prescription is given. A recent publication reported that, in patients treated with high-dose inhaled steroids for pulmonary disease, dermal thickness was reduced.[39] The effect was less than that of oral

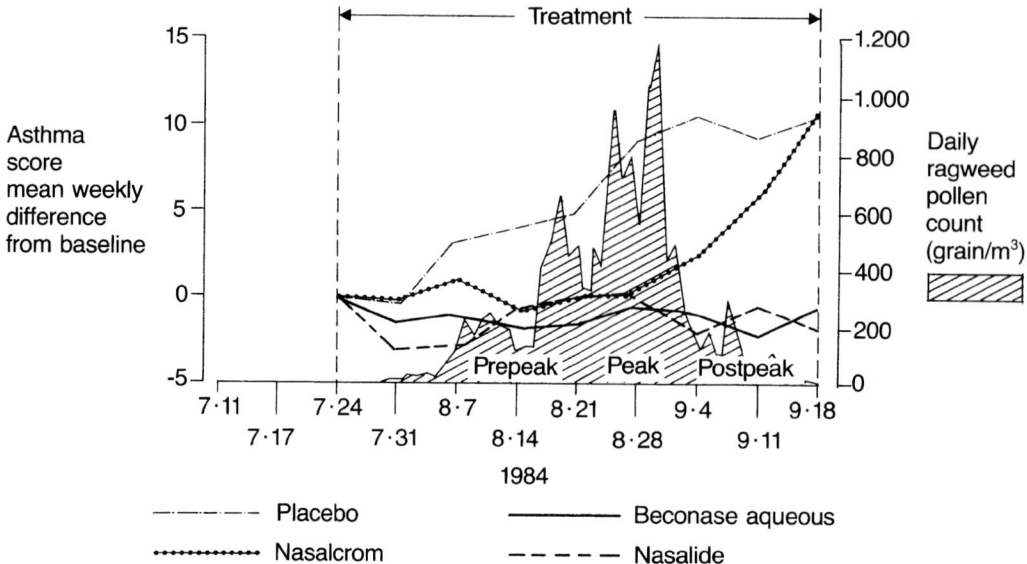

Fig. 14.9. Mean weekly scores for symptoms of asthma, adjusted for baseline values in 58 patients with seasonal asthma. Treatment groups and study period were as described in legend for Fig. 14.7. Daily seasonal ragweed pollen count is shown in shaded area. Expected increase in seasonal symptoms of asthma did not occur in glucocorticoid-treated groups. Reprinted with permission from *Mayo Clinic Proc* 1987; *62:* 125-24.

steroids and more than that of no treatment or low-dose inhaled steroids. An inhibitory effect of high-dose inhaled steroids on growth in severe asthmatic children has been reported, but interpretation of the results is confounded by the known effect of the disease itself on growth.[40] Case reports of posterior subcapsular cataracts following intranasal steroid usage have also appeared.[41] The applicability of these observations to the use of intranasal steroids in allergic rhinitis is unknown.

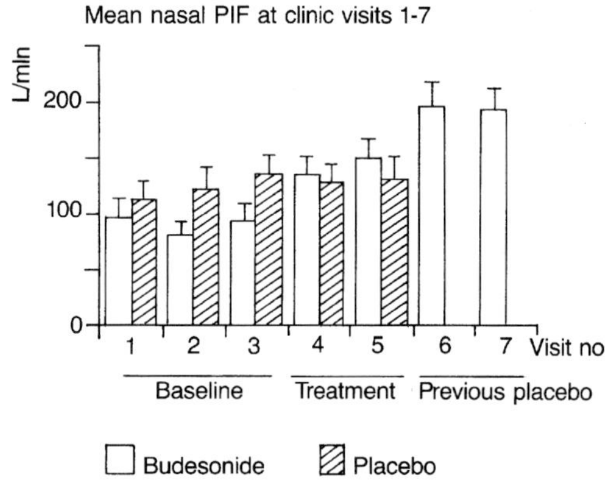

Questions

Two questions regarding intranasal steroids should be considered in future studies. First, do intranasal steroids, because of their antiinflammatory actions, alter the natural history of allergic rhinitis? The major difficulty in answering this question is the limited information available on the natural history of allergic rhinitis and its prognosis without treatment. The spontaneous resolution of allergic rhinitic symptoms with increasing age has been estimated to be between 5 and 10%. Remission occurs primarily in patients with mild seasonal disease of less than 5 years' duration. Contrariwise, the development of perennial asthma occurs in about 5 to 10% of subjects.[43] We do not know what percentage of allergic rhinitics progress to perennial nonallergic rhinitis or develop other complications of inadequately managed disease. We must obtain this information and determine which patients will progress to more refractory disease. Without this

Fig. 14.10. Mean values and SEM for nasal peak inspiratory flow rate (PIF) in patients with nasal polyps are presented. Baseline values in the placebo-treated group happened to be higher than for the budesonide-treated group. However, treatment with budesonide, but not placebo, elicited increases in PIF rates. Reprinted with permission from *J Allergy Clin Immunol* 1990; *86:* 946-53.

knowledge, recommendations for therapy vary from the minimum required to obtain symptomatic relief to an aggressive approach aimed at altering the natural history of the disease.

Secondly, since intranasal steroids have minimal side-effects and are potent, nonsedating and effective against multiple aspects of allergic inflammation, should they be recommended as first-line therapy? Opposing this notion are: 1) the fact that they do not provide as rapid an onset of action as antihistamines and decongestants, 2) the public bias against steroids, 3) patients preference for oral medication and 4) the need for continuous treatment in mild and episodic disease. If controlling inflammation, as proposed for asthma, becomes the major thrust for therapy, then the use of intranasal steroids will dramatically increase.

Conclusion

Intranasal steroids are a potent and highly effective treatment for patients with allergic rhinitis. Their intranasal efficacy exceeds that of antihistamines, decongestants and cromolyn. They are less efficacious on associated symptoms such as ocular irritation. Intranasal steroids, however, can be effectively combined with other therapies to achieve maximal individual relief. Studies in human subjects have demonstrated multiple antiinflammatory actions with no single mechanism fully explaining their efficacy. Multiple formulations exist with none demonstrating overwhelming superiority. Their major adverse effect is local irritation. Currently, intranasal steroids represent the gold standard to which other treatments should be compared.

References

1 Hillas J, Booth RJ, Somerfield S, Morton R, Avery J, Wilson JD. A comparative trial of intranasal beclomethasone dipropionate and sodium cromoglycate in patients with chronic perennial rhinitis. *Clin Allergy* 1980; *10:* 253-8.
2 Welsh PW, Stricker WE, Chu-Pin C, et al. Efficacy of beclomomethasone nasal solution, flunisolide, and cromolyn in relieving symptoms of ragweed allergy. *Mayo Clinic Proceedings* 1987; *62:* 125-34.
3 Harding SM, Heath S. Intranasal steroid aerosol in perennial rhinitis: comparison with an antihistamine compound. *Clin Allergy* 1976; *6:* 369-72.
4 Juniper EF, Kline PA, Hargreave FE, Dolovich J. Comparison of beclomethasone dipropionate aqueous nasal spray, astemizole, and the combination in the prophylactic treatment of ragweed pollen-induced rhinoconjunctivitis. *J Allergy Clin Immunol* 1989; *83:* 627-33.
5 Schleimer RP. Glucocorticosteroids. In: Middleton E, Reed C, Ellis E, eds. *Allergy: Principles and Practice*. St. Louis: CV Mosby, 1988: 739-65.
6 Pelikan Z, de Vries K. Effects of some drugs applied topically to the nasal mucosa before nasal provocation tests with allergen. *Acta Allergol* 1974; *29:* 337.
7 Mygind N, Johnsen NJ, Thomsen J. Intranasal allergen challenge during corticosteroid treatment. *Clin Allergy* 1977; *7:* 69.
8 Vilsvik J, Jenssen A, Walstad R. The effect of beclomethasone dipropionate aerosol on allergen-induced nasal stenosis. *Clin Allergy* 1975; *5:* 291.
9 Pipkorn U. Budesonide and nasal allergen challenge testing in man. *Allergy* 1982; *37:* 129.
10 Okuda M, Senba O. Effects of beclomethasone dipropionate nasal spray on subjective and objective findings in perennial rhinitis. *Clin Otolaryngol* 1980; *53:* 15.
11 Pipkorn U. Budesonide and nasal histamine challenge. *Allergy* 1982; *37:* 129.
12 Pipkorn U, Andersson P. Budesonide and nasal mucosal histamine content and anti-IgE-induced histamine release. *Allergy* 1982; *37:* 1.
13 Otsuka H, Denburg J, Befus AD, et al. Effect of beclomethasone dipropionate on nasal metachromatic cell sub-populations. *Clin Allergy* 1986; *16:* 589-95.
14 Bende M, Lindqvist N, Pipkorn U. Effect of a topical glucocorticoid, budesonide, on nasal mucosal blood flow as measured with Xe33 wash-out technique. *Allergy* 1983; *38:* 461.
15 Pipkorn U, Proud D, Lichtenstein LM, Kagey-Sobotka A, Norman PS, Naclerio RM. Inhibition of mediator release in allergic rhinitis by pretreatment with topical glucocorticoids. *N Engl J Med* 1987; *316:* 1506-10.
16 Holmberg K, Pipkorn U. Influence of topical beclomethasone dipropionate suspension on human nasal mucociliary activity. *J Clin Pharmacol* 1986; *30:* 625-7.
17 Andersson M, Andersson P, Pipkorn U. Topical glucocorticosteroids and allergen-induced increase in nasal reactivity: relationship between treatment time and inhibitory effect. *J Allergy Clin Immunol* 1988; *82:* 1019-26.
18 Andersson M, Andersson P, Venge P, Pipkorn U. Eosinophils and eosinophil cationic protein in nasal lavages in allergen-induced hyperresponsiveness: effects of topical glucocorticosteroid treatment. *Allergy* 1989; *44:* 342-8.
19 Baroody F, Lichtenstein LM, Kagey-Sobotka A, Proud D, Naclerio RM. Topical steroids inhibit antigen-induced nasal hyperreactivity to histamine [abstract]. *J Allergy Clin Immunol* 1989; *82:* 163.

20 Naclerio RM, Creticos PS, Norman PS, Hamilton RG. Intranasal steroids suppress the seasonal rise in antigen-specific IgE [abstract]. *J Allergy Clin Immunol* 1991; *87:* 221.
21 Linder A, Venge P, Deutschl H. Eosinophil cationic protein and myeloperoxidase in nasal secretion as markers of inflammation in allergic rhinitis. *Allergy* 1987; *42:* 583-90.
22 Svensson C, Andersson M, Persson CGA, Venge P, Alkner U, Pipkorn U. Albumin, bradykinins, and eosinophil cationic protein on the nasal mucosa surface in patients with hay fever during natural allergen exposure. *J Allergy Clin Immunol* 1990; *85:* 828-33.
23 Norman PS, Winkenwerder WL, Murgatroyd GW Jr, Parsons JW. Evidence for the local action of intranasal dexamethasone aerosols in the suppression of hay fever symptoms. *J Allergy* 1966; *38:* 93-9.
24 Lindqvist N, Andersson M, Bende M, Loth S, Pipkorn U. The clinical efficacy of budesonide in hay fever treatment is dependent on topical nasal application. *Clin Exp Allergy* 1989; *19:* 71-6.
25 Juniper EF, Guyatt GH, O'Byrne PM, Viveiros M. Aqueous beclomethasone diproprionate nasal spray: Regular versus "as required" use in the treatment of seasonal allergic rhinitis. *J Allergy Clin Immunol* 1990; *86:* 380-6.
26 Juniper EF, Kline PA, Ramsdale EH, Hargreave FE. Comparison of efficacy and side effects of aqueous steroid nasal spray (budesonide) and allergen-injection therapy (Pollinex-R) in the treatment of seasonal allergic rhinoconjunctivitis. *J Allergy Clin Immunol* 1990; *85:* 606-11.
27 Toft A, Wihl J-Å, Toxman J, Mygind N. Double-blind comparison between beclomethasone dipropionate as aersol and as powder in patients with nasal polyposis. *Clin Allergy* 1982; *12:* 391-401.
28 Ruhno J, Andersson B, Denburg J, et al. A double-blind comparison of intranasal budesonide with placebo for nasal polyposis. *J Allergy Clin Immunol* 1990; *86:* 946-53.
29 Orgel HA, Meltzer EO, Bierman W, et al. Intranasal fluocortin butyl in patients with perennial rhinitis: A 12-month efficacy and safety study including nasal biopsy. *J Allergy Clin Immunol* 1991; *88:* 257-64.
30 Hallworth GW, Padfield JM. A comparison of regional deposition in a model nose of a drug discharged from metered aerosol and metered-pump nasal delivery system. *J Allergy Clin Immunol* 1986; *77:* 348-53.
31 Mygind N. Local effect of intranasal beclomethasone dipropionate aerosol in hay fever. *Br Med J* 1973; *4:* 464-6.
32 *Physicians Desk Reference*, 44th edn. New Jersey: Medical Economics Co, Inc, 1990.
33 Norman PS, Winkenwerder WL, Agbayani BF, Migeon CJ. Adrenal function during the use of dexamethasone aerosols in the treatment of ragweed hay fever. *J Allergy* 1967; *40:* 57-61.
34 Mygind N, Clark TJH, eds. *Topical steroid treatment for asthma and rhinitis*. London: Balliere Tindall, 1980.
35 Ackerman MN, Friedman RA, Doyle WJ, Bluestone CD, Fireman P. Antigen-induced eustachian tube obstruction: an intranasal provocative challenge test. *J Allergy Clin Immunol* 1984; *73:* 604.
36 Zwillich CW, Pickett C, Hanson FN, Weil JV. Disturbed sleep and prolonged apnea during nasal obstruction in normal men. *Am Rev Respir Dis* 1981; *124:* 158-60.
37 Holopainen E, Malmberg H, Binder E. Long-term follow-up of intra-nasal beclomethasone treatment, a clinical and histologic study. *Acta Otolaryngol (Stockh)* 1982; *386:* 270-3.
38 Sørensen H, Mygind N, Pedersen CB, Prytz S. Long term treatment of nasal polyps with beclomethasone dipropionate aerosol. III. Morphological studies and conclusions. *Acta Otolaryngol (Stockh)* 1976; *182:* 260-4.
39 Capwell S, Reynolds S, Shuttleworth D, Edwards C, Finlay AY. Purpura and dermal thinning associated with high dose inhaled corticosteroids. *Br Med J* 1990; *300:* 1548-51.
40 Stead RJ, Cooke NJ. Adverse effects of inhaled steroids. *Br Med J* 1989; *298:* 403-4.
41 Fraunfelder FT, Myer SM. Posterior subcapsular cataracts associated with nasal or inhalation corticosteroids. *Am J Ophthalmol* 1990; *109:* 489-90.
42 Mygind N. *Nasal allergy*. Oxford: Blackwell Scientific Publications, 1978.

Chapter 15

Antihistamines

F Estelle R Simons

Introduction

The relatively non-sedating second-generation H_1-receptor antagonists such as terfenadine,[39] astemizole,[52] loratadine,[12] and cetirizine[10] (Fig. 15.1) have replaced their more sedating predecessors such as chlorpheniramine in the treatment of allergic rhinoconjunctivitis. H_1-antagonists are not the most potent medications available for the treatment of this disorder, but they are usually the medications from which patients seek relief first. They are available in many countries without a physician's prescription. Newer H_1-antagonists such as levocabastine,[3,14] azelastine,[40,71] ebastine,[38] noberastine[18,31] and epinastine[56] are currently undergoing clinical trials in allergic rhinitis.

Mechanisms of action

H_1-blockade

At low concentrations, H_1-receptor antagonists are pharmacologic antagonists of histamine at H_1-receptor sites and act by binding to H_1-receptors and preventing histamine from binding to the H_1-receptors, thus blocking the H_1-response.[60] For most H_1-antagonists, this binding is readily reversible, an exception being astemizole, which is not easily displaced from receptor sites.[52] The number of receptors occupied by histamine and the number of receptors occupied by the H_1-antagonists depend on the relative concentrations of histamine and of H_1-receptor antagonists near the receptor site. In the immediate hypersensitivity reaction, after mediator release, histamine concentrations in tissue can attain levels of 10^{-5} to 10^{-3} M. The concentrations of H_1-receptor antagonists and their active metabolites achieved in tissues vary with the absorption, distribution, metabolism, and elimination of a particular antagonist, and peak tissue concentrations reach 5×10^{-6} M.[61] Many H_1-receptor antagonists have active metabolites and the local concentrations of the active metabolite are as relevant, or even more relevant, than the local concentrations of the parent compound.

Anti-allergic effects of H_1-receptor antagonists

In vitro and *in vivo*, many H_1-receptor antagonists have been found to have anti-allergic effects[7,11,44,45,49,53,69] (Fig. 15.2). Some, such as cetirizine, also have anti-inflammatory effects, better demonstrated to date *in vitro*[16,19,53] and in human skin[11] than in patients with allergic rhinoconjunctivitis[28,35] (Fig. 15.3).

In vitro, terfenadine, astemizole, loratadine, cetirizine, azelastine, ketotifen, chlorpheniramine, diphenhydramine, azatadine, and oxatomide inhibit immunogenic and non-immunogenic mediator release to varying degrees. Their anti-allergic effects differ, depending on the cell type and source (rodent mast cells, human tissue mast cells, or peripheral blood basophils), the concentration of the agonist and antagonist, and the mediator being measured. The precise mechanism of action of the anti-allergic effect is unknown; inhibition of intracellular calcium ion mobilization has been the best-studied mechanism to date.[53]

In patients with allergic rhinitis who are challenged intranasally with antigens to which they are sensitized, H_1-receptor antagonists such as azatadine[69] or levocabastine,[49] applied topically before challenge, or terfenadine,[7,44] loratadine,[7] cetirizine,[45] or diphenhydramine,[37] given by mouth before

Second generation H₁ receptor antagonists

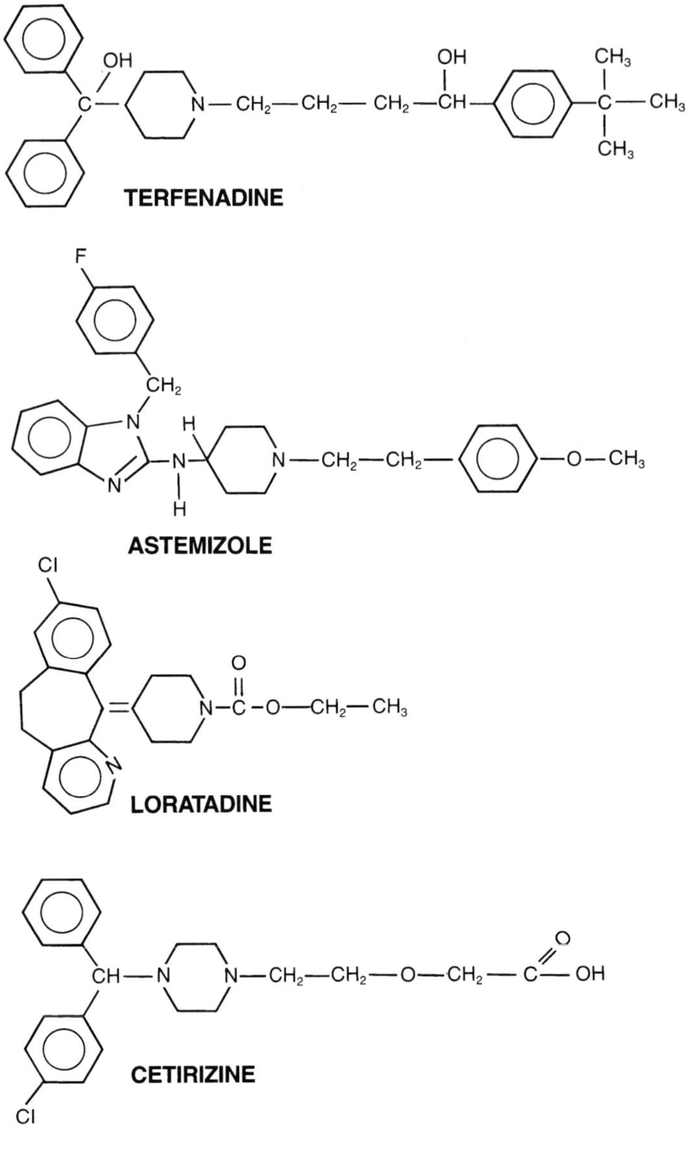

Fig. 15.1. Chemical structure of selected second-generation H₁-receptor antagonists.

challenge, effectively prevent the symptoms of sneezing, itching, and rhinorrhea during the immediate reaction to allergen. The H₁-receptor antagonists tested so far in a nasal challenge model also inhibit the increase in vascular permeability evidenced by increases in concentrations of albumin, kinins, and TAME-esterase activity recovered in nasal lavage fluid. Some, but not all, H₁-receptor antagonists prevent histamine release after antigen challenge. Terfenadine, 60 mg bid or 300 mg bid for 1 week before challenge prevents the increase in histamine seen in the nasal lavage fluid after challenge[44] (Fig. 15.2), as does loratadine pre-treatment.[7] Cetirizine, 20 mg daily for 2 days before challenge does not prevent histamine increase or prostaglandin D_2 increase, but it does prevent LTC_4 increase, the LTC_4 probably arising from cells other than mast cells.[45]

The late-phase reaction, manifest as nasal congestion and hyperirritability, is thought to be mediated chiefly by eicosanoids and by neutrophil and eosinophil chemotactic factors and other inflammatory factors; however, the role of histamine in the late-phase reaction has not been entirely ruled out. During the early response to antigen, increases in histamine levels appear to be associated with acti-

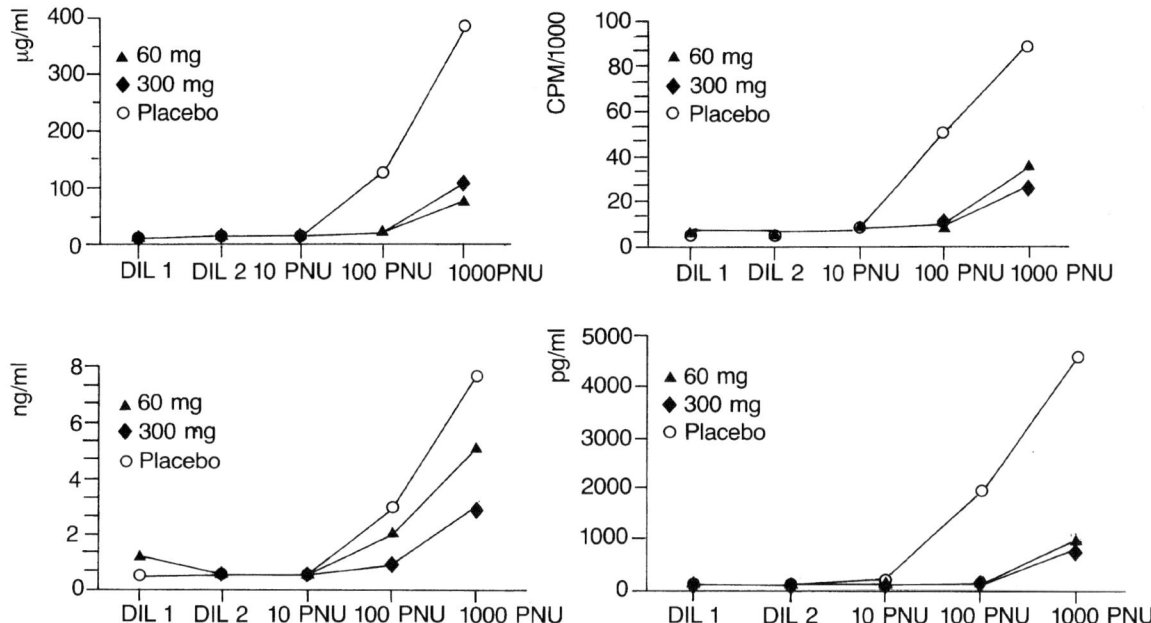

Fig. 15.2. In a double-blind, crossover study, 12 patients with allergic rhinitis and ragweed sensitization had intranasal ragweed challenges followed by nasal lavages. One-week pretreatment with terfenadine 60 mg twice daily *or* terfenadine, 300 mg twice daily was significantly more effective than placebo in reducing sneezing (not shown) and in reducing median levels of albumin (top right), TAME-esterase activity (top left), histamine (bottom right) and kinin (bottom left) activity in the lavage fluid. The nasal challenge protocol is shown on the horizontal axis: Dil = diluent for antigen extract; PNU = protein nitrogen units. From Naclerio et al.[44]

vation of mast cells. In the subset of patients who exhibit a late response to antigen, the rise in histamine is concomitant with an increase in the number of basophils in lavage fluid. Histamine alone does not induce a protracted inflammatory response in the nasal mucosa. H_1-receptor antagonists such as terfenadine and cetirizine have been found to inhibit the allergen-induced increased non-specific

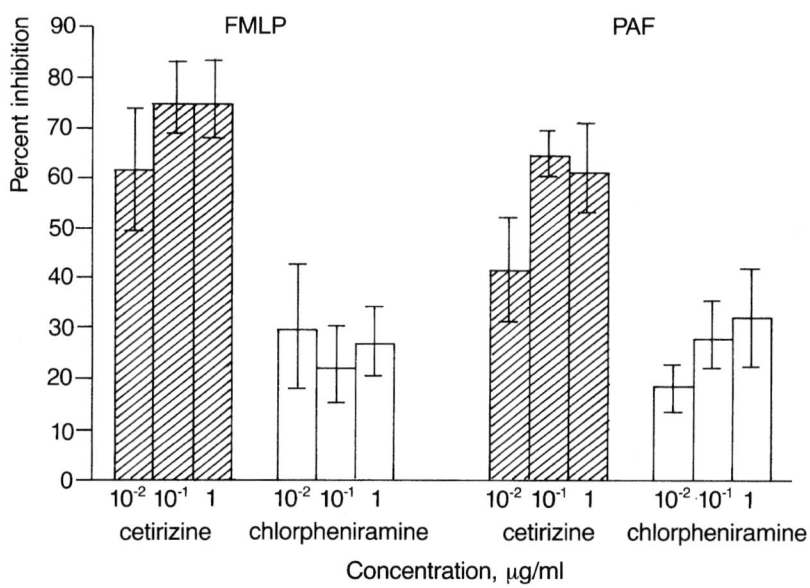

Fig. 15.3. Cetirizine, but not chlorpheniramine, significantly inhibited the eosinophil chemotactic response to N-formyl-Met-Leu-Phe (FMLP) 10^{-6} and to PAF-acether (PAF) 10^{-6} M *in vitro*. Each histogram represents the mean ± SEM of 14 experiments. From De Vos et al.[16]

nasal reactivity measured by methacholine challenge 24 hours after nasal allergen challenge[35] (Fig. 15.4). Additional studies are required to clarify the anti-allergic effects of H_1-receptor antagonists *in vivo*.

Pharmacokinetics and pharmacodynamics

Pharmacokinetics

H_1-receptor antagonists are well-absorbed when administered orally, with peak serum concentrations being reached approximately 2 hours after dosing in fasting patients. All the first-generation and most of the second-generation H_1-receptor antagonists currently available are metabolized extensively by the hepatic cytochrome P_{450} system.[12, 39, 40, 52] Cetirizine, the active carboxylic acid metabolite of the first-generation H_1-receptor antagonist hydroxyzine, and levocabastine are eliminated primarily by the renal route.[10, 14, 70] Clearance rates and serum elimination half-life values of H_1-antagonists are variable, with half-life values ranging from less than 24 hours for agents such as cetirizine (Fig. 15.5), and terfenadine, loratadine, and their active metabolites, to approximately 24 hours for chlorpheniramine, brompheniramine, hydroxyzine, and azelastine, to 9.5 days for astemizole and its active

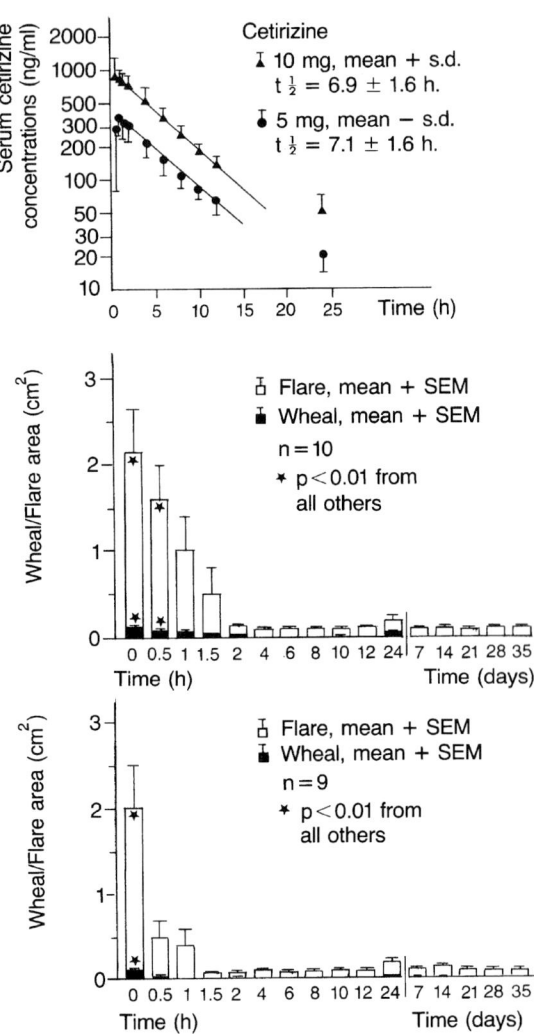

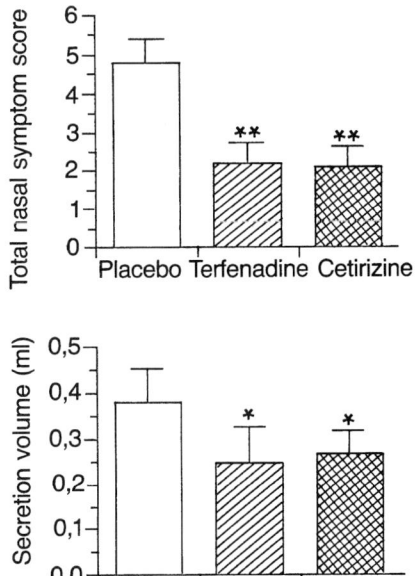

Fig. 15.4. In a double-blind, placebo-controlled study in 15 patients, terfenadine, 60 mg twice daily *or* cetirizine, 10 mg once daily for 5 days relieved symptoms, shown as a composite nasal score after allergen challenge, significantly better than placebo did** ($p<0.01$). Terfenadine or cetirizine also significantly reduced the allergen-induced increase in the secretory response to a methacholine challenge, performed 24 hours after intransal challenge with birch or timothy pollen in a dose of 10,000 BU* ($p<0.05$). From Klementsson et al.[35]

Fig. 15.5. In a double-blind, parallel group study of a single oral dose of cetirizine, 5 mg in 10 children versus a single oral dose of cetirizine, 10 mg in 9 children, the serum elimination half-life of cetirizine was approximately 7 hours (top panel). A single dose of cetirizine, 5 mg (middle panel) or 10 mg (bottom panel), significantly suppressed the mean wheal and flare areas resulting from epicutaneous tests with histamine phosphate, 1 mg/ml, from 1-24 hours post-dose. In the subsequent multiple-dose phase of the study, the wheal and flare suppression 12 hours post-cetirizine dose did not differ significantly on days 7, 14, 21, 28, and 35. From Watson et al.[70]

metabolites. The relatively low serum H_1-receptor antagonist concentrations measured following recommended single oral doses may indicate extensive distribution into tissues.[60, 65]

Serum elimination half-life values for H_1-receptor antagonists are generally shorter in children than in adults.[60, 63, 65, 70] The longer serum elimination half-life values and correspondingly slower clearance rates in elderly patients for H_1-receptor antagonists are attributed to age-related decreases in hepatic function, including decreased liver blood flow, smaller liver size, and diminished number and metabolizing capacity of hepatocytes. Serum elimination half-life values for H_1-receptor antagonists metabolized in the cytochrome P_{450} system may also be prolonged in patients with hepatic dysfunction[60, 65] and in patients concomitantly receiving ketoconazole or other cytochrome P_{450} inhibitors. Patients with prolonged serum elimination half-life values may develop elevated serum and tissue concentrations of H_1-antagonists and their active metabolites, and may be at increased risk from the adverse effects of H_1-antagonists. The serum elimination half-life value of cetirizine may be prolonged in elderly patients and in patients with impaired renal function.[10]

Pharmacodynamics

In efficacy studies of H_1-receptor antagonists in allergic rhinoconjunctivitis, symptoms such as nasal itching, rhinorrhea, blockage, and sneezing are subjectively scored; efficacy has not been correlated with serum concentrations and true pharmacodynamic information has not been obtained. In some studies, the efficacy of H_1-receptor antagonists has been assessed objectively using suppression of the histamine- or antigen-induced wheals and flares, a well-validated bioassay.[10, 12, 26, 31, 36, 39, 40, 52, 56 64, 70] Peak suppression of histamine-induced wheals and flares by H_1-receptor antagonists generally occurs 5 to 7 hours after oral administration[64] (Fig. 15.6) while peak serum concentrations occur somewhat earlier. The delay in response is probably not due to delay in the drug reaching the target organ since, throughout a dosing interval following a single dose, skin concentrations exceed serum concentraions.[61] Maximum antihistaminic effects of the H_1-receptor antagonists persist even when serum concentrations of the parent compound have declined to the lowest limits of analytical detection[70] (Fig. 15.5). This persistence of effect is probably due to the presence of active metabolites and/or high tissue/serum concentration ratios. H_1-receptor antagonists should therefore be given *before* an anticipated allergic reaction, if possible, in order to achieve maximum efficacy. The duration of action of a single dose of one of these medications, assessed subjectively by suppression of symptoms such as itching of the skin or nose, sneezing, and rhinorrhea, or objectively by suppression of the histamine- or allergen-induced wheal and flare in the skin, is much more prolonged than might be expected from consideration of the serum elimination half-life values. The duration of action may be surprisingly long in elderly patients or in patients with hepatic dysfunction.

Lack of subsensitivity

In recent long-term rhinoconjunctivitis studies, no evidence for induction of metabolism or decrease in efficacy over weeks or months has been found with second-generation H_1-receptor antagonists.[29, 33] In highly objective, long-term studies of the antihistaminic effect of terfenadine, loratadine, or ceterizine in the skin, no evidence of diminishing effect has been found in studies of 1-3 months duration[8, 66, 70] (Fig. 15.5). The apparent subsensitivity of the first-generation H_1-receptor antagonists reported years ago in allergic rhinitis and in the skin may have been partially due to lack of compliance because of low efficacy and adverse effects. Development of subsensitivity in H_1-receptors in the lower airways has not been ruled out.

H_1-receptor antagonists in allergic rhinoconjunctivitis

Rationale for use of H_1-receptor antagonists

While no one chemical mediator of inflammation is responsible for induction of all the signs and symptoms of allergic rhinitis, there is evidence that histamine is a mediator of major importance in this disorder. Intranasal challenge with histamine in a dose of approximately 1 mg reproduces all the symptoms of allergic rhinitis. These include sneez-

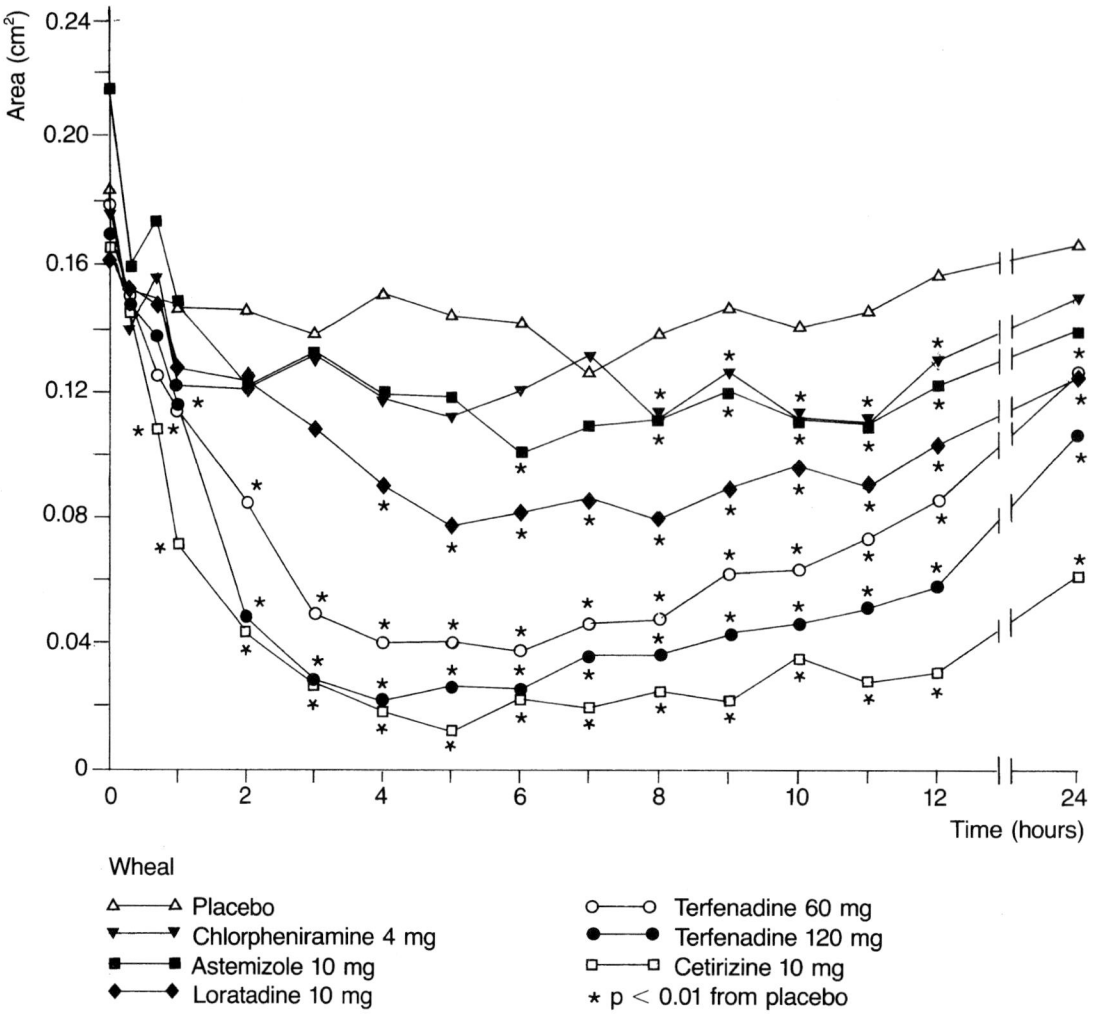

Fig. 15.6. In a single-dose, double-blind, seven-way, crossover study in 20 adults, mean wheal areas were measured after epicutaneous histamine phosphate (1 mg/ml) before and up to 24 hours after a single oral dose of placebo or H_1-receptor antagonist. The rank order of suppression was, from most effective to least effective: cetirizine 10 mg > terfenadine 120 mg > terfenadine 60 mg > loratadine 10 mg > astemizole 10 mg > chlorpheniramine 4 mg > placebo. From Simons et al.[64]

ing and pruritus, resulting from stimulation of sensory nerves; rhinorrhea or increased liquid on the surface of the nasal mucosa, resulting from reflex stimulation of the submucous glands; and nasal blockage, due to decreased tone in the capacitance vessels and leakage of plasma proteins.

Standards of excellence in clinical trials

Ideally, clinical trials of a new H_1-antagonist in allergic rhinoconjunctivitis should be double-blind, randomized, and placebo-controlled, and the initial trials of a new H_1-antagonist should contain a first-generation H_1-comparator such as chlorpheniramine. An adequate number of patients should be monitored, so that the study has sufficient power to show lack of differences, as well as differences between the treatment modalities, with certainty. Patients should be matched for sensitivity to the allergens likely to be encountered during the study. In seasonal allergic rhinoconjunctivitis studies, pollen counts should be monitored throughout the study and patients should get a similar amount and duration of exposure to the relevant pollens. The

Antihistamines

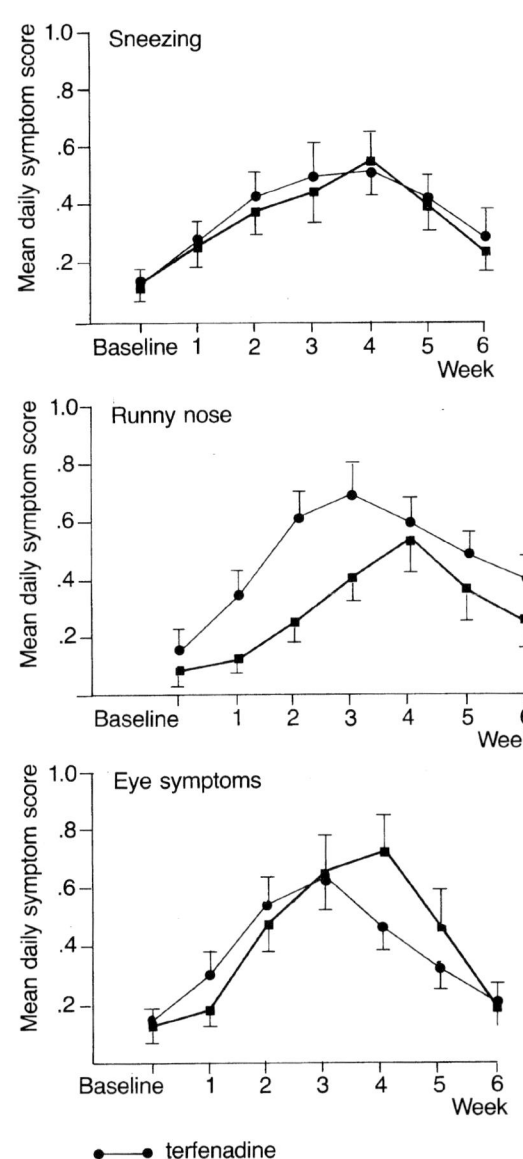

Fig. 15.7. In a double-blind, parallel-group, single-center study, 60 patients with a history of ragweed-induced rhinoconjunctivitis took either astemizole 10 mg daily *or* terfenadine 60 mg twice daily for 7 weeks, beginning 1 week before the ragweed pollen season. Astemizole was more effective than terfenadine in controlling rhinorrhea, but other nasal symptoms and eye symptoms were similar in the two groups of patients. From Juniper et al.[29]

amount of "rescue" medication(s) required, in addition to the treatment modalities being investigated, should be considered an important index of the therapeutic efficacy of the H_1-antagonist being compared.

Clinical trials of H_1-receptor antagonists

In numerous studies in which patients with allergic rhinitis have recorded symptom scores over weeks or months, H_1-receptor antagonists have been found to relieve sneezing, itching, and nasal discharge, and also to relieve ocular symptoms such as itching, tearing, and erythema[1, 2, 9, 10, 12, 15, 18, 20, 26-29, 32, 33, 36, 39, 40, 43, 47, 52, 58, 68, 70, 71] (Fig. 15.7). Neither first-generation nor second-generation H_1-receptor antagonists are very effective in relieving nasal blockage; hence, decongestants such as pseudoephedrine may be added to H_1-antagonists in fixed-dose formulations in order to provide better relief of this symptom[2, 58, 68] (Fig. 15.8).

In randomized, prospective, double-blind studies in patients with seasonal or perennial rhinitis, the second-generation H_1-receptor antagonists have been generally found to be superior to placebo and comparable to a first-generation H_1-receptor antagonist such as chlorpheniramine. Terfenadine, 60 mg twice daily or 120 mg once daily;[39, 43] astemizole, 10 mg daily;[52] loratadine, 10 mg daily;[12] cetirizine, 10 mg daily;[10] and azelastine, 2 mg twice daily[40] are the doses recommended by the manufacturers as providing optimal efficacy with minimal likelihood of causing sedation or other adverse effects. In seasonal allergic rhinitis treatment, these medications are said to have comparable efficacy but no direct comparisons of their effectiveness are available. Terfenadine seems to provide faster onset of symptom relief than astemizole, but in studies of 1 or 2 months duration astemizole gives superior relief. In the treatment of seasonal allergic rhinitis, terfenadine is optimally effective *if* started before peak pollen counts occur.[9]

Topical application of H_1-receptor antagonists in allergic rhinoconjunctivitis

It has been known for years that topical application of an H_1-receptor antagonist to the nasal mucosa can prevent or relieve allergic rhinitis symptoms.[34] There is renewed interest in topical H_1-receptor antagonist treatment. Intranasally administered azelastine and levocabastine are effective in relieving pruritus, sneezing, and rhinorrhea in short-term studies in patients with allergic rhinoconjunctivitis,[3, 14, 40, 71] but, like H_1-receptor antagonists ad-

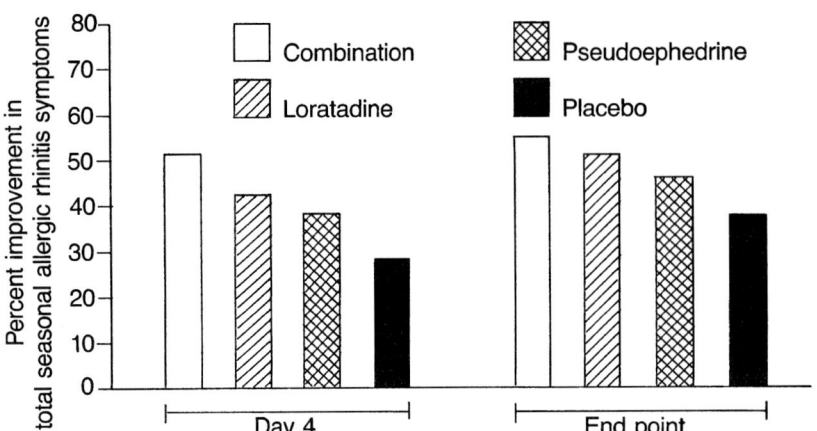

Fig. 15.8. In a double-blind, parallel-group, multi-center study in 435 patients with seasonal allergic rhinitis, a combination tablet containing loratadine 5 mg and pseudoephedrine 120 mg given bid effected a 50% decrease in total symptom scores on day 4 and was significantly ($p<0.03$) more effective than the components alone or placebo. Loratadine alone or pseudoephedrine alone, with 43% and 33% decline in symptom scores, respectively, also were more effective than placebo ($p<0.05$). The scores represent the sum of nasal discharge, stuffiness, itching, sneezing, eye itching, burning, tearing, redness, and ear itching. At end point, the combination was not significantly better than loratadine alone, but was significantly better than pseudoephedrine or placebo ($p<0.05$). From Storms et al.[68]

ministered orally, they are not highly effective in relieving blockage.

Efficacy of H_1-receptor antagonists versus intranasal cromolyn or intranasal corticosteroids

The H_1-receptor antagonist terfenadine provides relief of allergic rhinitis comparable to that provided by intranasal cromolyn (sodium cromoglycate) in a 4% solution administered four times daily[48] (Fig. 15.9). Topical application of levocabastine nasal spray may provide better relief of allergic rhinitis than topical application of intranasal cromolyn.[55] The second-generation H_1-receptor antagonists are generally found to be less potent than intranasal corticosteroids in the treatment of allergic rhinitis symptoms. Patients treated with an H_1-receptor antagonist alone or with an H_1-receptor antagonist in combination with an intranasal corticosteroid have had superior relief of ocular symptoms, when compared with patients treated with an intranasal corticosteroid alone[4, 30] (Fig. 15.10). While H_1-receptor antagonists are extremely useful in the treatment of mild or moderate allergic rhinoconjunctivitis, patients with severe allergic rhinitis will require an intranasal corticosteroid for complete relief of symptoms.

Coadministration of H_1- and H_2-receptor antagonists in allergic rhinoconjunctivitis

H_2-receptor antagonists administered simultaneously with H_1-receptor antagonists topically or by mouth are significantly more effective in decreasing nasal airflow resistance induced by topical histamine provocation than either H_1- or H_2-antagonists are alone, but the added effects are small and have not been found in all studies.[23, 57] Topical pretreatment with an H_2-receptor antagonist alone decreases rhinorrhea, but not sneezing, in contrast to pretreatment with the H_1-receptor antagonist, which decreases both rhinorrhea and sneezing.[25]

Diminishing role of first-generation H_1-receptor antagonists

Many first-generation H_1-receptor antagonists such as triprolidine and tripelennamine, as expected, are disappearing from clinical use because of their short serum elimination half-life values and requirement for three or four times daily administration combined with relative lack of efficacy and a high incidence of sedation and other adverse effects. The first-generation H_1-receptor antagonists such as chlorpheniramine[63] and diphenhydramine[37] will continue to be used by some patients because of their relatively high benefit-risk ratio compared to

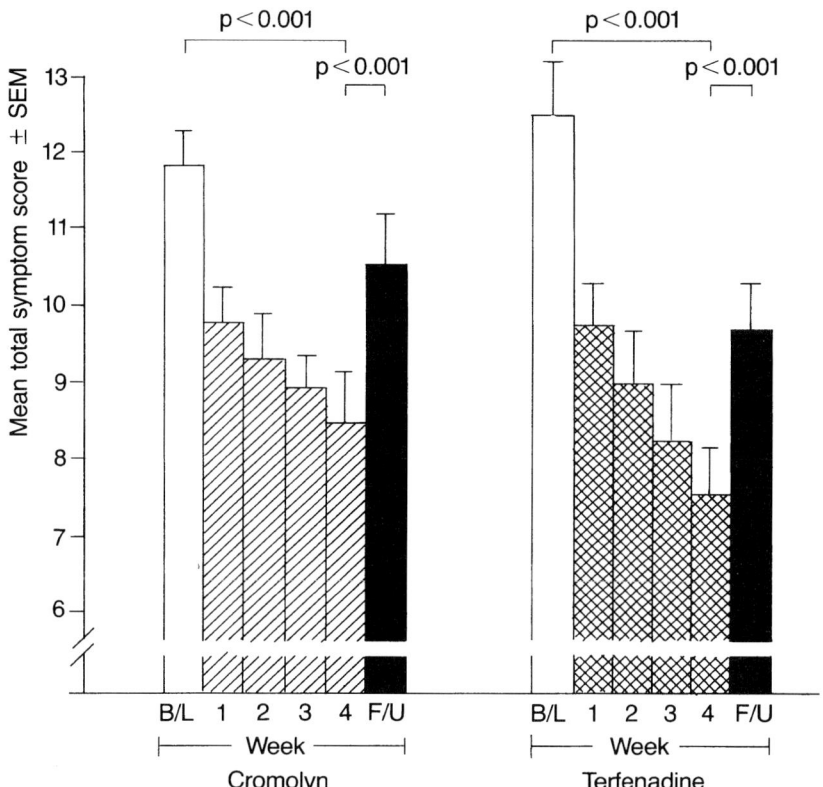

Fig. 15.9. In a double-blind, double-dummy study, 79 patients with allergic rhinitis received either cromolyn sodium 4%, 1 spray in each nostril qid *or* terfenadine 60 mg bid, along with the appropriate placebo spray or tablet for 4 weeks, following a 1-week baseline qualification period. Baseline scores were similar for severity of allergic rhinitis symptoms. Both treatments resulted in significant improvement; at the end of 4 weeks, no statistically significant difference was found for total symptom scores. From Orgel et al.[48]

other first-generation H_1-antagonists, and their low cost.[60] Based on new pharmacokinetic and pharmacodynamic information, once-daily dosing at bedtime may provide relief of symptoms with less interference with central nervous system function.[37, 63]

H_1-receptor antagonists in upper respiratory tract infections

In contrast to their efficacy in allergic rhinoconjunctivitis, in viral infection-induced rhinitis (the common "cold"), H_1-antagonist treatment results in the same rate of improvement in respiratory symptoms as placebo does.[21] There is little scientific rationale for H_1-antagonist use in the treatment of "colds"; histamine concentrations are not increased in nasal secretions in persons with symptomatic experimental rhinovirus upper respiratory tract infections, in contrast to the increased levels of kinins, TAME-esterase activity, and albumin which are found.[50]

Adverse effects of H_1-receptor antagonists

Improved benefit risk ratio of second-generation H_1-antagonists

Most first-generation H_1-receptor antagonists cross the so-called blood-brain barrier, which consists of the endothelial lining of the capillaries of the central nervous system. These medications have a variable propensity to cause central nervous system (CNS) effects, and this has limited their use. First-generation H_1-receptor antagonists may also block alpha-adrenergic receptors, 5-hydroxytryptamine (serotonin) receptors, and/or cholinergic muscarinic receptors.[41]

The second-generation H_1-receptor antagonists such as terfenadine, astemizole, loratadine, and cetirizine are relatively lipophobic, and penetrate poorly into the CNS because of their larger molecular size, electrostatic charge, or the addition of a chemical group that is ionized at physiologic pH.

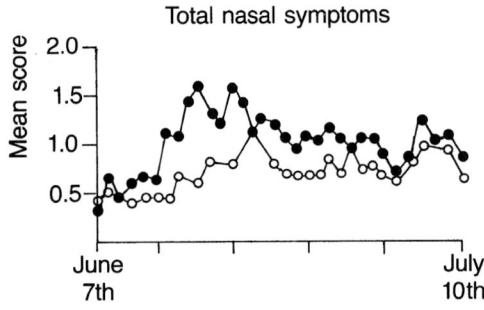

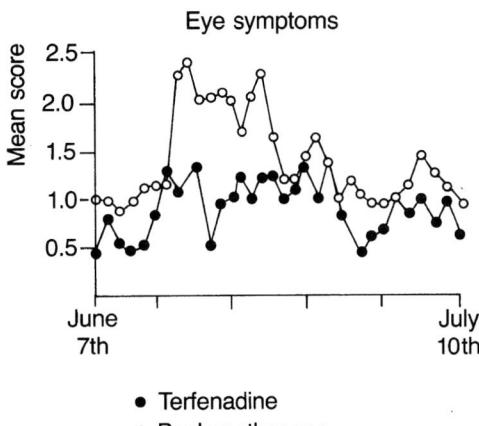

- Terfenadine
- Beclomethasone

Fig. 15.10. Forty-nine patients participated in a randomized, double-blind, parallel-group comparison of beclomethasone dipropionate aqueous nasal spray with terfenadine tablets 60 mg bid for 1 month. Both treatments were effective in controlling hay fever symptoms. The beclomethasone-treated patients had lower nasal symptom scores than the terfenadine-treated patients and this reached statistical significance on high pollen count days. In contrast, terfenadine-treated patients had lower eye symptom scores than beclomethasone-treated patients, statistically significant during the first half of the study. From Beswick et al.[4]

The relative contributions of these factors are unknown. The second-generation H_1-receptor antagonists have much less affinity for cholinergic and 5-hydroxytryptaminergic receptors than their predecessors do, and this may contribute to the relative absence of adverse CNS effects following their administration.[67] The second-generation H_1-receptor antagonists also have relatively greater affinity for peripheral H_1-receptors than for central receptors.[41, 53]

The CNS effects of H_1-receptor antagonists do not necessarily parallel their potency as peripheral H_1-receptor antagonists. The incidence of sedation and impairment of CNS function associated with

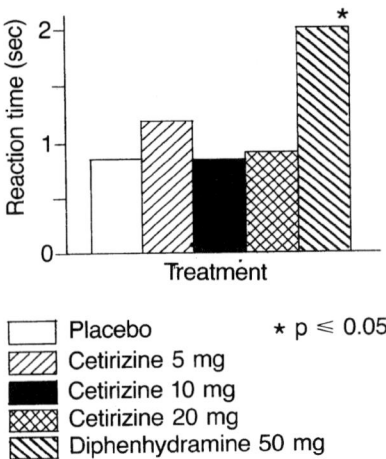

Fig. 15.11. In a double-blind, single-dose, five-way crossover study, 15 male volunteers ingested placebo, cetirizine 5, 10, or 20 mg, and diphenhydramine, 50 mg. Numerous subjective measurements of drowsiness and objective measurements of mental performance were made 2 hours after dosing. During simulated accident avoidance in a simulated automobile-driving situation, diphenhydramine, 50 mg, slowed the reaction time significantly more than placebo or cetirizine, 5, 10, and 20 mg did. From Gengo et al.[22]

manufacturers' recommended doses of the second-generation H_1-receptor antagonists (terfenadine 60 or 120 mg, astemizole 10 mg, loratadine 10 mg, and cetirizine 10 mg) is similar to that seen with placebo and is significantly lower than that produced by first-generation H_1-receptor antagonists such as chlorpheniramine or diphenhydramine[5, 6, 22, 38, 41, 46, 54, 59] (Fig. 15.11). Higher doses of loratadine, cetirizine, or terfenadine may be associated with an increased incidence of sedation and CNS dysnfunction.[6, 10, 12, 20] Assessment of CNS function is based not only on subjective reporting, but also on objective studies which are not influenced by subjects' motivation level, boredom level, or amount of practice; for example, the multiple sleep-latency test, in which the time to stage I electroencephalogram sleep is measured when subjects are given repeated opportunities to fall asleep under standardized conditions.[59] In many studies, although patients deny sedation, objective evidence of impairment of CNS function can be documented.[41]

Occasional patients ingesting a massive terfenadine overdose have experienced cardiac arrest secondary to ventricular arrhythmia (torsade de pointes).[13] Terfenadine may also have a cardiotoxic effect when administered concomitantly with a cytochrome P_{450} inhibitor such as ketoconazole.[42]

A few patients, most of whom have admitted to taking 10 or more times the recommended dose of astemizole, have experienced ventricular tachycardia, torsade de pointes, and cardiac arrest after ingestion of astemizole.[62] Also, astemizole, like the first-generation H_1-receptor antagonist cyproheptadine, may cause appetite stimulation and inappropriate weight gain.[26]

Following oral azelastine administration, altered taste perception has been reported in up to 58% of patients, while following intranasal azelastine administration, nasal "burning" has been reported by 5% and altered taste perception by 3.5% of patients.[40] Intranasal levocabastine seldom produces nasal irritation.[14] During short-term use, intranasal azelastine and levocabastine have not resulted in local sensitization.

The concept of a "non-sedating" H_1-receptor antagonist is proving to be an oversimplification. Preferably, the magnitude of the beneficial effects of each H_1-receptor antagonist should be related to the magnitude of the unwanted effects in the central nervous system and in other systems. In the broadest sense, a "benefit-risk ratio" should be developed for each H_1-receptor antagonist.

Medication interactions

While potentiation of the sedative and anticholinergic adverse effects of first-generation H_1-receptor antagonists by central nervous system active substances such as alcohol, sedatives, hypnotics and antidepressants has been a major concern, in manufacturers' recommended doses, the second-generation H_1-receptor antagonists, unlike their predecessors, produce a low incidence of sedation which is not increased by the coadministration of alcohol, diazepam, or other central nervous system-active substances.[6, 38]

When a decongestant is added to a relatively non-sedating second-generation H_1-receptor antagonist such as terfenadine, loratadine, or cetirizine, the fixed-dose combination formulation may produce a higher incidence of adverse effects, chiefly central nervous system stimulation and insomnia, than the second-generation H_1-receptor antagonist alone produces.

Lack of adverse effects of H_1-antagonists in patients with asthma

The second-generation H_1-receptor antagonists have some anti-asthma effect and may relieve mild seasonal asthma symptoms when taken over weeks or months.[17, 51] In patients with grass pollen-induced asthma, terfenadine 180 mg three times daily was superior to placebo in a double-blind crossover study of 8 weeks duration, as assessed by symptom scores (cough and wheeze significantly reduced by 77% and 47%, respectively), and a modest increase in peak expiratory flow rates, despite a 40% reduction in inhaled beta-agonist use.[51]

H_1-receptor antagonists are not drugs of first choice for asthma; however, previous concerns about their potential adverse effects in asthma have not been substantiated. Patients with asthma who require H_1-receptor antagonists for treatment of concurrent rhinoconjunctivitis will not be harmed by H_1-receptor antagonist treatment, and may even gain some modest anti-asthma benefit from the H_1-receptor antagonist.

Use in pregnancy and lactation

Although teratogenic effects of first-generation H_1-receptor antagonists have been noted in animals and are a potential concern in humans, there is no evidence that second-generation H_1-antagonists cause fetal anomalies in humans. Neonatal withdrawal syndromes have been reported in infants born to women who have received large therapeutic doses of first-generation H_1-receptor antagonists such as diphenhydramine immediately before parturition, but withdrawal syndromes have not been reported in infants born to mothers receiving second-generation H_1-receptor antagonists. The newer medications should, nevertheless, be used with caution during pregnancy. H_1-receptor antagonists are excreted in breast milk.[24]

Conclusion

H_1-receptor antagonists effectively prevent and relieve mild or moderate allergic rhinoconjunctivitis symptoms and, even in patients with severe allergic rhinoconjunctivitis symptoms, addition of an H_1-antagonist to the treatment regimen with intranasal

Table 15.1. *Formulations and dosages of some representative H_1-receptor antagonists.*

Generic (proprietary) names of second-generation H_1-receptor antagonists	Formulation	Recommended dose
Terfenadine (Seldane®, Teldanex®)	Tablets 60 mg, 120 mg Suspension 30 mg/5 mL★	Adult: 60 mg bid *or* 120 mg od Pediatric: (3-6 yrs): 15 mg bid (7-12 yrs): 30 mg bid
Astemizole (Hismanal®)	Tablets 10 mg Suspension 5 mg/5 mL★	Adult: 10 mg od Pediatric: 0.2 mg/kg/24 hr
Loratadine (Claritin®)	Tablets 10 mg	Adult: 10 mg od
Cetirizine (Zyrtec®, Reactine®)	Tablets 10 mg★	Adult: 10 mg od
Azelastine (Astelin®)	Tablets 2 mg★	Adult: 2 mg bid

★ not available in the U.S. at time of writing.

corticosteroids may enhance relief of symptoms, particularly ocular symptoms.

The second-generation H_1-receptor antagonists such as terfenadine, astemizole, loratadine, and cetirizine have supplanted most of the first-generation H_1-receptor antagonists such as chlorpheniramine in the treatment of allergic rhinoconjunctivitis because of their more favorable benefit/risk ratios. If a first-generation H_1-antagonist such as chlorpheniramine or diphenhydramine is used in allergic rhinoconjunctivitis, a single large dose at bedtime may provide relief of symptoms and reduce perceived sedation.[37, 60]

Formulations and recommended dosages of representative second-generation H_1-receptor antagonists are listed in Table 15.1. Most of the second-generation H_1-antagonists are suitable for once-daily dosing, e.g., terfenadine, 120 mg once daily;[1, 39, 43] astemizole, 10 mg once daily;[26, 27, 29, 33, 36, 47, 52] loratadine, 10 mg once daily;[12, 15, 47] or cetirizine, 10 mg once daily,[1, 10, 20, 28, 36, 70] despite their differences in pharmacokinetics and pharmacodynamics.

References

1. Backhouse CI, Renton R, Fidler C, Rosenberg RM. Multicentre, double-blind comparison of terfenadine and cetirizine in patients with seasonal allergic rhinitis. *Br J Clin Pract* 1990; *44:* 88-91.
2. Backhouse CI, Rosenberg RM, Fidler C. Treatment of seasonal allergic rhinitis: a comparison of a combination tablet of terfenadine and pseudoephedrine with the individual ingredients. *Br J Clin Pract* 1990; *44:* 274-9.
3. Bende M, Pipkorn U. Topical levocabastine, a selective H_1 antagonist, in seasonal allergic rhinoconjunctivitis. *Allergy* 1987; *42:* 512-5.
4. Beswick KBJ, Kenyon GS, Cherry JR. A comparative study of beclomethasone dipropionate aqueous nasal spray with terfenadine tablets in seasonal allergic rhinitis. *Curr Med Res Opin* 1985; *9:* 560-7.
5. Betts T, Markman D, Debenham S, Mortiboy D, McKevitt T. Effects of two antihistamine drugs on actual driving performance. *Br Med J* 1984; *288:* 281-2.
6. Bhatti JZ, Hindmarch I. The effects of terfenadine with and without alcohol on an aspect of car driving performance. *Clin Exp Allergy* 1989; *19:* 609-11.
7. Bousquet J, Lebel B, Chanal I, Morel A, Michel F-B. Antiallergic activity of H_1-receptor antagonists assessed by nasal challenge. *J Allergy Clin Immunol* 1988; *82:* 881-7.
8. Bousquet J, Chanal I, Skassa-Brociek W, Lemonier C, Michel FB. Lack of subsensitivity to loratadine during long-term dosing during 12 weeks. *J Allergy Clin Immunol* 1990; *86:* 248-53.
9. Brooks CD, Karl KJ, Francom SF. Profile of ragweed hay fever symptom control with terfenadine started before or after symptoms are established. *Clin Exp Allergy* 1990; *20:* 21-6.
10. Campoli-Richards DM, Buckley MM-T, Fitton A. Cetirizine: a review of its pharmacological properties and clinical potential in allergic rhinitis, pollen-induced asthma and chronic urticaria. *Drugs* 1990; *40:* 762-81.
11. Charlesworth EN, Kagey-Sobotka A, Norman PS, Lichtenstein LM. Effect of cetirizine on mast cell-mediator release and cellular traffic during the cutaneous late-phase reaction. *J Allergy Clin Immunol* 1989; *83:* 905-12.
12. Clissold SP, Sorkin EM, Goa KL. Loratadine. A preliminary review of its pharmacodynamic properties and therapeutic efficacy. *Drugs* 1989; *37:* 42-57.
13. Davies AJ, Harindra V, McEwan A, Ghose RR. Cardiotoxic effect with convulsions in terfenadine overdose. *Br Med J* 1989; *298:* 325.

14. Dechant KL, Goa KL. Levocabastine. A review of its pharmacological properties and therapeutic potential as a topical antihistamine in allergic rhinitis and conjunctivitis. *Drugs* 1991; *41:* 202-24.
15. Del Carpio J, Kabbash L, Turenne Y, et al. Efficacy and safety of loratadine (10 mg once daily), terfenadine (60 mg twice daily), and placebo in the treatment of seasonal allergic rhinitis. *J Allergy Clin Immunol* 1989; *84:* 741.
16. De Vos C, Joseph M, Leprevost C, et al. Inhibition of human eosinophil chemotaxis and of the IgE-dependent stimulation of human blood platelets by cetirizine. *Int Arch Allergy Appl Immunol* 1989; *88:* 212-5.
17. Dijkman JH, Hekking PRM, Molkenboer JF, et al. Prophylactic treatment of grass pollen-induced asthma with cetirizine. *Clin Exp Allergy* 1990; *20:* 483-90.
18. Drouin MA, Knight A, Yang WH, Alexander M, Del Carpio J, Arnott WS. Multicentre clinical evaluation of the efficacy and safety of noberastine, a new H_1-antagonist, in seasonal allergic rhinitis. *J Allergy Clin Immunol* 1991; *87:* 154.
19. Fadel R, David B, Herpin-Richard N, Borgnon A, Rassemont R, Rihoux J-P. In vivo effects of cetirizine on cutaneous reactivity and eosinophil migration induced by platelet-activating factor (PAF-acether) in man. *J Allergy Clin Immunol* 1990; *86:* 314-20.
20. Falliers CJ, Brandon ML, Buchman E, et al. Double-blind comparison of cetirizine and placebo in the treatment of seasonal rhinitis. *Ann Allergy* 1991; *66:* 257-62.
21. Gaffey MJ, Kaiser DL, Hayden FG. Ineffectiveness of oral terfenadine in natural colds: evidence against histamine as a mediator of common cold symptoms. *Pediatr Infect Dis J* 1988; *7:* 223-8.
22. Gengo FM, Gabos C, Mechtler L. Quantitative effects of cetirizine and diphenhydramine on mental performance measured using an automobile driving simulator. *Ann Allergy* 1990; *64:* 520-6.
23. Havas TE, Cole P, Parker L, Oprysk D, Ayiomamitis A. The effects of combined H_1 and H_2 histamine antagonists on alterations in nasal airflow resistance induced by topical histamine provocation. *J Allergy Clin Immunol* 1986; *78:* 856-60.
24. Hilbert J, Radwanski E, Affrime MB, Perentesis G, Symchowicz S, Zampaglione N. Excretion of loratadine in human breast milk. *J Clin Pharmacol* 1988; *28:* 234-9.
25. Holmberg K, Pipkorn U, Bake B, Blychert L-O. Effects of topical treatment with H_1 and H_2 antagonists on clinical symptoms and nasal vascular reactions in patients with allergic rhinitis. *Allergy* 1989; *44:* 281-7.
26. Howarth PH, Emanuel MB, Holgate ST. Astemizole, a potent histamine H_1-receptor antagonist: effect in allergic rhinoconjunctivitis, on antigen and histamine-induced skin weal responses and relationship to serum levels. *Br J Clin Pharmacol* 1984; *18:* 1-8.
27. Howarth PH, Holgate ST. Comparative trial of two non-sedative H_1 antihistamines, terfenadine and astemizole, for hay fever. *Thorax* 1984; *39:* 668-72.
28. Howarth PH, Wilson SJ, Brewster H. The influence of cetirizine on symptom generation and nasal eosinophilia in seasonal allergic rhinitis. *J Allergy Clin Immunol* 1991; *87:*151.
29. Juniper EF, White J, Dolovich J. Efficacy of continuous treatment with astemizole (Hismanal) and terfenadine (Seldane) in ragweed pollen-induced rhinoconjunctivitis. *J Allergy Clin Immunol* 1988; *82:* 670-5.
30. Juniper EF, Kline PA, Hargreave FE, Dolovich J. Comparison of beclomethasone dipropionate aqueous nasal spray, astemizole, and the combination in the prophylactic treatment of ragweed pollen-induced rhinoconjunctivitis. *J Allergy Clin Immunol* 1989; *83:* 627-33.
31. Kamali F, Emanuel M, Rawlins MD. A double-blind placebo controlled dose response study of noberastine on histamine induced weal and flare. *Eur J Clin Pharmacol* 1991; *40:* 83-5.
32. Kemp JP, Buckley CE, Gershwin ME, et al. Multicenter, double-blind, placebo-controlled trial of terfenadine in seasonal allergic rhinitis and conjunctivitis. *Ann Allergy* 1985; *54:* 502-9.
33. Kemp JP, Meltzer EO, Orgel HA, Ostrom NK, Welch MJ. Evaluation of tolerance during 8 weeks of astemizole or terfenadine therapy in patients with perennial allergic rhinitis. *J Allergy Clin Immunol* 1990; *85:* 243.
34. Kirkegaard J, Secher C, Borum P, Mygind N. Inhibition of histamine-induced nasal symptoms by the H_1 antihistamine chlorpheniramine maleate: demonstration of topical effect. *Br J Dis Chest* 1983; *77:* 113-22.
35. Klementsson H, Andersson M, Pipkorn U. Allergen-induced increase in nonspecific nasal reactivity is blocked by antihistamines without a clear-cut relationship to eosinophil influx. *J Allergy Clin Immunol* 1990; *86:* 466-72.
36. Lobaton P, Moreno F, Coulie P. Comparison of cetirizine with astemizole in the treatment of perennial allergic rhinitis and study of the concomitant effect on histamine and allergen-induced wheal responses. *Ann Allergy* 1990; *65:* 401-5.
37. Majchel AM, Proud D, Kagey-Sobotka A, Lichtenstein LM, Witek TJ, Naclerio RM. Persistent efficacy of a combination antihistamine / analgesic / decongestant product the morning after a bedtime dose. *J Allergy Clin Immunol* 1991; *87:* 151.
38. Mattila MJ, Kuitunen T. Ebastine, a non-sedative H_1-antihistamine without alcohol interaction. *Eur J Pharmacol* 1990; *183:* 1653-4.
39. McTavish D, Goa KL, Ferrill M. Terfenadine: an updated review of its pharmacological properties and therapeutic efficacy. *Drugs* 1990; *39:* 552-74.
40. McTavish D, Sorkin EM. Azelastine: a review of its pharmacodynamic and pharmacokinetic properties, and therapeutic potential. *Drugs* 1989; *38:* 778-800.
41. Meltzer EO. Antihistamine- and decongestant-induced performance decrements. *J Occup Med* 1990; *32:* 327-34.
42. Monahan BP, Ferguson CL, Killeavy ES, Lloyd BK, Troy J, Cantilena LR. Torsades de pointes occurring in association with terfenadine use. *JAMA* 1990; *264:* 2788-90.
43. Murphy-O'Connor JC, Renton RL, Westlake DM. Comparative trial of two dose regimens of terfenadine in patients with hay fever. *J Int Med Res* 1984; *12:* 333-7.
44. Naclerio RM, Kagey-Sobotka A, Lichtenstein LM, Freidhoff L, Proud D. Terfenadine, an H_1 antihistamine, inhibits histamine release in vivo in the human. *Am Rev Respir Dis* 1990; *142:* 167-71.
45. Naclerio RM, Proud D, Kagey-Sobotka A, Freidhoff L, Norman PS, Lichtenstein LM. The effect of cetirizine on early allergic response. *Laryngoscope* 1989; *99:* 596-9.
46. Nicholson AN, Stone BM. Performance studies with the H_1-histamine receptor antagonists, astemizole and terfenadine. *Br J Clin Pharmacol* 1982; *13:* 199-202.
47. Oei HD. Double-blind comparison of loratadine (SCH 29851), astemizole, and placebo in hay fever with special regard to onset of action. *Ann Allergy* 1988; *61:* 436-9.
48. Orgel HA, Meltzer EO, Kemp JP, Ostrom NK, Welch MJ. Comparison of intranasal cromolyn sodium, 4%, and oral terfenadine for allergic rhinitis: symptoms, nasal cytology, nasal ciliary clearance, and rhinomanometry. *Ann Allergy* 1991; *66:* 237-44.
49. Pécoud A, Zuber P, Kolly M. Effects of a new selective H_1 receptor antagonist (levocabastine) in a nasal and conjunctival provocation test. *Int Arch Allergy Appl Immunol* 1987; *82:* 541-3.
50. Proud D, Naclerio RM, Hendley JO, Gwaltney JM Jr. Kinins are generated in nasal secretions during natural rhinovirus colds. *J Infect Dis* 1990; *161:* 120-3.
51. Rafferty P, Jackson L, Smith R, Holgate ST. Terfenadine, a potent histamine H_1-receptor antagonist in the treatment of grass pollen sensitive asthma. *Br J Clin Pharmacol* 1990; *30:* 229-35.

52. Richards DM, Brogden RN, Heel RC, Speight TM, Avery GS. Astemizole: a review of its pharmacodynamic properties and therapeutic efficacy. *Drugs* 1984; *28:* 38-61.
53. Rimmer SJ, Church MK. The pharmacology and mechanisms of action of histamine H_1-antagonists. *Clin Exp Allergy* 1990; *20:* 3-17.
54. Roth T, Roehrs T, Koshorek G, Sicklesteel J, Zorick F. Sedative effects of antihistamines. *J Allergy Clin Immunol* 1987; *80:* 94-8.
55. Schata M, Jorde W, Richarz-Barthauer U. Levocabastine nasal spray is better than sodium cromoglycate and placebo in the topical treatment of seasonal allergic rhinitis. *J Allergy Clin Immunol* 1991; *87:* 873-8.
56. Schilling JC, Adamus WS, Kuthan H. Antihistaminic activity and side effect profile of epinastine and terfenadine in healthy volunteers. *Int J Clin Pharmacol Ther Toxicol* 1990; *28:* 493-7.
57. Secher C, Kirkegaard J, Borum P, Maansson A, Osterhammel P, Mygind N. Significance of H_1 and H_2 receptors in the human nose: rationale for topical use of combined antihistamine preparations. *J Allergy Clin Immunol* 1982; *70:* 211-8.
58. Segal A, Boggs F, Falliers C, et al. A placebo-controlled, doubleblind, randomized, parallel study comparing the safety and efficacy of Seldane-D and Tavist-D in the treatment of patients with seasonal allergic rhinitis. *J Allergy Clin Immunol* 1991; *87:* 152.
59. Seidel WF, Cohen S, Bliwise NG, Dement WC. Cetirizine effects on objective measures of daytime sleepiness and performance. *Ann Allergy* 1987; *59:* 58-62.
60. Simons FER. H_1-receptor antagonists: clinical pharmacology and therapeutics. *J Allergy Clin Immunol* 1989; *84:* 845-61.
61. Simons FER, Chen X, Fraser T, Simons KJ. H_1-receptor antagonist concentrations are higher in skin than in serum following IV dosing. *J Allergy Clin Immunol* 1991; *87:* 225.
62. Simons FER, Kesselman MS, Giddins NG, Pelech AN, Simons KJ. Astemizole-induced torsade de pointes. *Lancet* 1988; *2:* 624.
63. Simons FER, Luciuk GH, Simons KJ. Pharmacokinetics and efficacy of chlorpheniramine in children. *J Allergy Clin Immunol* 1982; *69:* 376-81.
64. Simons FER, McMillan JL, Simons KJ. A double-blind, single-dose, crossover comparison of cetirizine, terfenadine, loratadine, astemizole, and chlorpheniramine versus placebo: suppressive effects on histamine-induced wheals and flares during 24 hours in normal subjects. *J Allergy Clin Immunol* 1990; *86:* 540-7.
65. Simons FER, Simons KJ. Second-generation H_1-receptor antagonists. *Ann Allergy* 1991; *66:* 5-21.
66. Simons FER, Watson WTA, Simons KJ. Lack of subsensitivity to terfenadine during long-term terfenadine treatment. *J Allergy Clin Immunol* 1988; *82:* 1068-75.
67. Snyder SH, Snowman AM. Receptor effects of cetirizine. *Ann Allergy* 1987; *59:* 4-8.
68. Storms WW, Bodman SF, Nathan RA, et al. SCH 434: A new antihistamine/decongestant for seasonal allergic rhinitis. *J Allergy Clin Immunol* 1989; *83:* 1083-90.
69. Togias AG, Naclerio RM, Warner J, et al. Demonstration of inhibition of mediator release from human mast cells by azatadine base: in vivo and in vitro evaluation. *JAMA* 1986; *255:* 225-229.
70. Watson WTA, Simons KJ, Chen XY, Simons FER. Cetirizine: a pharmacokinetic and pharmacodynamic evaluation in children with seasonal allergic rhinitis. *J Allergy Clin Immunol* 1989; *84:* 457-64.
71. Weiler JM, Meltzer EO, Dockhorn R, Widlitz MD, D'Eletto TA, Freitag JJ. A safety and efficacy evaluation of azelastine nasal spray in seasonal allergic rhinitis. *J Allergy Clin Immunol* 1991; *87:* 219.

Chapter 16

Immunotherapy

JEAN BOUSQUET
FRANCOIS-B MICHEL

Specific immunotherapy (SIT) was introduced in 1911 for the treatment of pollinosis by Noon & Freeman.[1] The most common form of administration is the subcutaneous route,[2, 3] but oral,[4, 5] sublingual[6] or nasal SIT[7, 8] might also be effective. Immunotherapy is still controversial since many protocols have been devised empirically, some allergens are still poorly defined, the mechanisms of action are not yet clear, the duration is poorly characterized and allergen injections expose subjects to systemic reactions that, in rare cases, become life-threatening.[9-11] However, SIT is one of the most common treatments in children and adolescents in many parts of the world[10] and is effective under optimal conditions which include a demonstrated IgE-mediated disease, a high-quality extract, an optimal allergen dose and a correct indication.[12] In the future, new technologies and the improvement of our knowledge of the basic mechanisms of allergic diseases may completely change the scope of immunotherapy.

Efficacy

Subcutaneous pollen immunotherapy

The efficacy of pollen-SIT suggested by the decrease of target organ sensitivity during nasal allergen challenge[13-21] (Table 16.1) is widely documented in optimally designed double-blind placebo-controlled trials performed in rhinitis due to grass pollen[13-15, 22-32] (Table 16.2), ragweed pollen[33-47] (Table 16.3) and mountain cedar pollen.[48] Grass and ragweed pollen extracts are effective in rhinoconjunctivitis and recent studies have confirmed the efficacy of SIT in grass pollen asthma (for review see[49]). However, although studies comparing the efficacy of immunotherapy and pharmacotherapy are urgently required, there is only one such study. Juniper et al[50] compared the efficacy of budesonide, a highly effective topical steroid, with Pollinex®, in the treatment of ragweed hay fever and observed that the pharmacologic treatment was superior in efficacy and safety. However, this study cannot be extended owing to the low efficacy of Pollinex® in ragweed pollen allergy.[35] In a recent double-blind placebo-controlled study, Varney et al[32] evaluated the efficacy and safety of immunotherapy in patients with severe grass pollen allergy not controlled by standard antiallergic drugs and showed that immunotherapy was effective in reducing symptoms and need for medications including the use of systemic corticosteroids. Double-blind placebo-controlled trials have not been done to evaluate other pollens and although it is postulated to be effective,[12] proper trials have to be done. Moreover, SIT is effective in optimal conditions, but fails when inappropriately used and SIT is not equally effective in all patients. Several parameters, therefore, have to be examined including the quality of the extracts used, and the SIT schedule; cross-reactivities between allergens and the sensitization of patients are critical.

Extracts used. Standardized extracts are now available for many pollen species[51] but are still lacking for important regional allergens such as cypress pollen. Many different extracts have been proposed since the introduction of SIT. Aqueous extracts are effective, especially when standardized, but they expose the patient to a high rate of systemic reac-

Table 16.1. Results of controlled and double-blind placebo-controlled and open studies of the effect of immunotherapy on nasal allergen challenge.

Author	Ref	Allergen	Number A	Number P	Number C	Extract	Schedule	Duration	Nasal challenge epr	Nasal challenge lpr
Bousquet	13	grass	15	10		formald. allergoid	rush	6 wk	$p<0.001$	
Bousquet	14	grass	39	18		HMW formald. allergoid	clustered		$p<0.0001$	
Bousquet	15	grass*	16	17		standardized	rush	6 wk	$p<0.01$	
		multiple species*	16	17		standardized	rush	6 wk	NS	
Frostad	17	grass	41		30	standardized	rush	2 yr	$p<0.001$	
Iliopoulos	18	ragweed	21		20	standardized	classical	8 mo	$p<0.003$	NS for symptoms $p<0.05$ for mediators
Osterballe	20	grass	20		14	partially purified antigen 19,25	classical	1 yr	improved	
	21		20				classical	1 yr	improved	
Viander	21	birch	38		19	Allpyral®	classical	2 yr	improved?	

A: Active treatment. P: Placebo. C: Controls. epr: early phase reaction, lpr: late phase reaction. formald. allergoid: formalinized allergoid, HMW: high molecular weight.
*: patients were polysensitized and treated with multiple pollen extracts but challenge was done with grass pollen.

tions so attempts have been made to prepare extracts having a decreased allergenicity (reduction of side-effects) without reduction of immunogenicity (efficacy). Among the various preparations, adsorbed extracts on aluminium, tyrosine or calcium phosphate are commercially available and were shown to decrease the incidence of side reactions, but they only represent a first attempt and their efficacy has only rarely been reported in placebo-controlled studies with unstandardized extracts.[31] Extracts polymerized by formaldehyde[13, 14, 22, 23, 42, 47, 52] or glutaraldehyde[25, 35, 36, 53, 54] are effective, but high molecular weight preparations are safer and as effective as the aqueous extracts or the low molecular weight ones. PEG-modified extracts represent another interesting approach but they did not completely confirm in humans the hopes raised by animal studies.[55]

Maintenance dose. The maintenance dose is still a matter of debate. Initially, it was proposed to give a high dose to patients but, owing to severe reactions (for review see[2, 3]), other investigators followed the concept of Rinkel[56] who proposed low doses after the so-called skin test titration. However, this technique has been found ineffective during placebo-controlled studies[37, 43] and should not be used any more. Then, it was proposed to give to patients the "highest tolerated dose" with potent extracts[2, 57] but, again, severe systemic reactions were observed in many patients.[2, 58] We[14, 15] proposed to use an *optimal maintenance dose*, i.e. a dose inducing a change in cell reactivity but giving a low and acceptable rate of mild systemic reactions. We started by serially studying skin tests after SIT and defined a dose inducing a decrease in the skin test end-point in over 80% of patients treated. Then, we confirmed that this dose was able to increase the provocative allergen dose during nasal challenge.[13-15] Finally, we also demonstrated that this optimal dose achieved a significant protection in patients suffering from grass pollen-induced rhinoconjunctivitis and asthma.[13-16, 22, 23] Using a 10-fold greater dose, the number of systemic side reactions was increased without major changes in efficacy.[15] However, a much greater increase might have enhanced the effectiveness of SIT but side reactions are likely to be greater in number and unacceptable in severity. For ragweed pollen allergens, Turkeltaub et al took a similar approach.[59]

Table 16.2. Results of double-blind placebo-controlled studies in grass pollen allergy.

Author	Ref	Allergen	Number A	Number P	Extract	Schedule	Protocol	Duration	Effect on skin test	Effect on symptom-medication score	
Bousquet	22	grass	15	11	standardized	rush	pre+co-season	1 yr	$p<0.01$	N	$p<0.01$
		grass	16		formald. allergoid	rush	pre+co-season	1 yr	$p<0.02$	N	$p<0.05$
Bousquet	13	grass	15	10	formald. allergoid	clustered	pre+co-season	1 yr	$p<0.001$	N	$p<0.005$
Bousquet	23	grass	18		standardized	rush	pre+co-season	1 yr	$p<0.01$	N,O,B	$p<0.01$
		grass	15	14	formald. allergoid	clustered	pre+co-season	1 yr	$p<0.04$	O,B	$0.05<p<0.01$
		grass	13		HMW-allergoid	clustered	pre+co-season	1 yr	$p<0.005$	N,O,B	$p<0.01$
Bousquet	14	grass	39	18	HMW-allergoid	clustered	pre+co-season	1 yr	$p<0.05$	N,B	$0.05<0<0.01$
Bousquet	15	grass	16	17	standardized	rush	pre+co-season	1 yr	$p<0.02$	N	$p<0.02$
		multiple species	16	17	standardized	rush	pre+co-season	1 yr	NS	N	NS
Frankland	24	grass	50	50	"pollaccine"	classical		1 yr		N	$p<0.001$
		grass	50	50	purified antigen	classical		1 yr		N	$p<0.001$
Grammer	25	grass	18	18	polymer. glutarald.	classical	12 injections	12 wk		N	$p<0.02$
Grammer	26	grass	22	22	polymer. glutarald.	accelerated	13 injections	9 wk		N	$p<0.05$
McAllen	27	grass	47	23	Allpyral®	classical	?	1 yr		N,B	NS
			40		depot preparation	classical	?	1 yr		N,B	$p=0.05$
Machiels	28	grass	7	8	Ag-Ab complexes	classical	pre+co-season	3 mo		N	NS
Machiels	29	grass	37	12	Ag-Ab complexes	classical	pre+co-season	3 mo		N,B	$p<0.03$ & $p<0.001$
Ortolani	30	grass	8	8	standardized	classical	pre-season	1 yr		N	$p<0.001$
Starr	31	grass	42	10	alum-pyridine	classical	pre-season	1 yr		N	79% improved
Varney	32	grass	20	20	standardized, alum	classical	pre+co-season	1 yr		N, B	$p<0.01$
Weyer	33	grass	17	16	aqueous then Al(OH)$_3$	classical	pre-season	1 yr		N	peak of season, $p<0.03$

N: nasal, O: ocular, B: bronchial.
Ag-Ab: antigen-antibody.

Table 16.3. Results of double-blind placebo-controlled studies in ragweed pollen rhinitis.

Author	Ref	Number P	Number A	Extract	Schedule	Protocol	Dose	Duration	Effect on symptom-medication scores
Arbesman	34	19	19	repository	12 injection	pre-season	M: 4,000 PNU	2 yr	NS vs placebo
			22	aqueous	12 injection	pre-season	M: 10,000 PNU	2 yr	improved
Cockroft	35	21	22	Pollinex®	4 injections	pre-season	M: 4,000 Noon U	1 yr	improved: A: 67%, P: 38%
Grammer	36	19	21	polymer. glutarald.	classical	15 injections	M: 6,250 PNU, C: 50,000 PNU	15 wk	$p<0.02$
Hirsch	37	74	81	aqueous	Rinkel	pre + co-season	M: 27-41 PNU, 0.1-0.15 µg Ag E	2 yr	NS for ragweed
Lichtenstein	40	24	24	antigen E	classical	pre-season	C: 17-800 µg	1 yr	$p<0.01$
Lichtenstein	39	30	18	antigen E	classical	pre-season	1,0 mg	1 yr	$p<0.01$
			21	antigen E + K	classical	pre-season	1,4 mg	1 yr	$p<0.01$
			19	crude rw, aqueous	classical	pre-season	C: 8,800 PNU	1 yr	$p<0.01$
Lowell	41	12	12	aqueous	classical	pre-season	not stated	1 yr	$p<0.01$
Meriney	42	10	10	formald. allergoid	classical	pre-season	C: 10,710 PNU	20 wk	$p<0.01$
Van Metre	43	12	12	aqueous	Rinkel	pre + co-season	C: 94 ng AgE	3 mo	NS
Van Metre	44	17	15	aqueous	classical	pre + co-season	C: 70µg AgE	1 yr	$p<0.01$
			18	aqueous	clustered	pre + co-season	C: 17.5 µg AgE	1 yr	$p<0.01$
Norman	45	21	21	aqueous whole rw	classical	pre-season	C: 9,483 PNU per yr	4 yr	3rd, 4th yr; $p<0.02$
			21	antigen E	classical	pre-season	C: 195,530 PNU per yr	4 yr	3rd, 4th yr; $p<0.04$
Norman	46	21	20	alum-precipitate	classical	pre-season	C: 13,746 PNU (yr 1)	3 yr	$p<0.006$
Norman	47	22	22	formald. allergoid	clustered	pre-season	C: 63,600 PNU (yr 1)	2 yr	$p<0.01$
			22	aqueous	classical	pre-season	C: 2,000 PNU (yr 1)	2 yr	$p<0.01$

M: maximal dose, C: cumulative dose.

Cross-reactivities between allergens. Many related or unrelated allergens share common epitopes leading to cross-reactivities that complicate the diagnosis and the treatment of allergic diseases. Important cross-reactivities exist among pollens of grasses or Oleaceae, or some of the Ambrosiaceae or deciduous trees or, to a lesser extent, Compositeae. Patients allergic to grass pollens usually have positive skin tests and serum-specific IgE towards many if not most species. Thus, it should be determined whether patients need to be treated by all the relevant species or only a few of them, or only one. During the early years of SIT in Europe, timothy (*Phleum pratense*) was commonly used as it was supposed to have a broad allergen content. To improve the efficacy of SIT a mixture of five to six common grasses, including timothy, was then proposed in the middle of the century. During the last 10 years, the use of a single allergen species has tended to be favored in Northern Europe. This may not, however, relate to the entire world since pollens of some species such as Bermuda grass (*Cynodon dactylon*) or cereals do not completely cross-react with timothy. Allergen mixtures present many defects. They may be less stable in an aqueous extract than single species since interactions between allergens exist and enzymatic degradation of allergens has already been demonstrated. It is more difficult to standardize mixtures, and the dilution of major epitopes in mixtures may lead to a low-dose SIT regimen. On the other hand, single allergen species may be less effective because some relevant epitopes may be lacking. Løwenstein et al[60] using cross-immunoelectrophoresis proposed that rye grass possesses epitopes that might be relevant for most other grass pollen species and that SIT with single allergens may be effective. This was at least partly confirmed by Frostad et al[61] and Bousquet et al (unpublished observations) who observed that SIT with a single allergen species (rye grass or orchard grass) was as effective as SIT with four or five species. Similar findings were observed with birch and deciduous tree pollens.[62,63]

Patients sensitized to birch pollen often present cross-reactive epitopes with many raw fruits and vegetables and, in theory, birch pollen-SIT might reduce fruit allergy. Møller[64] examined the efficacy of birch pollen SIT in apple sensitivity but failed to observe any efficacy for fruit allergy.

Polysensitized patients. The IgE immune response to environmental allergens depends both on genetic and environmental factors and is highly heterogeneous.[65, 66] It was shown that patients only allergic to grass pollens differ clinically and immunologically[66] from those allergic to many pollen species (Fig. 16.1-2). These present symptoms earlier in the season than those allergic to grass pollens only, due to the combined effects of priming of the nasal mucosa and to an earlier onset of the allergen exposure. Polysensitized patients have a qualitatively and quantitatively increased IgE immune response towards grass pollen allergens, suggesting that SIT efficacy may differ between individuals allergic to grass pollen only or to multiple pollen species. Two controlled studies comparing the efficacy of SIT in these two groups of patients were performed. Grass pollen-allergic patients were treated with an optimal maintenance dose of a standardized orchard grass pollen extract whereas those allergic to multiple pollen species received the same biologically equivalent dose of all standardized allergens to which they were sensitized.[15, 67] The results of both studies indicated that grass pollen-allergic patients had significantly fewer symptom and medication scores during the pollen season than either the placebo group[15] or the control group.[67] On the other hand, SIT in polysensitized individuals was variably effective and mean symptom-medication scores were not significantly different in treated and placebo or control groups. Moreover, nasal challenge was significantly improved in the grass pollen group only.[15] These two studies suggest that the efficacy of SIT is greater in monosensitized grass pollen-allergic individuals as compared with polysensitized patients, possibly because the optimal dose differs between these groups.

Age of the patients. For theoretical reasons based on the mechanisms of the immune response, it is usually recommended to start SIT in children and adults and to avoid it in elderly subjects. In ragweed pollen allergy, Hedlin et al[68] compared results of allergen immunotherapy in pediatric and adult populations. Biological responses were measured by nasal challenges, skin tests and the evolution of antigen-specific immunoglobulins. They observed that ragweed immunotherapy leads to immunolo-

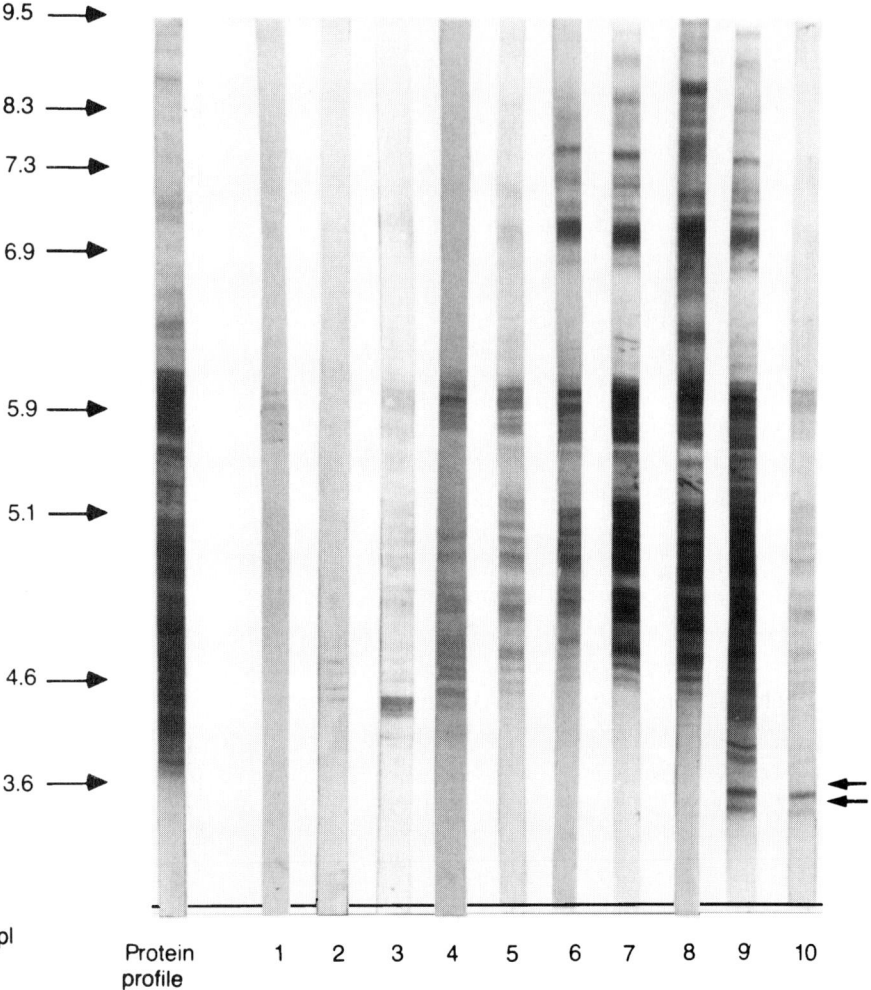

Fig. 16.1. IgE immunoblots against orchard grass pollen allergens. Patients only allergic to grass pollen are in group 1-4. Patients sensitized to multiple pollen species are in group 5-10. From Bousquet J, Becker WM, Hejjaoui A, Cour P, Chanal I, Lebel B, Dhivert H, Michel FB. Clinical and immunological reactivity of patients allergic to grass pollens and to multiple pollen species. Efficacy of a double-blind, placebo-controlled, specific immunotherapy with standardized extract. *J Allergy Clin Immunol* 1991; *88:* 43-53.

gical and biological consequences that are comparable in children and adults. However, this study does not give clear information on older patients who usually improve spontaneously.

Before 5 years of age, SIT may be started but it is desirable to evaluate more closely its benefits since SIT leads to a greater number of systemic reactions. Systemic reactions, especially asthma, may be more severe and most young children did not fully develop their allergenic sensitization. On the other hand, a retrospective study has suggested that SIT in pollen-allergic patients may prevent the onset of asthma.

During pregnancy, the severity of allergic diseases is often modified and, SIT should not be started but may be continued if effective.[69]

Other routes for allergen administration in pollen rhinitis

The usual route of administration of SIT is the subcutaneous one. Recent studies have, however, shown that oral[4, 5, 20, 70-75] or nasal SIT[7, 8, 76, 77] are inconstantly effective even when the appropriate extracts are given at a high dose. Systemic or focal reactions were rather low with local administration of extracts. However, oral SIT with current extracts is not cost-effective since very large doses of extracts are required for its effectiveness. The addition of oral SIT to boost parenteral SIT may be effective but more data are needed.[78, 79] Sublingual SIT is currently under investigation but definite results are not yet available.

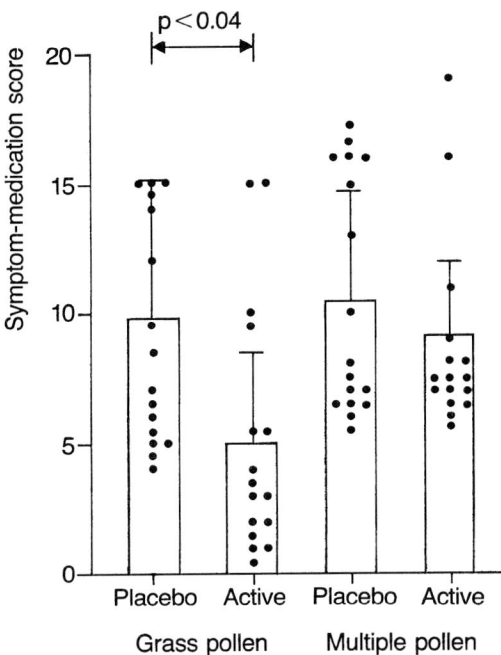

Fig. 16.2. Symptom-medication scores during the pollen season. From Bousquet J, Becker WM, Hejjaoui A, Cour P, Chanal I, Lebel B, Dhivert H, Michel FB. Clinical and immunological reactivity of patients allergic to grass pollens and to multiple pollen species. Efficacy of a double-blind, placebo-controlled, specific immunotherapy with standardized extract. *J Allergy Clin Immunol* 1991; 88: 43-53.

Efficacy of SIT with other allergens

Few double-blind placebo-controlled studies have been performed with house dust mites (Table 16.4),[80-85] animal proteins[86] or molds[87,88] (Fig. 16.3) in the treatment of rhinitis. Most studies revealed that the actively-treated group was significantly improved and these results were confirmed by nasal challenge. SIT was shown to be effective in optimal conditions but this treatment completely fails when inappropriately used. The quality of the extracts used and the SIT schedules are again of paramount importance in daily practice.

Side reactions

Life-threatening reactions are not uncommon with very potent extracts and deaths have been reported.[9-11] The rate of systemic reactions is greater with potent pollen extracts than with either less potent extracts[89-92] or high molecular weight

Table 16.4. *Results of double-blind placebo-controlled studies in house dust mite rhinitis.*

Author	Ref	Placebo number	Active number	Extract	Protocol	Dose	Duration	Symptom-medication score	Nasal challenge
Blainey	80	18	17	tyrosine adsorbed	classical	400 Noon U	14 mo	?	improved
Corrado	81	33	33	Conjuvac®	classical		2 yr	$p<0.001$	$p<0.01$
D'Souza	82	48	48	aqueous	classical	variable	12 inj	improved for A + R	$p<0.025$
Ewan	83	19	16	standardized	classical	M: 17,000 BU	3 mo	$p<0.01$	$p<0.05$
Gabriel	84	33	33	aqueous	classical		1 yr	improved	NS
McHugh	85	30	30	standardized	classical	M: 100,000 BU	1 yr	NS (3 mo) $p<0.01$ (12 mo)	$p<0.05$* (3 mo) NS (12 mo)
		20		alum-pyridine		M: 10,000 PNU		NS (3 and 12 mo)	$p<0.05$** (12 mo)

M: maximal dose.
A: asthma, R: rhinitis.
*: statistical difference from baseline and placebo, **: statistical difference from baseline only.
inj: injections.

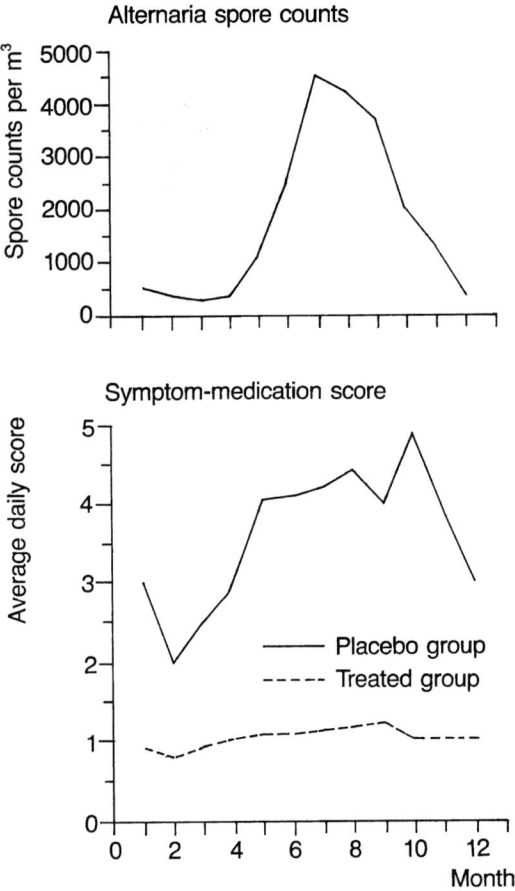

Fig. 16.3. Symptom-medication scores of patients receiving immunotherapy with a standardized Alternaria extract or placebo. From Horst M, Hejjaoui A, Horst V, Michel FB, Bousquet J. Double-blind, placebo-controlled rush immunotherapy with a standardized Alternaria extract. *J Allergy Clin Immunol* 1990; 85: 460-72.

preparations.[14, 15, 23, 25, 35, 54] Bousquet et al[92] examined the occurrence of systemic reactions in pollen-allergic individuals who received the same rush protocol with the same standardized extracts. They observed that the rate of systemic reactions was increased in patients who had presented asthma (and rhino-conjunctivitis) during the previous pollen season compared with those who had had rhino-conjunctivitis alone. The incidence of generalized urticaria and anaphylaxis was similar in both groups, but bronchial symptoms occurred mostly in asthmatic patients. This study indicates that asthmatic patients are at higher risk during SIT.

Before any injection, patients should be monitored carefully and the treatment delayed if the patient presents any symptom of asthma or respiratory infection. Injections should only be given under the close supervision of a trained physician, in settings where anaphylactic reactions can be immediately corrected. The patient should be monitored for up to 30 minutes after the shot. Systemic reactions occurring after allergen injection should be regarded as possibly serious and adrenaline (and oxygen therapy) should be immediately administered if necessary.

Duration

Duration of SIT is another matter of debate. In the case of inhalant allergy in atopic individuals data are lacking to support any definite conclusion, but it appears that a long-term treatment, at least 3 years, is required. In a retrospective study, Mosbech et al[93] observed that the effect of grass pollen-SIT was still lasting several years after its cessation. Grammer et al[94] using high molecular weight polymerized extracts reached similar conclusions. For perennial allergens, the duration of SIT may even be longer.

Indications

Double-blind placebo-controlled studies have therefore confirmed the efficacy of SIT but clinical efficacy does not mean clinical indication, especially as 1) controlled trials of SIT are optimally designed and may not always be applicable to daily medical practice and 2) a safe and effective pharmacologic treatment is also available for the treatment of allergic diseases. Thus, before starting SIT it is essential to consider several factors to appreciate the respective value of allergen avoidance, pharmacotherapy and SIT. 1) Demonstration that the disease is due to an IgE-mediated allergy and that high-quality extracts are available. 2) Complete allergen avoidance is impossible. 3) Potential severity of the affection to be treated. 4) Efficacy of available treatments, including quality of allergen extracts that are used. 5) Cost and duration of each type of treatment. 6) Risk incurred by the patient due to the allergic disease and the treatments.

In patients receiving SIT, both SIT and pharmacotherapy should be used in combination since very few patients will be completely free of symptoms when treated with SIT, but, on the other hand, SIT reduces the need for medications in severe cases.[32] Moreover, allergen avoidance should always be attempted even if it cannot be complete.

Specific immunotherapy needs to be prescribed by specialists and done by physicians who are trained to use emergency techniques if anaphylaxis occurs. Before starting SIT each patient should be carefully informed of risks, duration and effectiveness of this treatment and cooperation and compliance to the treatment are absolute requirements before starting it.

The specific indications have been extensively studied and the Position Papers of the European Academy of Allergy and Clinical Immunology[95] and WHO/IUI[12] have proposed some guidelines.

Pollen rhinitis

It is commonly accepted, and recently confirmed by Varney et al,[32] that SIT is indicated in severe pollinosis, especially when asthma complicates rhino-conjunctivitis. On the other hand, SIT should not be started in mild to moderately severe rhino-conjunctivitis responding favorably to antihistamines and topical drugs, except if the season is long-lasting as is the case in Southern Europe, South Africa and California. Varney et al[32] pointed out that patients with perennial asthma should be specifically excluded, but this recommendation appears to be important only if asthma is moderately severe to severe.

House dust mite rhinitis

House dust immunotherapy should not be used any more. With mite allergens, the indications of SIT are still vague but can be envisaged especially if the patient presents asthma. In rhinitis, a course of topical steroids is often required at the beginning of SIT since symptoms are due to both allergy and inflammation.

Allergy to animal proteins

Although it has been recommended by the Position Papers[12, 95] that allergen avoidance be preferred to SIT in animal dander allergy, SIT may be envisaged, especially for occupational exposure.

Allergy to molds

Molds are major allergens in allergic rhinitis but they often induce polysensitizations and most extracts are not standardized yet. SIT using standardized extracts of *Alternaria* and *Cladosporium* was shown to be effective.[87, 88] However, SIT with many mold species or with extracts of unknown quality should not be administered.

Immunotherapy with other extracts

Specific immunotherapy with extracts of undefined allergens (bacteria, foods, *Candida albicans*, insect dusts) should not be used any longer.

Contraindications

Absolute contraindications include patients with other serious immunopathological conditions, malignancies, poor compliance, severe psychological disorders and/or treatment by β-blocking agents.

Monitoring

After the first pollen season, or 6 months for perennial allergens, patients receiving SIT should be reassessed and the treatment stopped if not effective. *In vivo* and *in vitro* methods have been proposed to evaluate the efficacy of SIT. The evolution of IgG, IgG subclasses or IgE against whole allergens or purified antigens does not give any valuable information.[96] Provocative challenges are often correlated with the efficacy of SIT but only when a group of patients is considered.[14-16, 22, 34] They are less predictive for an individual patient and are difficult to do routinely in clinical practice. The evolution of the cutaneous late-phase reaction may also be considered since relationships between late cutaneous responses and specific antibody responses have been positively correlated with outcome of immunotherapy for seasonal allergic rhinitis.[97]

Conclusion

Specific immunotherapy is a common treatment of allergic rhinitis. With high quality standardized extracts, SIT is effective when optimally administered in seasonal and perennial rhinitis. However, SIT is a treatment that should be prescribed by a specialist and administered by or under the close supervision of a physician trained to treat anaphylactic reactions that may occur with very potent extracts. The reduction of systemic reactions may be attempted by improving extracts (high molecular weight preparations) and designing an *optimal dose* that leads to efficacy with a low rate of mild systemic reactions. Patients receiving SIT often require an additional pharmacological treatment but the immunologic treatment often makes it possible either to reduce drugs or to improve the control of the disease. In the future, it is likely that allergen-specific and/or allergen-non-specific *immunological drugs* will be available and, among the several approaches attempted, many are promising.

Acknowledgment

The authors thank Dr W Becker, H Dhivert, F Djoukhadar, A Dotte, E Frank, P Godard, B Guérin, A Hejjaoui, B Hewitt, J Knani, HJ Maasch, JL Ménardo, W Skassa-Brociek, R Wahl, and Mrs M Deltour for their help.

References

1 Noon L, Cantab BC. Prophylactic inoculation against hay fever. *Lancet* 1911; i: 1572-3.
2 Norman PS, Kunkel G, Weeke B. Immunotherapy. In: Mygind N, Weeke B, eds. *Allergic and vasomotor rhinitis: clinical aspects.* Copenhagen: Munksgaard 1986: 132-9.
3 Van Metre TE Jr, Adkinson NF J. Immunotherapy for aeroallergen disease. In: Middleton E Jr, Reed CE, Ellis EF, Adkinson NF Jr. Yunginger JW, eds. *Allergy. Principles and practice*, 3rd edn. St Louis: The CV Mosby Co 1989: 1327-44.
4 Björksten B, Moeller C, Broberger U, et al. Clinical and immunological effects of oral immunotherapy with a standardized birch pollen extract. *Allergy* 1986; 41: 290-5.
5 Platts-Mills TAE. Oral immunotherapy: a way forward. *J Allergy Clin Immunol* 1987; 80: 129-31.
6 Scadding GK, Brostoff J. Low dose sublingual therapy in patients with allergic rhinitis due to house dust mite. *Clin Allergy* 1986; 16: 483-92.
7 Georgitis JW, Reisman RE, Clayton WF, Mueller UR, Wypych JI, Arbesman CE. Local intranasal immunotherapy for grass-allergic rhinitis. *J Allergy Clin Immunol* 1983; 71: 71-6.
8 Johansson SGO, Deuschl H, Zetterström O. Use of glutaraldehyde-modified timothy grass pollen extract in nasal hyposensitization treatment of hay fever. *Int Archs Allergy Appl Immunol* 1979; 60: 447-60.
9 Lockey RF, Benedict LM, Turkeltaub PC, Bukantz SC. Fatalities from immunotherapy (IT) and skin testing. *J Allergy Clin Immunol* 1987; 79: 660-77.
10 Norman PS. Fatal misadventures. *J Allergy Clin Immunol* 1987; 79: 572-3.
11 Committee on Safety of Medicine. Desensitizing vaccines. *Br Med J* 1986; 293: 948.
12 Thompson RA, Bousquet J, Cohen S, et al. Allergen specific immunotherapy. Report of a WHO-IUIS working group. *Lancet* 1989; i: 259-61.
13 Bousquet J, Maasch HJ, Martinot B, et al. Double-blind placebo-controlled immunotherapy with mixed grass pollen allergoids. II. Comparison between parameters assessing the efficacy of immunotherapy. *J Allergy Clin Immunol* 1988; 82: 439-46.
14 Bousquet J, Hejjaoui A, Soussana M, Michel FB. Double-blind, placebo-controlled immunotherapy with mixed grass-pollen allergoids. IV. Comparison of the safety and efficacy of two dosages of a high-molecular-weight allergoid. *J Allergy Clin Immunol* 1990; 85: 490-7.
15 Bousquet J, Becker WM, Hejjaoui A, et al. Clinical and immunological reactivity of patients allergic to grass pollens and to multiple pollen species. Efficacy of a double-blind, placebo-controlled, specific immunotherapy with standardized extract. *J Allergy Clin Immunol* 1991; 88: 43-53.
16 Creticos PS, Marsh DG, Proud D, et al. Responses to ragweed-pollen nasal challenge before and after immunotherapy. *J Allergy Clin Immunol* 1989; 84: 197-205.
17 Frostad AB, Bolle R, Grimmer Ø, Aas K. A new, well-characterized, purified allergen preparation from timothy pollen. II. Allergenic in vivo and in vitro properties. *Int Archs Allergy Appl Immunol* 1978; 55: 35-40.
18 Ilioupoulos O, Proud D, Adkinson ND, et al. Effects of immunotherapy on the early, late and rechallenge nasal reaction to provocation with allergen: Changes in inflammatory mediators and cells. *J Allergy Clin Immunol* 1991; 87: 855-66.
19 Hedlin G, Silber G, Schieken L, et al. Attenuation of allergen sensitivity early in the course of ragweed immunotherapy. *J Allergy Clin Immunol* 1989; 84: 390-9.
20 Østerballe O. Immunotherapy in hay fever with two major allergens 19, 25 and partially purified extracts of timothy pollen. A controlled double-blind study. In vivo variables, season. I. *Allergy* 1980; 35: 473-89.
21 Viander M, Koivikko A. The seasonal symptoms of hyposensitized and untreated hay fever patients in relation to birch pollen counts: correlations with nasal sensitivity, prick tests and RAST. *Clin Allergy* 1978; 8: 387-96.
22 Bousquet J, Hejjaoui A, Skassa-Brociek W, et al. Double-blind placebo-controlled immunotherapy with mixed grass pollen allergoids. I. Rush immunotherapy with allergoids and standardized orchard grass pollen. *J Allergy Clin Immunol* 1987; 80: 591-8.
23 Bousquet J, Maasch H, Hejjaoui A. Double-blind placebo-controlled immunotherapy with mixed grass pollen allergoids. III. Comparison with an unfractionated allergoid, a fractionated allergoid and a standardized orchard grass pollen extract in rhinitis, conjunctivitis and asthma. *J Allergy Clin Immunol* 1989; 84: 546-56.
24 Frankland AW, Augustin R. Prophylaxis of summer hay fever and asthma: a controlled trial comparing crude grass-pollen extracts with the isolated main protein components. *Lancet* 1954; i: 1055-8.
25 Grammer LC, Shaughnessy MA, Suszko IM, Shaugnessy JJ, Patterson R. A double-blind histamine placebo-controlled trial of polymerized whole grass for immunotherapy of grass allergy. *J Allergy Clin Immunol* 1983; 72: 448-53.

26 Grammer LC, Shaughnessy MA, Finkle SM, Shaugnessy JJ, Patterson R. A double-blind placebo-controlled trial of polymerized whole grass administered in an accelerated dosage schedule for immunotherapy of grass pollinosis. *J Allergy Clin Immunol* 1986; *78:* 1180-4.

27 Mc Allen M. Hyposensitization in grass pollen hay fever. *Acta Allergol* 1969; *24:* 421-31.

28 Machiels JJ, Buche M, Somville MA, Jacquemin MG, Saint-Remy JM. Complexes of grass pollen allergens and specific antibodies reduce allergic symptoms and inhibit the seasonal increase of IgE antibody. *Clin Exp Allergy* 1990; *20:* 653-60.

29 Machiels JJ, Somville MA, Jacquemin MG, Saint-Rémy JMR. Allergen-antibody complexes can efficiently prevent seasonal rhinitis and asthma in grass pollen hypersensitive patients. *Allergy* 1991; *46:* 335-48.

30 Ortolani C, Pastorello E, Moss R, et al. Grass pollen immunotherapy: a single year double-blind placebo-controlled study in patients with grass pollen-induced asthma and rhinitis. *J Allergy Clin Immunol* 1984; *73:* 283-9.

31 Starr MS, Weinstock M. Studies in pollen allergy. III. The relationship between blocking antibody levels, and symptomatic relief following hyposensitization with Allpyral in hay fever subjects. *Int Arch Allergy Appl Immunol* 1970; *38:* 514-21.

32 Varney VA, Gaga M, Aber VR, Kay AB, Durham SR. Usefulness of immunotherapy in patients with severe summer hay fever uncontrolled by antiallergic drugs. *Br Med J* 1991; *302:* 265-9.

33 Weyer A, Donat N, L'Heritier C, et al. Grass pollen hyposensitization versus placebo therapy. I. Clinical effectiveness and methodological aspects of a pre-seasonal course of desensitization with a four-grass pollen extract. *Allergy* 1981; *36:* 309-17.

34 Arbesman CE, Reisman RE. Hyposensitization therapy including repository: a double-blind study. *J Allergy* 1964; *35:* 12-7.

35 Cockroft DW, Cuff MT, Tarlo SM, Dolovich J, Hargreave FE. Allergen injection therapy with glutaraldehyde-modified-ragweed pollen-tyrosin adsorbate. A double-blind trial. *J Allergy Clin Immunol* 1977; *60:* 56-62.

36 Grammer LC, Zeiss CR, Suszko IM, Shaughnessy MA, Patterson R. A double-blind, placebo-controlled trial of polymerized whole ragweed for immunotherapy of ragweed allergy. *J Allergy Clin Immunol* 1982; *69:* 494-9.

37 Hirsch SR, Kalbfleisch JH, Golbert TM, et al. Rinkel injection therapy: a multicenter controlled study. *J Allergy Clin Immunol* 1980; *68:* 133-45.

38 Juniper EF, O'Connor J, Roberts RS, Evans S, Hargreave FE, Dolovich J. Polyethylene glycol-modified ragweed extract: comparison of two treatment regimens. *J Allergy Clin Immunol* 1986; *78:* 851-6.

39 Lichtenstein LM, Norman PS, Winkenwerder L. A single year of immunotherapy of ragweed hay fever. *Ann Intern Med* 1971; *75:* 663-70.

40 Lichtenstein LM, Norman PS, Winkenwerder WL. Clinical and in vitro studies on the role of immunotherapy in ragweed hay fever. *Am J Med* 1968; *44:* 514-24.

41 Lowell FC, Franklin W. A double-blind study of the effectiveness and specificity of injection therapy in ragweed hay fever. *N Engl J Med* 1965; *273:* 675-9.

42 Meriney DK, Kothari H, Chinoy P, Grieco MH. The clinical and immunologic efficacy of immunotherapy with modified ragweed extract (allergoid) for ragweed hay fever. *Ann Allergy* 1986; *56:* 34-8.

43 Van Metre TE, Adkinson NF, Lichtenstein LM, et al. A controlled study of the effectiveness of the Rinkel method of immunotherapy for ragweed pollen hay fever. *J Allergy Clin Immunol* 1980; *65:* 288-97.

44 Van Metre TE, Adkinson NF Jr, Amodio FJ, et al. A comparative study of the effectiveness of the Rinkel method and the current standard method of immunotherapy for ragweed pollen hay fever. *J Allergy Clin Immunol* 1981; *66:* 500-13.

45 Norman PS, Winkelwerder WL, Lichtenstein L. Immunotherapy of hay fever with ragweed antigen E: comparisons with whole extracts and placebo. *J Allergy* 1968; *42:* 93-108.

46 Norman PS, Lichstenstein LM. Comparison of alum-precipitated and unprecipitated aqueous ragweed pollen extracts in the treatment of hay fever. *J Allergy Clin Immunol* 1978; *61:* 384-9.

47 Norman PS, Lichtenstein LM, Kagey-Sobotka A, Marsh DG. Controlled evaluation of allergoids in the immunotherapy of ragweed hay fever. *J Allergy Clin Immunol* 1982; *70:* 248-60.

48 Pence HL, Mitchell DQ, Greenly RL, Updegraff BR, Selfridge HA. Immunotherapy for mountain cedar pollinosis. A double-blind controlled study. *J Allergy Clin Immunol* 1976; *58:* 39-50.

49 Bousquet J, Hejjaoui A, Michel FB. Specific immunotherapy in asthma. *J Allergy Clin Immunol* 1990; *86:* 292-305.

50 Juniper EF, Kline PA, Ramsdale EH, Hargreave FE. Comparison of the efficacy and side effects of aqueous steroid nasal spray (budesonide) and allergen-injection therapy (Pollinex-R) in the treatment of seasonal allergic rhinoconjunctivitis. *J Allergy Clin Immunol* 1990; *85:*606-11.

51 Reed CE, Yunginger JW. Quality assurance and standardization of allergy extracts in allergy practice. *J Allergy Clin Immunol* 1989; *84:* 4-8.

52 Marsh DG, Norman PS, Roebber M, Lichtenstein LM. Studies on allergoids from naturally occurring allergens. III. Preparation of ragweed pollen allergoids by aldehyde modification in two steps. *J Allergy Clin Immunol* 1981; *68:* 449-59.

53 Grammer LC, Shaughnessy MA, Shaugnessy JJ, Silvestri L, Patterson R. Allergenicity, immunogenicity, and safety of immunotherapy with various molecular weight ranges of polymerized ragweed. *J Allergy Clin Immunol* 1985; *76:* 195-200.

54 Grammer LC, Silvestri L, Suszko IM, Shaughnessy MA, Patterson R. Evaluation and standardization of polymerized ragweed extracts by chromatography, radioimmunoassay inhibition, and endpoint cutaneous titration. *J Allergy Clin Immunol* 1983; *72:* 160-7.

55 Dreborg S, Åkerblom EB. Immunotherapy with monomethoxypolyethylene glycol modified allergens. *Crit Rev Ther Drug Carrier Syst* 1990; *6:* 315-65.

56 Rinkel HJ. Inhalant Allergy. II. The coseasonal application of serial dilutions. *Ann Allergy* 1949; *7:* 639-45.

57 Creticos PS, Van Metre TE, Mardiney MR, et al. Dose response of IgE and IgG antibodies during ragweed immunotherapy. *J Allergy Clin Immunol* 1984; *73:* 94-104.

58 Lessof M, Chandler B. Experience with spectralgen™ / pharmalgen™. A new kind of allergen preparation. Proceedings of an International Allergy Workshop. Amsterdam: Excerpta Medica, 1983: 1-88.

59 Turkeltaub PC, Campbell G, Mosimann JE. Comparative safety and efficacy of short ragweed extracts differing in potency and composition in the treatment of fall hay fever. Use of allergenically bioequivalent doses by parallel line bioassay to evaluate comparative safety and efficacy. *Allergy* 1990; *45:* 528-46.

60 Löwenstein H, Wihl J-Å, Bache Billesbølle K, Bøwadt H. Rationale for specific immunotherapy of grass pollen allergy with extracts of rye pollen. *Allergy* 1984; *39:* 421-32.

61 Frostad AB, Grimmer Ø, Sandvik L, Moxnes A, Aas K. Clinical effects of hyposensitization using a purified allergen preparation from timothy pollen as compared to crude aqueous extracts from timothy pollen and a four-grass pollen mixture respectively. *Clin Allergy* 1983; *13:* 337-57.

62 Møller C, Dreborg S. Cross-reactivity between deciduous trees during immunotherapy. I. In vivo results. *Clin Allergy* 1986; *16:* 135-44.

63 Petersen BN, Janniche H, Munch EP, et al. Immunotherapy with partially purified and standardized tree pollen extracts. I. Clinical results from a three-year double-blind study of patients with pollen extracts either of birch or combination of alder, birch and hazel. *Allergy* 1988; *43:* 353-62.

64. Møller C. Effect of pollen immunotherapy on food hypersensitivity in children with birch pollinosis. *Ann Allergy* 1989; *62:* 343-5.
65. Peltre G, Lapeyre J, David B. Heterogeneity of grass pollen allergens (*Dactylis glomerata*) recognized by IgE antibodies in human patients sera by a new nitrocellulose immunoprint technique. *Immunol Lett* 1982; *5:* 127-31.
66. Bousquet J, Hejjaoui A, Becker WM, et al. Clinical and immunological reactivity of patients allergic to grass pollens and to multiple pollen species clinical and immunological reactivity. *J Allergy Clin Immunol* 1991; *87:* 737-46.
67. Hejjaoui A, Braquemond P, Bousquet J, Demaille J, Michel FB. Efficacy of pollen immunotherapy according to the allergenic profile of the patients. *J Allergy Clin Immunol* 1985; *75:* 164.
68. Hedlin G, Silber G, Naclerio R, et al. Comparison of the in-vivo and in-vitro response to ragweed immunotherapy in children and adults with ragweed-induced rhinitis. *Clin Exp Allergy* 1990; *20:* 491-500.
69. Metzger JW, Turner E; Patterson R. The safety of immunotherapy during pregnancy. *J Allergy Clin Immunol* 1978; *61:* 268-75.
70. Björksten B, Croner S, Dreborg S, et al. A double-blind study of oral immunotherapy in children allergic to birch pollen using high doses of allergen. *J Allergy Clin Immunol* 1986; *77:* 214-8.
71. Taudorf E, Laursen LC, Djurup R, et al. Oral administration of grass pollen to hay fever patients. *Allergy* 1985; *40:* 321-35.
72. Taudorf E, Laursen LC, Lanner A, et al. Oral immunotherapy in birch pollen hay fever. *J Allergy Clin Immunol* 1987; *80:* 153-61.
73. Van Niekerk CH, De Wet JI. Efficacy of grass-maize pollen oral immunotherapy in patients with seasonal hay fever: a double-blind study. *Clin Allergy* 1987; *17:* 507-14.
74. Cooper PJ, Darbyshire J, Nunn AJ, Warner JO. A controlled trial of oral hyposensitization in pollen asthma and rhinitis in children. *Clin Allergy* 1984; *14:* 541-50.
75. Mosbech H, Dreborg S, Madsen F, et al. High dose grass pollen tablets used for hyposensitization in hay fever patients. A one-year double-blind placebo-controlled study. *Allergy* 1987; *42:* 451-6.
76. Georgitis JW, Nickelsen JA, Wypych JI, et al. Local intranasal immunotherapy with high dose polymerized ragweed extract. *Int Archs Allergy Appl Immunol* 1986; *81:* 170-9.
77. Welsh PW, Butterfield JH, Yunginger JW, Agarwal MK, Gleich GJ. Allergen-controlled study of intranasal immunotherapy for ragweed hay fever. *J Allergy Clin Immunol* 1983; *71:*454-60.
78. Trede NS, Urbanek R. Combination of parenteral and oral immunotherapy in grass pollen-allergic children. A double-blind controlled study of clinical and immunological efficacy. *Allergy* 1989; *44:* 272-80.
79. Horak F, Wheeler AW. Oral hyposensitization with enteric-coated allergens as extension therapy following a basic subcutaneous course of injections. *Int Archs Allergy Appl Immunol* 1987; *84:* 74-8.
80. Blainey AD, Phillips MJ, Ollier S, Davies RJ. Hyposensitization with a tyrosine adsorbed extract of *Dermatophagoides pteronyssinus* in adults with perennial rhinitis. *Allergy* 1984; *39:* 521-8.
81. Corrado OJ, Pastorello E, Ollier S, et al. A double-blind study of hyposensitization with an alginate conjugate extract of *D. pteronyssinus* (Conjuvac®) in patients with perennial rhinitis. *Allergy* 1989; *44:* 108-15.
82. D'Souza MF, Pepys J, Wells ID, et al. Hyposensitization with *Dermatophagoides pteronyssinus* in house dust allergy: a controlled study of clinical and immunological effects. *Clin Allergy* 1973; *3:* 177-93.
83. Ewan PW, Alexander MM, Snape C, Ind PW, Agrell B, Dreborg S. Effective hyposensitization in allergic rhinitis using a partially purified extract of house dust mite. *Clin Allergy* 1988; *18:* 501-8.
84. Gabriel M, Ng HK, Allan WGL, Hill LE, Nunn AJ. Study of prolonged hyposensitization with *D. pteronyssinus* extract in allergic rhinitis. *Clin Allergy* 1977; *7:* 325-36.
85. McHugh SM, Lavelle B, Kemeny DM, Patel S, Ewan PW. A placebo-controlled trial of immunotherapy with two extracts of *Dermatophagoides pteronyssinus* in allergic rhinitis, comparing clinical outcome with changes in antigen-specific IgE, IgG and IgG subclasses. *J Allergy Clin Immunol* 1990; *86:* 521-32.
86. Alvarez Cuesta E, Cuesta J. Animal dander immunotherapy. In: Bonifazi F, Antonicelli L, eds. Proceedings of the Symposium "Immunotherapy". Ancona, Italy: Il Lavoro Editoriale 1991: 86-93.
87. Horst M, Hejjaoui A, Horst V, Michel FB, Bousquet J. Double-blind, placebo-controlled rush immunotherapy with a standardized Alternaria extract. *J Allergy Clin Immunol* 1990; *85:* 460-72.
88. Dreborg S, Agrell B, Foucard T, et al. A double-blind, multicenter immunotherapy trial in children using a purified and standardized *Cladosporium herbarum* preparation. I. Clinical results. *Allergy* 1986; *41:* 131-40.
89. Vervloet D, Khairallal E, Arnaud A, Charpin J. A prospective national study of the safety of immunotherapy. *Clin Allergy* 1980; *10:* 59-64.
90. Greenberg MA, Kaufman CR, Gonzalez GE, Rosenblatt CD, Smith LJ, Summers RJ. Late and immediate systemic-allergic reactions to inhalant allergen immunotherapy. *J Allergy Clin Immunol* 1986; *77:* 865-70.
91. Bousquet J, Hejjaoui A, Dhivert H, Clauzel AM, Michel FB. Immunotherapy with a standardized *Dermatophagoides pteronyssinus* extract. III. Safety of rush immunotherapy in asthmatic patients. *J Allergy Clin Immunol* 1989; *93:* 797-802.
92. Hejjaoui A, Ferrando R, Michel FB, Bousquet J. Systemic reactions occurring during immunotherapy with standardized pollen extracts. *J Allergy Clin Immunol* (in press).
93. Mosbech H, Østerballe O. Does the effect of immunotherapy last after termination of treatment? *Allergy* 1988; *43:* 523-9.
94. Grammer LC, Shaughnessy MA, Suszko IM, et al. Persistence of efficacy after a brief course of polymerized ragweed allergens: A controlled study. *J Allergy Clin Immunol* 1984; *73:* 484-9.
95. Malling HJ, Basomba A, Bousquet J, et al. Specific Immunotherapy. Position paper of the European Academy of Allergy and Clinical Immunology. *Allergy* 1988; *43 (suppl 6):* 1-33.
96. Birkner T, Rumpold H, Jarolim E, et al. Evaluation of immunotherapy-induced changes in specific IgE, IgG and IgG subclasses in birch pollen allergic patients by means of immunoblotting. Correlation with clinical response. *Allergy* 1990; *45:* 418-26.
97. Parker WA Jr, Whisman BA, Apaliski SJ, Reid MJ. The relationships between late cutaneous responses and specific antibody responses with outcome of immunotherapy for seasonal allergic rhinitis. *J Allergy Clin Immunol* 1989; *84:* 667-77.

Chapter 17

Surgical treatment

IAN S MACKAY

Introduction

The management of allergic and non-allergic rhinitis is primarily a medical problem and some believe that surgery plays a minor role, if any at all. Medical treatment, however, apart from hyposensitization, offers no more chance of a 'cure' and is aimed at the control of symptoms. These symptoms may respond to medication alone or require a combination of medical and surgical treatment.

The philosophy of 'medical' *or* 'surgical' treatment should be discouraged. The patient complaining of nasal obstruction, sneezing and watery rhinorrhea may well respond to medical treatment alone, but if obstruction persists, surgery may be required to improve the airway while medical treatment will need to continue to control the other symptoms. It is necessary to explain this carefully to the patient prior to surgery to avoid the operation being deemed a failure.

It is important to make a careful diagnosis and treat the underlying condition and a dual medical and surgical approach can be applied both to making the diagnosis as well as the treatment in a 'combined clinic'. The intricacies of the immunological factors may well be better understood by the physician while the importance of an endoscopic diagnosis has been stressed in Chapter 6.

Symptoms

The symptoms of allergic and non-allergic rhinitis may be considered under two principal headings: 1) primary symptoms which include nasal obstruction, watery rhinorrhea, sneezing and itching; and 2) secondary symptoms, nasal congestion, post nasal drip, facial pain, headache and hyposmia.

The terms 'nasal obstruction' and 'nasal congestion' are not used synonymously here. 'Obstruction' in this situation, is applied to limitation of airflow, such as one might measure with rhinomanometry, while 'congestion' is reserved for the sensation which might result from obstruction of the ethmodial sinuses and the ostiomeatal complex. This definition is important, as many patients undergo surgical procedures to reduce the turbinates and straighten the septum in a failed attempt to improve their 'nasal block', when a more careful history, endoscopic examination and possibly imaging techniques may have revealed underlying ethmoidal sinus involvement.

As far as the primary symptoms are concerned, surgery plays no role in the management of sneezing and itching. Watery rhinorrhea, will usually respond to medical treatment, particularly now that topical ipratropium bromide is available for those patients who do not respond to other medications. If this fails to control the symptoms, however, ablation of the parasympathetic supply by vidian neurectomy may be justifiable. Nasal obstruction, where this is the main symptom, and particularly where this is the only symptom, frequently requires surgical intervention. The author, in reviewing over 1,000 patients in this group, found medical treatment alone beneficial in less than one-half.[1] Straightening of the nasal septum and/or the nose by septoplasty or septo-rhinoplasty can be undertaken and enlarged turbinates reduced. Nasal polyps may obstruct the airway and require surgical removal though this is covered in Chapter 20.

Secondary symptoms may result from the involvement of the paranasal sinuses. The mucosal lining of the nose and paranasal sinuses is continuous and it would be rare for inflammation, whether this be allergic or non-allergic, to affect one and not the other. Once the lining of the middle meatus is swollen it may block the osteomeatal complex and since the maxillary, anterior and middle ethmoidal and frontal sinuses all drain through this area the patient may be predisposed to sinus involvement resulting in congestion, facial pain and headache. Inflammation of the olfactory mucosa in the upper part of the nasal cavity may lead to problems with olfaction.

Surgery of the nasal septum and external nose

The unfortunate nasal septum has over the years probably been blamed for nasal obstruction rather more often than it deserved, the reasons for this in part being that deviation of this partition was easy to diagnose and the procedure of submucosal resection (SMR) was well-established many decades ago. The possible complications of a septal perforation, collapse of the dorsum or a flapping septum led to the more conservative approach of septoplasty aimed at repositioning, rather than removing the offending cartilage.[2] The introduction of the endoscope as a diagnostic tool, while improving the potential for unsurpassed visualization of the middle and inferior meatus, the posterior nasal cavity and inspecting nasal spurs has, paradoxically, made it easier to miss a generalized deviation of the septum, which is more easily appreciated with a nasal speculum.

The nose itself may be twisted as the result of trauma or mal-development and may require rhinoplasty or septorhinoplasty to correct the shape and function. Alar collapse may lead to valvular nasal block on inspiration. Most patients will develop some indrawing of the alar when breathing in through the nose and many can collapse the nostrils if they breathe in sufficiently forcibly. This in itself therefore is not abnormal and surgery should be reserved for those patients in whom collapse occurs at normal physiological flow rates. This can be achieved either by repositioning the existing lower lateral nasal cartilages[3] or grafting more cartilage harvested from the concha of the pinna.[4]

Surgical management of enlarged turbinates

Before embarking on a surgical procedure to reduce the bulk of turbinates, it is essential to make an accurate endoscopic anatomical diagnosis. Having excluded obstruction due to other causes such as nasal polyps and a sensation of congestion due to middle meatal pathology, the next task is to assess whether the limitation of airflow is due primarily to enlargement of the middle turbinates or the inferior turbinates. Middle turbinates may contain a large air cell (concha bullosa) which may be associated not only with blockage of the ostiomeatal complex but at times cause marked limitation of nasal airflow. This deformity can be corrected simply under local anesthesia with endoscopic control, incising the lower edge of the turbinate with a sickle knife and removing the thin lateral lamella of bone.[5]

The inferior turbinate, in allergic and non-allergic rhinitis, will often be grossly swollen due to inflammation of the overlying mucosa and in many cases this will respond to medication. At times, however, the swelling persists and some form of surgical procedure may be justified.

Many techniques have been described, some relying on scarring the mucosa by linear diathermy, cautery, laser, submucosal diathermy or freezing with a cryoprobe. Other techniques include partial trimming of the inferior border, anterior or posterior ends, radical excision or submucosal resection of the turbinate bone. No 'one-technique' is likely to be useful for all cases and an attempt should be made to assess which is likely to be most appropriate. If the enlarged turbinate does not respond to vasoconstriction it is likely that the problem is related to a bulky turbinate bone which should be reduced either by surgical trimming or submucosal excision (turbinoplasty) which aims at removing bone but retaining the medial and some of the lateral surface mucosa. Bulky posterior ends, which may be seen at endoscopy, may at times require excision. Where vasoconstrictors can produce a marked improvement in airway, a submucosal scarring technique should prove beneficial and the submucosal multiple outfracture has been shown to be helpful.

The improvement following surgical reduction of the turbinates may be short-lived. Warwick-Brown & Marks[6] followed up a large series of patients undergoing submucosal diathermy, partial trimming, or radical trimming – all with or without out-fracture of the turbinate bone – and found that although 82% felt their symptoms had improved at

1 month, only 41% remained symptom-free at 1 year, regardless of the technique used. These results were in accord with those of Jones & Lancer[7] following submucosal diathermy. Mabry,[8] however, was able to demonstrate a 75% success rate following 'turbinoplasty' with a follow-up time of 3 years or more. This technique involved a submucosal reduction of the turbinate bone.

There is poor correlation between the patient's symptoms and nasal resistance as measured by rhinomanometry. Wight et al.[9] compared the results of trimming the anterior portion of the inferior turbinate with a radical turbinectomy. The anterior end of the turbinate protrudes into the nasal valve area where it causes maximum obstruction. Rhinomanometry confirmed that, although the resistance was satisfactorily reduced in both groups, the symptom score was significantly better in those patients undergoing the more radical procedure.

Sinus surgery

Nearly a century ago, Caldwell[10] demonstrated the possible importance of the middle meatus and anterior ethmoids as the key to sinus pathology. The work of Proetz,[11] Hilding,[12] Proctor[13] and Messerklinger[14] have supported this view and nowhere is this more true than with sinus problems arising secondarily to rhinitis where inflammation of the mucosa overlying the middle and inferior turbinates may obstruct the middle meatus, predisposing to sinus infection which in turn causes more inflammation, and a vicious circle ensues.

Obstruction of this ostiomeatal complex is particularly suited to functional endoscopic sinus surgery (FESS). Nasal polypectomy, routine intransal ethmoidectomy, trimming the middle turbinate, opening the sinuses posteriorly and progressing anteriorly, can all be undertaken with an endoscope. FESS, however, was a term introduced by Kennedy[15] to distinguish 'sinus surgery with endoscopes' from the Messerklinger technique, popularized by Stammberger[16], which aims at restoring the natural mucociliary clearance mechanism, drainage and aeration of the sinuses by a minimally invasive technique maintaining as much of the normal anatomy as possible. Using an endoscope, the surgery commences anteriorly and progresses posteriorly, superiorly and laterally, but only as far as is necessary, concentrating particularly on the ostiomeatal complex, the anterior ethmoid, its infundibulum and the middle ethmoids. The endoscope affords the surgeon an exceptionally clear and well illuminated field of vision, with the added advantage of the ability to inspect recesses with angled distal lenses. Very encouraging results of endoscopic sinus surgery have been reported by many authors.[16, 17, 18]

Wigand,[17] in common with others, reported that certain patient groups could be identified as being associated with a poor prognosis, e.g. patients with cystic fibrosis, asthmatics and, in particular, aspirin-sensitive asthmatics – 31% of whom were reported as 'no change' or 'worse' – and there is still an important role for more radical procedures, which may still be undertaken endoscopically when dealing with more aggressive disease.

Vidian neurectomy

With the introduction of topical steroids, more effective and less sedating H_1 antagonists and topical anticholinergics, the need for surgery to treat watery rhinorrhea has progressively decreased. Notwithstanding this, there is a very small number of patients who, despite all attempts with medication, will continue to complain of this trying condition and for whom a surgical option may be considered.

Stimulation of the parasympathetic supply to the nasal mucosa results in watery rhinorrhea; dividing this supply should, and in many instances does, reduce nasal secretions. Malcomson[19] introduced resection of the vidian nerve via a transantral approach and this method was popularised by Golding-Wood.[20] Various other approaches have been described including a septal approach[21] and a direct transnasal approach.[22] Whatever technique is used, any improvement may be short-lived, probably due to reinnervation.

The transnasal technique has the advantage of being relatively quick and simple to undertake and can be repeated if necessary. In a series of 22 patients on whom this technique was used by the author and who were followed up for between 21 and 36 months, 13 (59%) remained better, 3 (14%) were the same, but 6 (27%) regarded their symptoms as worse.

Conclusion

Both medical and surgical treatment aim to control the symptoms of allergic and non-allergic rhinitis and can be complementary to one another. Surgical treatment plays an important role in the management of the primary symptom of nasal blockage and may be useful for controlling obstinate watery rhinorrhea. Secondary symptoms which may result from obstruction of the paranasal sinuses in the middle meatus may be corrected by minimally invasive functional endoscopic sinus surgery.

While it is often reasonable to consider medication as the first line of action, surgical treatment will not necessarily be indicated simply because the former has failed. Some symptoms are *no more likely* to respond to surgery than to medical treatment. Conversely, many patients may best be managed by a combined medical and surgical approach and medical treatment may be particularly important in maintaining any improvement gained surgically, or in preventing recurrence.

A combined medical and surgical clinic staffed by physicians and surgeons who manage patients together has proved to be an effective alliance which has benefitted both the patients and the understanding of their practitioners.[23]

References

1. Mackay I, Cole P. Rhinitis, sinusitis and associated chest disease. In: Mackay IS, Bull TR, eds. *Scott-Brown's Otolaryngology* vol 4, London: Butterworths, 1987: 61-92.
2. Cottle MH. Corrective surgery on the nasal septum and external pyramid. Chicago: American Rhinologic Society, 1960.
3. Rettinger G, Masing H. Rotation of the alar cartilage in collapsed alae. *Rhinology* 1981; *19:* 81-86.
4. Walter C. Survey of the use of composite grafts in the head and neck region. *Otolaryngolol Clin N Am* 1972; *10:* 571-602.
5. Stammberger H. *Functional Endoscopic Sinus Surgery.* Toronto:. BC Decker, 1991: 350-5.
6. Warwick-Brown NP, Marks NJ. Turbinate surgery; how effective is it? A long-term assessment. *ORL* 1987; *49:* 314-20.
7. Jones AS, Lancer JM. Does submucosal diathermy to the inferior turbinates reduce nasal resistance to airflow in the long term? *J Larygol Otol* 1987; *101:* 448-52.
8. Mabry RL. Inferior turbinoplasty: patient selection, technique and long-term consequences. *Otolaryngol Head Neck Surg* 1988; *98:* 60-6.
9. Wight RG, Jones AS, Clegg RT. A comparison of anterior and radical trimming of the inferior nasal turbinates and the effects on nasal resistance to airflow. *Clin Otolaryngol* 1988; *13:* 223-6.
10. Caldwell GW. Disease of the accessory sinuses of the nose and an improved method of treatment for suppuration of the maxillary antrum. *NY Med J* 1893; *58:* 526-8.
11. Proetz AW. *Essays on the applied physiology of the nose*, 2nd edn. St. Louis: Annals Publishing Company, 1953.
12. Hilding AC. Physiologic basis of nasal operations. *California Med* 1950; *72:* 103-7.
13. Proctor DF, Andersen I. eds. *The Nose: upper airway physiology and the atmospheric environment*. Amsterdam: Elsevier Biomedical, 1982.
14. Messerklinger W. *Endoscopy of the nose*. Baltimore: Urban & Schwarzenberg, 1978.
15. Kennedy DW. Functional endoscopic sinus surgery: technique. *Arch Otolaryngol* 1985; *111:* 646-9.
16. Stammberger H, Posawetz W. Functional endoscopic sinus surgery. Concept, indications and results of the Messerklinger technique. *Eur Arch Otorhinolaryngol* 1990; *247:* 63-76.
17. Wigand WE. *Endoscopic surgery of the Paranasal Sinuses and Anterior Skull Base*. Stuttgart, New York: Georg Thieme Verlag, 1990.
18. Kennedy DW, Zinreich SJ, Shalaan H, Kuhn F, Naclerio R, Loch E. Endoscopic middle meatal antrostomy: theory, technique and patency. *Laryngoscope* 1987; *97:* 1-9.
19. Malcomson KG. The vasomotor activities of the nasal mucous membrane. *J Laryngol Otol* 1959; *73:* 73-98.
20. Golding-Wood PH. Pathology and surgery of chronic vasomotor rhinitis. *J Laryngol Otol* 1962; *76:* 969-77.
21. Minnis NL, Morrison AW. Trans-septal approach for vidian neurectomy. *J Laryngol Otol* 1971; *85:* 255.
22. Kirtane MV, Prabhu VS, Karnik PP. Transnasal preganglionic vidian nerve section. *J Laryngol Otol* 1984; *98:* 481-9.
23. Mackay IS, Stanley P, Greenstone M, Holmes P, Cole P. A nose clinic: initial results. *J Laryngol Otol* 1983; *97:* 925-31.

CHAPTER 18

Allergic rhinitis

MICHAEL A KALINER

Allergic rhinitis is the commonest immunologic disease and is the commonest chronic disease experienced by humans. About 10-17% of the American population experiences allergic rhinitis.[1] Most patients develop allergic rhinitis during childhood and young adulthood, although at least 30% of patients develop symptoms beyond age 30. Anecdotally, patients have been seen in their 8th decade who have developed new allergies. It is estimated that at least 25-30 million Americans suffer from allergic rhinitis.[2] The disease is chronic and requires frequent physician visits. Astoundingly, allergic rhinitis accounts for 2.5% of all physician visits for all diseases. It is estimated that another 0.5% of all visits is for the purpose of immunotherapy.

Clues to the allergic nature of the disease, and to the underlying causes, can be ascertained by the periodicity of the symptoms, precipitating events or exposures, and by what helps the patient to treat the symptoms. Suspicions generated by the history are strengthened by the signs of allergic rhinitis: swollen conjunctiva, swollen and boggy nasal mucosa with clear watery secretions, and the presence of extra creases and folds below the eyes (caused by the edema and rubbing). Skin testing is an invaluable confirmatory (not diagnostic) tool useful in helping establish the precise identity of aeroallergens causing the disease complex.

The pattern of the disease is determined in part by the spectrum of sensitivities exhibited by the patient. Thus, the most common symptom complex involves seasonal allergies, worse in the spring and fall of each year. These seasonal exacerbations correspond to the pollinating seasons of the trees (early spring), grasses (late spring and early summer) and weeds, especially ragweed (late summer through early fall). Conversely, year-round allergens such as dust mites, animal emanations, cockroaches, and household molds can cause perennial symptoms.

The development of sensitivity to an offending allergen requires the synthesis of IgE antibodies directed at the antigenic epitope. IgE production is carefully regulated and requires recognition of the allergen, development of IgE-producing plasma cells and the synthesis and secretion of IgE. All of these events are regulated by T lymphocyte-derived factors, with IL-4 increasing IgE production and interferon-gamma suppressing it. The capacity to produce IgE in increased amounts is genetically controlled, and therefore allergies run in families.

Once sufficient exposure to allergen has resulted in increased IgE production with sensitization of mast cells, subsequent exposure to allergen can elicit an allergic response. In humans, the mast cell is found in the loose connective tissue of all organs, especially around blood vessels, nerves, and lymphatics. They are most abundant in the skin, upper and lower respiratory tract, and in the gastrointestinal and reproductive mucosa.[3] In the nasal mucosa, most mast cells are found in the superficial 200 μm, generally clustered just beneath the basement membrane and in the epithelium. The number of mast cells increases during the allergy season, and the number of intra-epithelial mast cells may increase dramatically. In electron micrographs of resting nasal mast cells, the ubiquitous, densely stained, secretory granules are roughly spherical, and most are 0.2 to 0.5 μm in diameter (Fig. 18.1). Most granules comprise a dense, amorphous matrix material with embedded or interspersed crystalline constituents in the form of scrolls, gratings, or lattices.[4] Scrolls are found most commonly in cells undergoing degranulation. It should be noted that, even in experimentally unstimulated nasal

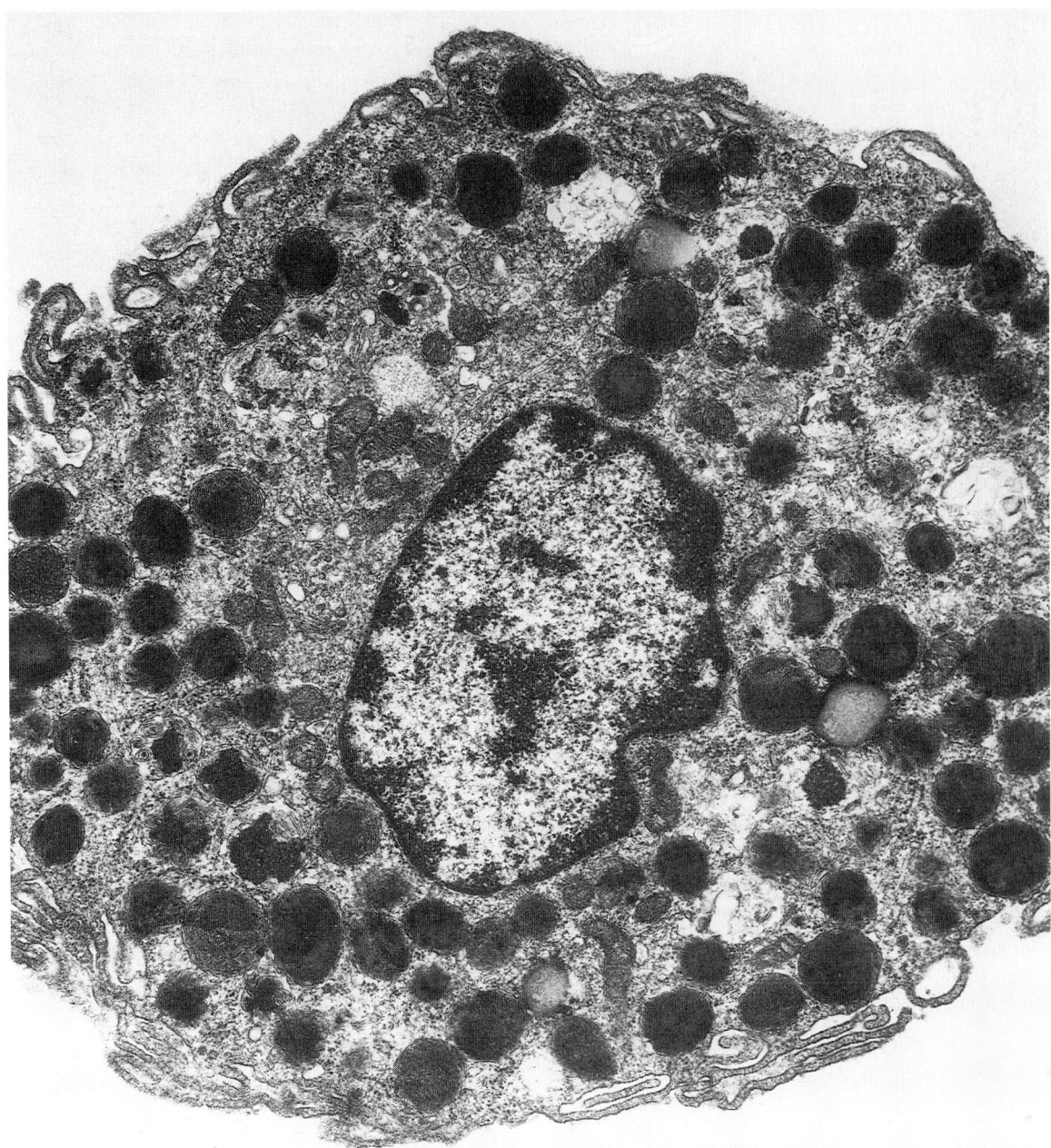

Fig. 18.1. Resting nasal mast cell. This cell is typical of the mast cells found in the most superficial 200 μm of the nasal mucosa. Each cell contains about 1,000 granules in its cytoplasm. In its resting state, the granules are amorphous in character. This cell has been exposed to the IgE found in the plasma from an atopic patient for 2 hours, but has not been exposed to antigen. Printed with permission from Friedman MM, Kaliner MA. In situ degranulation of human nasal mucosal mast cells: ultrastructural features and cell-cell interactions. *J Allergy Clin Immunol* 1985; *76:* 70-82.

tissue, variable numbers of degranulating mast cells are present. In unstimulated nasal epithelium, one-third of mast cells may be degranulated and the percentage progressively increases from the lamina propria to the mucosal surface.[4]

Early events following IgE-mediated stimulation of human lung mast cells include granule swelling with loss of stainable matrix, an increase in the proportion of granules demonstrating a scroll pattern, and the appearance of electron-dense clumps in the granules (Fig. 18.2). Granules progressively become more rope-like, with eventual solubiliza-

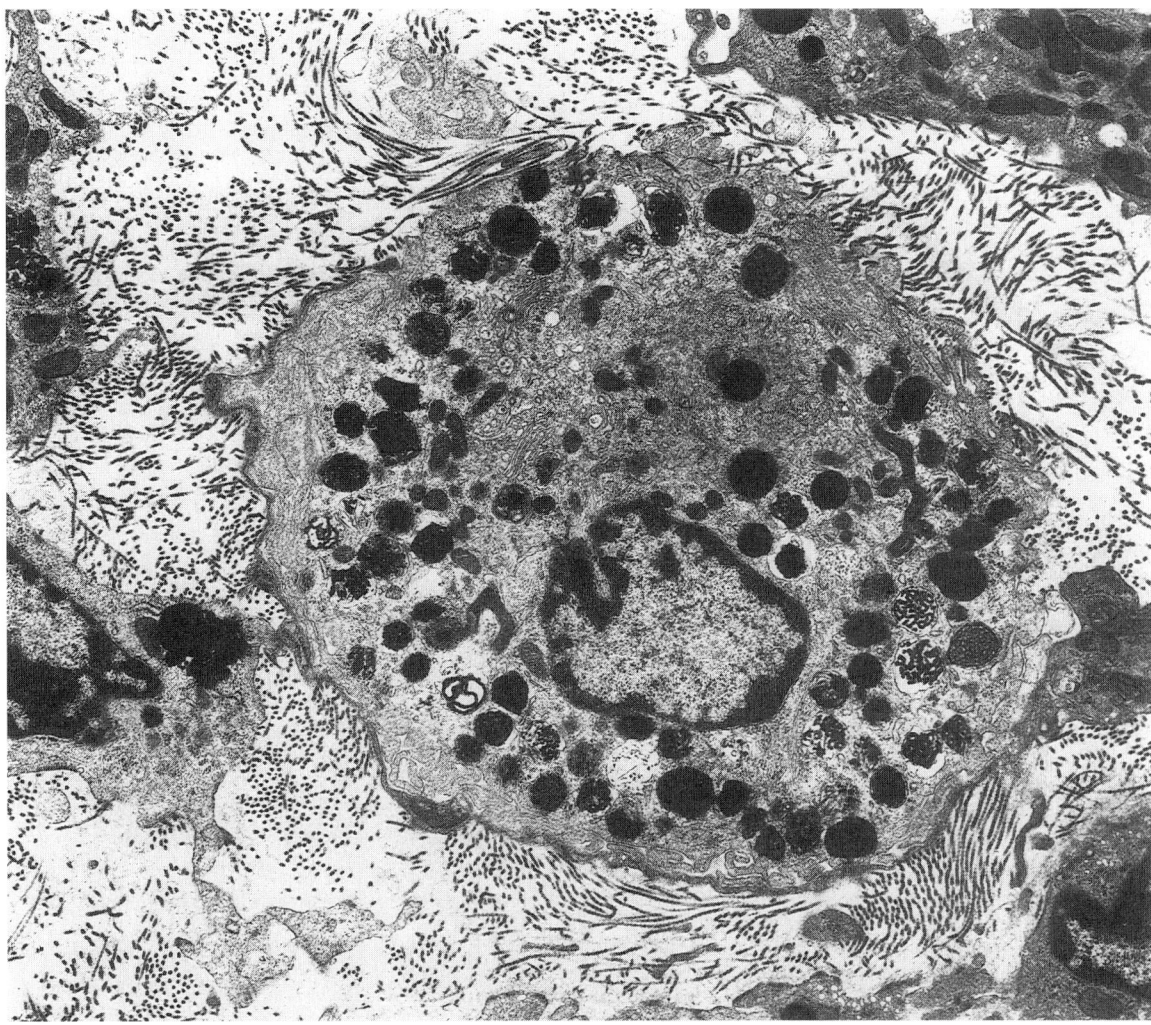

Fig. 18.2. Mast cell during the process of antigen-induced degranulation. This mast cell is undergoing degranulation initiated by a 15-minute exposure to ragweed allergen. The granules are taking on reticular and scroll-like appearances, some are entirely dissolved, and no extruded granular material is visible around the mast cell. The apparent number of granules has been reduced by their solubilization and release to the surrounding interstitial fluid. Printed with permission from Friedman MM, Kaliner MA. In situ degranulation of human nasal mucosal mast cells: ultrastructural features and cell-cell interactions. *J Allergy Clin Immunol* 1985; 76: 70-82.

tion of granule contents. In nasal and lung mast cells, extruded granules are never observed intact in the external environment of the degranulated nasal mast cell. Over the course of a few minutes, the degranulating mast cell may discharge the solubilized contents from 1,000 secretory granules into the surrounding interstitial fluid. Mast cells are found near superficial post-capillary venules (which respond with increased vascular permeability), sensory nerves (which respond by initiating the sensation of itching and elicit the sneeze reflex), and glands which respond by secretion.

The mechanism by which these responses are elicited involves the actions of the mediators of allergy, some of which are enumerated in Table 18.1.[6] The pattern of allergic reponse in the nasal mucosa usually exhibits one of two syndromes: episodic sneezing, itching and rhinorrhea; or nasal congestion. These two syndromes may overlap, although most patients will describe one or the other pattern as their primary problem. Associated symptoms include palatal and eye itching, conjunctival swelling, post-nasal drip, coughing, and the irrepressible need to sneeze.

The symptoms of allergic rhinitis are caused by the following processes (Table 18.2): 1) Vascular

Table 18.1. *Mediators of allergy selected for relevance to allergic rhinitis.*

Histamine

Chemotactic factors

Kininogenase

Prostaglandins

HETE's

Leukotrienes

Prostaglandin-generating factor

Bradykinin

Platelet-activating factor (PAF)

Tryptase and chymase

Inflammatory factors

Modified from Kaliner M, Eggleston P, Mathews K. Rhinitis and asthma. *JAMA* 1987; *258:* 2851-73.

Table 18.2. *Allergic rhinitis: major symptoms and putative mediators.*

Symptom	Mediator
Pruritus	histamine (H_1 receptor) prostaglandins
Sneezing	histamine (H_1 receptor) eicosanoids
Mucous secretion	histamine (reflex through H_1 receptor) eicosanoids PAF kinins
Swelling	histamine (H_1 receptor) eicosanoids kinins PAF
Nasal irritability	inflammatory factors chemotactic factors eicosanoids cytokines

Modified from Druce HM, Kaliner MA. Allergic rhinitis. In: Cherniack RM, ed. *Current therapy of respiratory disease,* 3rd edn. Toronto: BC Decker Inc, 1989: 16-8.

permeability causes edema fluid to collect in the mucosa causing nasal congestion and also contributing to the secretions in the nasal lumen. Permeability (Table 18.3) is caused by the actions of vasoactive amines including histamine (through its H_1 receptor), prostaglandins and leukotrienes, bradykinin, platelet-activating factor (PAF) and secondarily by the release of neuropeptides on the endothelial cells in the superficial post-capillary venules.[8, 9] 2) Mucous secretion contributes important molecules serving host-defense functions to the secretions. Glands are stimulated directly by prostaglandins, and reflexly by histamine which acts by causing the discharge from nerves of acetylcholine and several neuropeptides.[9, 10] 3) Neural reflexes stimulated by histamine (through its H_1 receptor) and possibly by other mast cell mediators cause the pruritus and sneezing reflexes, as well as glandular secretion.[9, 11] 4) Late-phase reactions (LPR) contribute to the edema and irritability of the nose. LPR are caused by inflammatory factors released from mast cells and include chemotactic factors, PAF, eicosanoids, and a number of inflammatory cytokines (which are also synthesized and released by lymphocytes).[12] These factors lead to the expression of adhesion molecules, the attraction of inflammatory cells and the infiltration of the mucosa with neutrophils, eosinophils, lymphocytes, mast cells, and basophils. This inflammation plays a major role in the increased irritability of the nose characteristically seen during the allergy season.

In general, allergic reactions occur at the interface between humans and their environments. These surfaces are endowed with a rapidly deployable host defense mechanism, the production of a copious supply of mucus, for which the mucous membrane was named. Many of the symptoms of allergic reactions are due to the glandular secretion, vascular permeability, edema and vasodilation which are really expressions of this primitive host defense mechanism.[13]

Nasal airway secretions and their constituent proteins derive from epithelial cells (including gob-

Table 18.3. *Mediators thought to cause microvascular permeability in allergic reactions.*

Mast cell mediators
   histamine
   bradykinin
   leukotrienes
   several prostaglandins
   chymase
   PAF
   reactive oxygen species

Neuropeptides
   substance P
   neurokinin A
   calcitonin gene-related peptide

Table 18.4. *Constituents of nasal secretions.*

Mucous cell products

    mucous glycoproteins

Serous cell products

    lactoferrin
    lysozyme
    secretory IgA and secretory component
    neutral endopeptidase
    aminopeptidase
    uric acid
    peroxidase
    secretory leukoprotease inhibitor

Plasma proteins

    albumin
    IgG, monomeric IgA, IgM, IgE
    carboxypeptidase N
    angiotensin-converting enzyme
    kallikrein

Indeterminate sources

    calcitonin gene-related peptide
    urea

Inflammatory mediators

    histamine
    TAMe esterase
    prostaglandin D_2
    bradykinin
    leukotriene C_4
    tryptase
    major basic protein
    eosinophil-derived neurotoxin
    eosinophil cationic protein

From Kaliner MA. Human respiratory secretions and host defence. *Am Rev Respir Dis* 1991; *144:* S52-64.

Table 18.5. *Roles and functions of human nasal secretions.*

Protective functions

    antioxidant (uric acid)
    humidification
    lubrication
    waterproofing
    insulation
    provide proper medium for ciliary actions

Barrier functions

    macromolecular sieve
    entrapment of microorganisms and particulates
    transport media for elimination of entrapped material

Host defence functions

    extracellular source of IgA/IgG
    extracellular site for multiple enzyme actions
    antimicrobial functions
        lysozyme
        lactoferrin
        IgA/IgG
        rapid development of multiple plasma proteins

From Kaliner MA. Human respiratory secretions and host defence. *Am Rev Respir Dis* 1991; *144:* S52-64.

let cells), submucosal glands (including both serous and mucous cells), blood vessels, and secretory cells resident in the mucosa (including plasma cells, mast cells, lymphocytes, and fibroblasts). Respiratory secretions consist of a mixture of mucous glycoproteins, glandular products and plasma proteins (Table 18.4). Baseline, resting secretions include the following major proteins: albumin (representing about 15% of total protein), IgG (2-4%), secretory IgA (15%), lactoferrin (2-4%), lysozyme (15-30%), non-secretory IgA (about 1%), IgM (< 1%), secretory leukoprotease inhibitor (10%) and mucous glycoproteins (about 10-15%).[10, 14-16] The functions of these secretory proteins are summarized on Table 18.5.

Increasing reactivity to inhaled allergens is one of the characteristics of allergic rhinitis. In other words, during the course of a pollen season it requires less and less pollen exposure to elicit symptoms. This phenomenon was observed by Connell many years ago and became known as "allergic priming".[17] The underlying causes of airway hyperreactivity are not clear as yet, but it is clear that LPR significantly contributes to increases in reactivity.[12, 18] LPR denotes the inflammatory response noted some hours after allergen challenge which may be manifest by airflow obstruction and the presence of increased infiltrating cells including eosinophils, neutrophils, basophils, and lymphocytes.[12] Nasal allergen challenge, under specific experimental conditions, may result in both an immediate and late-phase allergic response.[19, 20] Repeated allergen challenge increases both specific and non-specific nasal reactivity.[21] The mechanism by which LPR actually changes airway reactivity is under investigation. One recent study in a monkey model of asthma suggested that mast cell activation and elaboration of tumor-necrosis factor (TNF) led to the generation of adhesion molecules which then facilitated eosinophil infiltration and the generation of increased airway reactivity. Pretreatment with antibodies directed at TNF prevented the response.[22] Compelling arguments, however, can also be made for a role for neutral endopeptidase, increased or decreased amounts of neuropeptides, and specific actions of mediators derived from mast cells, lymphocytes or eosinophils.

The spectrum of symptoms of allergic rhinitis is therefore caused by both acute and chronic events. Therapy is aimed at these two targets, reversing the acute events and preventing the late responses which cause the chronic inflammatory changes. Although allergic rhinitis is not a life-threatening disease, it causes an unbelievable amount of morbidity, affecting the lives of nearly a fifth of the population. It has often been said that allergic rhinitis is a minor problem, unless you suffer from it yourself! Only an affected individual is aware of the distraction caused by episodes of sneezing or the irrepressible need to sneeze; the bother of chronic rhinorrhea (and what to do with the soggy tissues generated); the unbearable itching of eyes, nose and palate; and the fatigue elicited by these recurrent symptoms which may occur daily for months on end. Physicians need to be aware that we now understand this disease quite well, that excellent short-term and long-term therapeutic approaches are now available, and that the disease can be controlled quite effectively. It is a rare circumstance where therapeutic advances can make the lives of 1 out of every 5 people more comfortable! Certainly all physicians should be made aware of these advances.

Conclusions

Allergic rhinitis is the commonest immunologic disease in human experience and accounts for as many as 3% of all physician office visits for all diseases in the United States. Intense research over the past 2 decades has uncovered the underlying mechanisms reponsible for the symptomatology and appropriate treatment for the disease. Appreciation of the inflammatory component of the late phase of the nasal allergic reaction has allowed us to gain insights into airway hyperreactivity and its proper treatment. Thus, allergic rhinitis can be diagnosed and treated effectively and great improvement in the lifestyles of nearly 20% of the inhabitants of the temperate zones of Earth can be enhanced.

References

1. Broder I, Barlow PP, Hortin RJM. The epidemiology of asthma and hay fever in a total community, Tecumseh, Michigan. *J Allergy Clin Immunol* 1974; *54:* 100-10.
2. Druce H, Kaliner M. Allergic rhinitis. *JAMA* 1988; *259:* 260-3.
3. Metcalfe DD, Kaliner MA, Donlon MA. The mast cell. *CRC Crit Rev Immunol* 1981; *3:* 23-74.
4. Friedman MM, Kaliner MA. In situ degranulation of human nasal mucosal mast cells: ultrastructural features and cell-cell interactions. *J Allergy Clin Immunol* 1985; *76:* 70-82.
5. White MV, Kaliner MA. Mast Cells and asthma. In: Kaliner MA, Persson C, Barnes P, eds. *Asthma. Its Pathology and Treatment.* New York: Marcel Dekker. 1990: 409-40.
6. Kaliner M, Eggleston P, Mathews K. Rhinitis and asthma. *JAMA* 1987; *258:* 2851-73.
7. Druce HM, Kaliner MA. Allergic rhinitis. In: Cherniack RM, ed. *Current Therapy of Respiratory Disease-3.* Toronto: BC Decker Inc, 1989: 16-8.
8. Persson CGA, Ejjefält I, Alkner U, et al. Plasma exudation as a first line mucosal defense. *Clin Exp Allergy* 1991; *21:* 17-24.
9. Raphael GD, Baraniuk JN, Kaliner MA. How the nose runs and why. *J Allergy Clin Immunol* 1991; *87:* 457-67.
10. Raphael GD, Jeney EV, Baraniuk JN, Kim I, Meredith SD, Kaliner MA. The pathophysiology of rhinitis: lactoferrin and lysozyme in nasal secretions. *J Clin Invest* 1989; *84:* 1528-36.
11. Raphael GD, Meredith SD, Baraniuk JN, Kaliner MA. Nasal reflexes. *Am J Rhinol* 1988; *2:* 109-16.
12. Lemanske RF, Kaliner M. Late phase allergic reactions. In: Middleton E, Reed CE, Ellis EF, Adkinson NF Jr, Yunginger JW, eds. *Allergy: Principles and Practice,* 3rd edn. St Louis: The CV Mosby Co, 1988: 224-46.
13. Kaliner MA. Human respiratory secretions and host defense. *Am Rev Respir Dis* 1991; *144:* S52-64.
14. Raphael GD, Meredith SD, Baraniuk JN, Druce HM, Banks SM, Kaliner MA. The pathophysiology of rhinitis. II. Assessment of the sources of protein in histamine-induced nasal secretions. *Am Rev Respir Dis* 1989; *139:* 791-800.
15. Raphael GD, Druce HM, Baraniuk JN, Kaliner MA. Pathophysiology of rhinitis. I. Assessment of the sources of protein in methacholine-induced nasal secretions. *Am Rev Respir Dis* 1988; *138:* 413-20.
16. Meredith SD, Raphael GD, Baraniuk JN, Banks SM, Kaliner MA. The pathogenesis of rhinitis. III. The control of IgG secretion. *J Allergy Clin Immunol* 1989; *84:* 920-30.
17. Connell JT. Quantitative intranasal pollen challenges. III. The priming effect of allergic rhinitis. *J Allergy* 1969; *43:* 33-44.
18. Kaliner M. The late phase reaction and its clinical implications. *Hosp Pract* 1987; *22:* 73-83.
19. Naclerio RM, Meier HL, Kagey-Sobotka A, et al. Mediator release after nasal airway challenge with allergen. *Am Rev Respir Dis* 1983; *128:* 597-602.
20. Naclerio RM, Proud D, Togias A, et al. Inflammatory mediators in late antigen-induced rhinitis. *N Engl J Med* 1985; *313:* 65-70.
21. Iliopoulos O, Proud D, Adkinson NF, et al. Relationship between the early, late, and rechallenge reaction to nasal challenge with antigen: Observations on the role of inflammatory mediators and cells. *J Allergy Clin Immunol* 1990; *86:* 851-61.
22. Wegner CD, Gundel RH, Reilly P, Haynes N, Letts LG, Rothlein R. Intercellular adhesion molecule-1 (ICAM-1) in the pathogenesis of asthma. *Science* 1990; *247:* 456-9.

CHAPTER 19

Non-allergic rhinitis

ALKIS G TOGIAS

Definition and classification

Nonallergic rhinitis is a term that can be applied to any disease of the nose presenting with obstructive, hypersecretory and hyperirritable symptoms, without having an allergic etiology. This definition can be narrowed by allowing only chronic conditions to be included and, therefore, excluding acute viral and acute bacterial infections (Table 19.1).

A subcategory of treatable conditions which have specific etiologies can be further defined. Some, such as hypothyroidism, granulomatous and autoimmune diseases and tumors, are rather rare. Others, such as rhinitis of pregnancy and anatomic abnormalities of the nasal passages, are much more frequent. Symptoms of rhinitis also appear as sideeffects of systemically administered pharmacologic agents such as vasodilator antihypertensives, reserpine, oral contraceptives and other estrogens, and various antidepressants. Nasal congestion can occur as the result of topical, ophthalmic treatment with beta adrenergic blockers. As part of the classic hypersensitivity syndrome, acetylsalicylic acid and all the nonsteroidal antiinflammatory drugs (NSAID) are frequently associated with nasal polyposis and chronic sinusitis and can cause severe asthma attacks; however, rhinitic attacks also occur.[1] The name rhinitis medicamentosa applies to the rebound nasal obstruction and the pharmacologic tolerance that the vasculature of the nose develops in a percentage of patients who, for some other reason, use topical decongestants (alpha adrenergic agonists) chronically.

A number of systemic illnesses directly affect different functional aspects of the nose and may lead to chronic rhinitis of infectious origin, frequently associated with chronic or recurrent acute sinusitis. This category includes immunodeficiencies, and the immotile cilia syndrome (primary ciliary dyskinesia), as well as cystic fibrosis.

An interesting group of nonallergic rhinitis syndromes involves physical stimuli as triggers. These include inhalation of cold and dry air, ingestion of hot food and exposure to bright light. Because the symptoms associated with these conditions can be experimentally reproduced, some knowledge as to the pathophysiology of cold, dry air- and hot food-induced rhinitis has recently been gained.[2, 3]

Atrophic rhinitis represents a distinct nonallergic syndrome.[4] The classic ozena characterized by severe crusting, epistaxis and fetor is not frequently encountered in industrial countries anymore, but a less severe form which involves crusting and atrophic mucosal changes is present. Excessive nasal tissue removal by surgery aimed to relieve obstruction can result in this condition. In Egypt, South America and some nonindustrialized countries, *Klebsiella ozena* can be cultured from the nasal mucosa of patients with atrophic rhinitis.

Little information is available on the effects of pollutants and chemical sensitizers on the human nasal mucosa. Because of the well-known effects on the lower respiratory system we should assume that some forms of nonallergic rhinitis may be causally related to or exacerbated by such stimuli. More detailed information is presented in Chapter 4.

What remains is a number of poorly defined nasal conditions of unknown etiology and pathophysiology which are generally difficult to treat. Most patients with nonallergic rhinitis will be categorized under these conditions. Diagnostic workup is required to differentiate these syndromes from perennial allergic rhinitis because of similarities in the clinical presentation. The term 'vasomotor rhinitis' is frequently used for this category

Table 19.1.

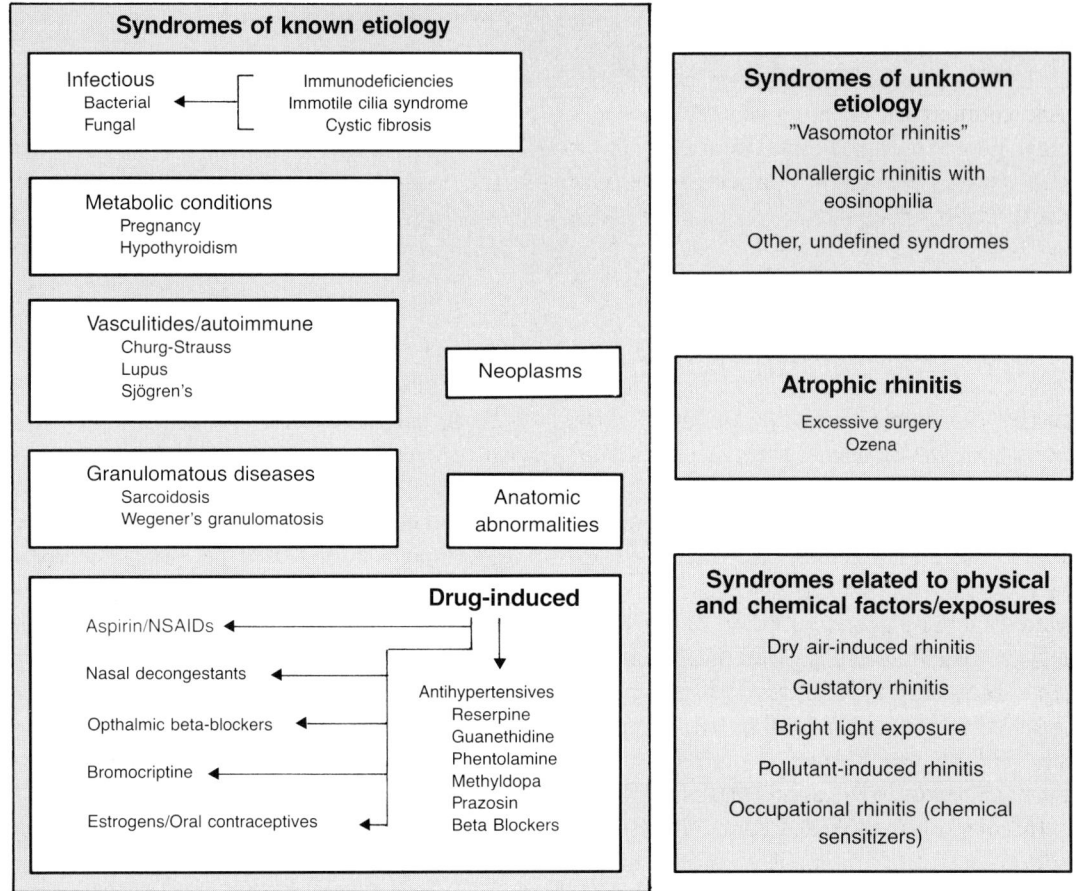

implying that the cause is a vascular/neurologic dysfunction of the mucosa. There are no scientifically sound data to support this notion and, therefore, the term is rather misleading.[5] Within the same subcategory, a syndrome that is characterized by nasal eosinophilia has been described.[6,7] Even if this criterion separates a number of patients from the rest of the group, it is not clear that the clinical presentation of the "nonallergic rhinitis with eosinophilia syndrome" (NARES) has any consistent pattern.

Epidemiology

Because of the lack of clear definitions it is very difficult to obtain epidemiologic data. Nevertheless, it is interesting to note that the U.S. National Health Interview Survey data from 1983-85 placed "chronic sinusitis" first in rank among the most common chronic conditions[8] with a prevalence of 13.5%. Since these surveys express the personal view of randomly selected individuals and since the symptomatology does not even allow physicians to distinguish between chronic sinusitis and the nonallergic rhinitis syndromes, a large number of cases reported as "chronic sinusitis" probably represent nonallergic rhinitis. Equally confusing is the report from the U.S. National Health and Nutrition Examination Survey II (1976-80) according to which the prevalence of "chronic rhinitis" is 20.4%.[9] Studies using allergy and otolaryngology clinic patient populations with chronic rhinitis report a 28-60% prevalence of nonallergic disease.[7,10-13] These numbers are based on skin testing and nonallergic rhinitis is an exclusion diagnosis. The high variability may be explained by the different techniques and reagents used in this procedure.

No sound data on the distribution of the different syndromes within the nonallergic rhinitis patient population are available.

An interesting observation relates to the age of onset of nonallergic rhinitis, in comparison to its allergic counterpart. In a retrospective study involving 362 randomly selected, new patients with rhinitis who were evaluated at the Johns Hopkins Medical School allergy clinic,[10] 70% of those diagnosed with nonallergic disease had developed their condition in adult life. In contrast, this figure was 31% for patients who were diagnosed with perennial and 26.7% with seasonal allergic rhinitis. From a different perspective, only 8.5% of patients who developed chronic rhinitis when younger than 20 years of age had nonallergic disease, this figure increasing to 34.5% for all adults and to 62.5% for patients who developed the condition when older than 40. These data are in agreement with previously published work by Mygind et al.[11] The nature of the sample does not allow us to conclude that the prevalence of nonallergic rhinitis is higher in older populations. However, it is tempting to speculate that causal relationships between some forms of nonallergic rhinitis and aging may exist, with aging-related changes of the nasal mucosa predisposing for the development of these conditions.

Clinical presentation and diagnosis

A nasal ailment can present with a rather restricted variety of symptoms. As a result, the symptoms of nonallergic rhinitis are similar to those of the allergic, perennial counterpart. One should, therefore, expect that patients will complain of nasal congestion, rhinorrhea, posterior nasal drainage, pressure or pain over the sinuses, and occasional sneezing or pruritus.

Conditions that involve neoplasms and anatomic abnormalities, as well as the topical decongestant-induced rhinitis syndrome, are mainly manifested with severe nasal obstruction and such presentation requires specific work-up. Flexible and rigid endoscopy have become the mainstay of such work-up. Notably, the suspicion for a neoplasm should increase if the obstructive symptoms are rather unilateral. Another important concept is that patients with anatomical obstruction may have nasal/sinus symptoms as a result of either sinus ostial blockade due to the primary obstructive process or as a result of changes in airflow pattern which increase local turbulence and can lead to hyperirritable areas on the mucosa. These areas may respond to nonspecific stimuli with diverse symptomatology.

The best way to differentiate between nonallergic and allergic rhinitis is to perform specific tests to rule out the latter. These can be either skin testing or quantification of IgE antibodies against suspected allergens in the patient's serum. These diagnostic methods are discussed in Chapter 9. One should emphasize, however, that a good history will prove valuable in diagnosing nonallergic rhinitis (Table 19.2).

By definition, nonallergic rhinitis is a chronic, perennial condition and the seasonal exacerbations classically seen in allergic disease are not generally encountered. However, virtually all individuals with chronic rhinitis, regardless of etiology, complain of symptoms related to abrupt changes in atmospheric conditions; the mechanism of this complaint is not understood. Also, patients suffering from cold, dry air-induced rhinitis will have a rather seasonal, winter-related, presentation.

In general, individuals who suffer from nonallergic rhinitis, other than those in whom a distinct physical stimulus is the culprit, cannot indicate specific precipitating factors. Those who do, however, will blame nonspecific irritants such as smoke, strong odors, perfumes, exposure to chemicals. This is in contrast with individuals with allergic rhinitis the majority of whom can relate acute episodes of rhinitis to a specific allergen exposure (mowing the lawn, pets, dusting, etc). The pitfall of such differentiation is that, secondary to chronic inflammation, patients with allergic rhinitis may also have a nonspecifically hyperirritable mucosa.

As mentioned previously, information on the age of onset of chronic rhinitis can tip the balance toward the diagnosis of either nonallergic or allergic disease. The clinical presentation may also be somewhat different. Our retrospective study of the clinic patient population[10] has generated some additional information on this matter: compared to perennial allergic rhinitis, a significantly lower percentage of patients with nonallergic disease complained of sneezing and conjunctival symptoms.

Table 19.2.

Differentiating nonallergic from allergic rhinitis

	History — Nonallergic	History — Allergic	Specific tests (for exclusion of allergic rhinitis)
Temporal pattern of symptoms	perennial	seasonal or perennial with seasonal exacerbations	Allergy Skin Testing Detection of specific IgE in patients' serum
Type of symptoms	congestion, rhinorrhea, posterior drainage, sinus pressure	sneezing, pruritus congestion, rhinorrhea, posterior drainage, sinus pressure	
Age of onset	70% are older than 20	70% are younger than 20	
Precipitating factors	nonspecific irritants	specific antigens ± nonspecific irritants	
Other atopic disease	not present	frequently present	
Family history of rhinitis	not frequent	frequent	

On the other hand, the complaints related to sinus disease (headaches, facial pressure) were significantly more commonly encountered in the nonallergic group. No difference could be found between the two conditions with respect to the prevalence of rhinorrhea and nasal congestion.

We also found that patients with perennial allergic rhinitis had a significantly higher association of their disease with asthma, compared to the nonallergic group. Inversely, a significantly higher percentage of patients with nonallergic rhinitis gave a history of one or more prior episodes of sinusitis.

Another finding was that a history of asthma or chronic rhinitis in a first-degree relative was reported by a significantly higher percentage of patients with allergic disease. Surprisingly, approximately 40% of patients with nonallergic rhinitis gave the same report, a much higher percentage than would be expected by random probability, based on the prevalence of rhinitis or asthma. This finding suggests that some of the nonallergic rhinitis syndromes may have a familial predisposition and is worth further research as it may help us unveil the etiologies of these conditions.

Pathophysiology

Our knowledge in this area is poor. Only in cases in which the naturally occurring symptoms are inducible by a relevant stimulus in an experimental setting can specific pathophysiologic information be obtained. In nonallergic rhinitis, these cases include cold, dry air-induced and hot food-related rhinitis, as well as the aspirin/NSAID hypersensitivity syndrome.

When patients who complain of cold air-induced rhinitis receive a 15-minute nasal cold, dry air (CDA) inhalation challenge they develop nasal symptoms, while nonsensitive individuals do not.[2] Our work in this field has demonstrated that mast cell-associated mediators are released in nasal secretions only in CDA responders after the challenge,[2,14] and that unilateral CDA provocation leads to a secretory response bilaterally, indicating the generation of a neuronal reflex. It seems that the CDA-induced rhinorrhea is to a large degree the result of glandular parasympathetic stimulation since it is partially blocked by local application of atropine.[15] The inflammatory mediators may have a contributing role in hypersecretion and may be even more important in the development of nasal congestion. In an attempt to explain the reason why only this group develops reactions to CDA we demonstrated that only these patients show an increase in the osmolality of nasal secretions after the provocation.[16] At the same time, compared with controls, these individuals release more histamine in response to a hyperosmolal nasal challenge, while they do not differ with regard to nonspecific nasal reactivity assessed by provocation with histamine.[17] Finally, we found that these patients shed a large number of epithelial cells in nasal lavage fluids following CDA challenge, compared with a nonsignificant effect in controls.[18] Taken together, these observations suggest that, for a so far unknown reason, the nasal mucosa of CDA-sensitive patients has a defect in humidifying inhaled air at extreme conditions. As a result, the osmolality of the epithelial lining fluid increases, epithelial desiccation and detachment occurs, mast cells and irritant sensory nerves are activated and a mucosal reaction ensues to restore the homeostasis of the tissue.

The picture is simpler in individuals who develop excessive rhinorrhea when eating spicy food. The reaction is purely neurogenic and parasympathetically mediated in that it is blocked by topical pretreatment with atropine[3] or ipratropium bromide.[19] It is not clear, however, whether the afferent arm of the reflex begins in the oral mucosa or in the nose by inhalation of a volatile ingredient of hot food. In pepper-spiced foods, the stimulatory substance is capsaicin.

A discussion on aspirin hypersensitivity goes beyond the scope of this chapter but it is interesting to note that recent studies involving aspirin-sensitive patients show increased sulfidopeptide leukotriene generation in nasal lavage fluids following oral aspirin challenge.[20] These and other data[21] seem to confirm the hypothesis that, by blocking the cyclooxygenase pathway, aspirin shifts the arachidonate metabolism to its lipoxygenase arm and leads to excessive generation of leukotrienes which may play a central role in causing the acute respiratory symptoms. It is still unknown, however, why only some individuals are affected by this biochemical event.

One important pathophysiologic question applying to patients with nonallergic rhinitis who do not belong in any of the above syndrome categories is whether the nasal mucosa is in a hyperreactive state and, therefore, responds vigorously to all forms of nonspecific stimulation, resulting in rhinitic symptomatology. A study by Borum[22] using nasal provocation with methacholine suggests that this is the case. Recently, in studies involving nasal provocation with capsaicin, Stjärne et al[23] suggest that patients with nonallergic rhinitis have a higher secretory response than normal controls. This effect is more evident in those presenting with the main complaint of rhinorrhea.[24] In a recent study comparing the effect of nasal provocation with histamine on patients with nonallergic rhinitis to those with perennial allergic rhinitis and to normal controls, we found that the nonallergic group falls between the allergic and the normal individuals with respect to sneezing, as well as to the vascular permeability response to the stimulus (Figure 19.1).[25] Our results suggest that a number of patients with nonallergic rhinitis have hyperreactive nasal disease and that the nonuniformity of the underlying problem in patients with this condition may explain the difference between the two rhinitic groups. It appears, therefore, that nasal hyperreactivity is a factor in nonallergic rhinitis. This observation can lead to more specific investigation into the causes of hyperreactivity which, at least in allergic disease, are largely attributable to chronic inflammation. In addition, it helps explain the symptoms that patients with nonallergic rhinitis develop when exposed to nonspecific atmospheric irritants.

Management

In the subgroup of patients with well-documented etiologies such as anatomic abnormalities, tumors, systemic diseases and drug-induced rhinitis, treatment should be aimed at the underlying problem. Therefore, discontinuation of the offending agent, surgical tumor removal, or anatomic correction may offer the solution to the problem.

Unfortunately, due to our general lack of knowledge regarding the etiologies and the pathophysiology of most nonallergic rhinitis syndromes, the treatment of these conditions tends to be largely symptomatic and not very efficacious. However, the relative efficacy of antiinflammatory treatment

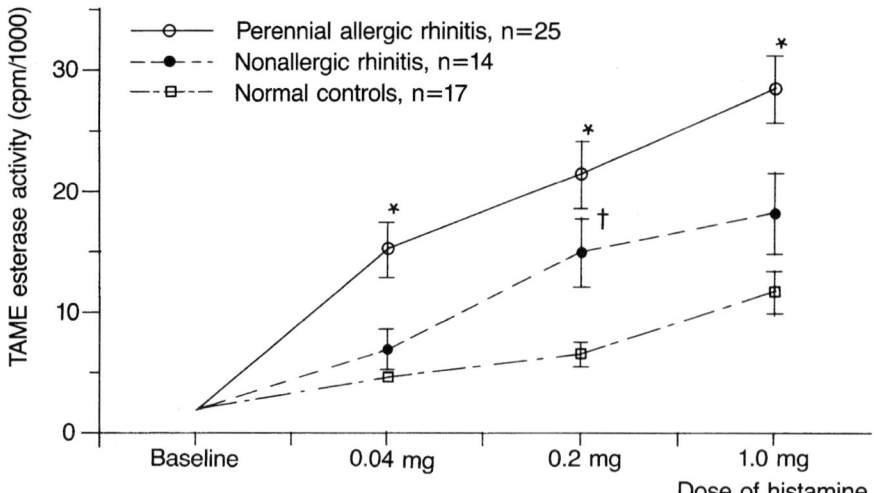

Fig. 19.1. The effect of nasal provocation with histamine on 3 distinct groups of subjects. TAME esterase activity mostly represents the activity of plasma killikrein and is, therefore, a marker of vascular permeability. cpm/1000: counts per minute $\times 10^{-3}$; *: $p < 0.001$, comparing the group with perennial allergic rhinitis to the normals; †: $p < 0.05$, comparing the group with nonallergic rhinitis to the normals.

with topical steroids has raised this modality to "first-line".

Mygind[26, 27] suggests that patients with perennial rhinitis should be generally categorized as "sneezers", "blockers" and "nose-blowers". In nonallergic rhinitis, the first group is rather rare. It appears, however, that these patients may benefit from antihistamine treatment, as suggested in a study by Wihl et al.[27] It is totally unknown how histamine is released to cause sneezing in these patients. On the other hand, the "blockers" should benefit by systemic or local decongestant preparations. The details of this form of treatment are presented in Chapter 10. Individuals who complain of excessive rhinorrhea have been treated in several studies with the local anticholinergic agent, ipratropium bromide.[28-30] This modality, which has a demonstrated efficacy, is discussed in Chapter 12. One should note that the efficacy of this agent has also been demonstrated in elderly patients with nonallergic rhinorrhea, a problem that probably affects large numbers in this age group.[31] Posterior nasal drainage is much less responsive to treatment, compared to anterior rhinorrhea. Part of this problem may be secondary to the fact that we do not understand whether this uncomfortable symptom is the result of increased volume of secretions which follow the mucociliary clearance path in the nasopharynx, or whether it occurs as a result of thicker secretions that disturb mucociliary clearance and irritate sensory nerves. In the latter case, anticholinergic agents may exacerbate, rather than improve, the problem.

Excessive rhinorrhea is sometimes dealt with by the surgical approach of vidian neurectomy, based on the series by Golding-Wood in 1961.[32] Although this approach is effective, the use of ipratropium bromide may eliminate its need. Furthermore, vidian nerve regeneration, leading to recurrence of rhinorrhea, appears to be a significant problem.

Topical steroids were probably tried in nonallergic rhinitis because of the enthusiasm generated by their efficacy in allergic disease. Although several studies have demonstrated clinical efficacy of these agents,[33, 34] a significant number of patients do not respond to this treatment. In trials involving both patients with perennial allergic and nonallergic rhinitis, it is clear that the majority of responders belong to the allergic group whereas nonresponders tend to be nonallergic.[35, 36] This finding emphasizes the diversity of nonallergic rhinitis which probably includes patients whose problem is related to underlying mucosal inflammation (most of these should respond to steroids) and patients whose pathophysiology is noninflammatory. An important finding from these studies is that the presence of eosinophilia in nasal secretions or scrapings, regardless of allergic status, is a positive prognostic factor for the efficacy of topical steroids.[36, 37] In this respect, it appears that nasal cytology may have a clinical application in nonallergic rhinitis, to provide information on whether intranasal steroids are worth a therapeutic trial. One should be cautious, however, with cytologic findings of neutrophilia. These cells may be abundant in all forms of inflammation, including infections, and corticosteroids will not be helpful in the latter situation.

Recently, some European groups have published their initial experience on the effect of sensory desensitization with capsaicin, the pungent component in pepper, in patients with intractable, nonallergic rhinitis.[23, 38, 39] The efficacy results are encouraging but potential long-term toxicity problems should be carefully addressed. Capsaicin activates mainly unmyelinated c-fiber polymodal nociceptors and generates pain sensation and CNS reflexes.[40] Repetitive local applications result in short-term neuronal desensitization which can affect several forms of stimuli (other chemicals, warmth, mechanical stimulation). In the human nose, the duration of this desensitization appears to range from a few days to a few weeks.[24, 41] The mechanism of this desensitization is not clear, although histologic evaluation in animal tissues shows depletion of the sensory nerve content of neuropeptides, particularly tachykinins.[40] In animal models, systemic administration of capsaicin leads to degeneration of some sensory nerves but, because of the reversibility of the desensitization phenomenon, there is no evidence that such neurotoxicity occurs with topical capsaicin administration in humans.[24, 41] However, this has to be more carefully investigated and confirmed.

Conclusion

Nonallergic rhinitis is a rather common diagnosis which covers several nasal conditions. In the majority, the etiology is unknown. The physician's task is to detect those syndromes that are treatable with measures aimed at the underlying cause and to differentiate the other forms of nonallergic rhinitis from its allergic, perennial counterpart. The type of symptomatology may be helpful in selecting an appropriate treatment modality. Topical steroids, which are now used abundantly in nonallergic rhinitis, may be more effective if their selection is based on the presence of nasal eosinophilia. Researchers and practitioners should follow closely the ongoing clinical studies of long-term neuronal desensitization with capsaicin. Overall, nonallergic rhinitis is not understood and the available treatments are far from optimal. More research will be required to achieve an impact on this condition.

References

1. Mathison DA, Stevenson DD. Hypersensitivity to nonsteroidal antiinflammatory drugs: Indications and methods for oral challenges. *J Allergy Clin Immunol* 1979; 64: 669-74.
2. Togias AG, Naclerio RM, Proud D, et al. Nasal challenge with cold, dry air results in the production of inflammatory mediators: Possible mast cells involvement. *J Clin Invest* 1985; 76: 1375-81.
3. Raphael GD, Hauptschein-Raphael M, Kaliner MA. Gustatory rhinitis. *Am J Rhin* 1989; 3: 145-9.
4. Holopainen E. Nasal mucous membrane in atrophic rhinitis with reference to symptom free nasal mucosa. *Acta Otolaryngol (Stockh)* 1967; Suppl 227: 26-47.
5. Mullarkey MF. The classification of nasal disease: An opinion. *J Allergy Clin Immunol* 1981; 67: 251-2.
6. Jacobs RL, Freedman PM, Boswell RN. Nonallergic rhinitis with eosinophilia (NARES syndrome). *J Allergy Clin Immunol* 1981; 67: 253-62.
7. Mullarkey MF, Hill JS, Webb DR. Allergic and nonallergic rhinitis: Their characterization with attention to the meaning of nasal eosinophilia. *J Allergy Clin Immunol* 1980; 65: 122-6.
8. Collins JG. Prevalence of selected chronic conditions, United States, 1983-85. *National Center for Health Statistics Advancedata* 1988; 155: 1-16.
9. Turkeltaub PC, Gergen PJ. The prevalence of allergic and nonallergic respiratory symptoms in the U.S. population: Data from the second national health and nutrition examination survey, 1976-80 (NHANES II). *J Allergy Clin Immunol* 1988; 81: 305.
10. Togias A. Age relationships and clinical features of nonallergic rhinitis. *J Allergy Clin Immunol* 1990; 85: 182.
11. Mygind N, Dirksen A, Johnsen NJ, et al. Perennial rhinitis: an analysis of skin testing, serum IgE, and blood and smear eosinophilia in 201 patients. *Clin Otolaryngol* 1978; 3: 189-96.
12. Viner A, Jackman N. Retrospective survey of 1271 patients diagnosed as perennial rhinitis. *Clin Allergy* 1976; 6: 251-9.
13. Wittig HJ, McLaughlin ET, Leifer KL, et al. Risk factors for the development of allergic disease: Analysis of 2,190 patient records. *Ann Allergy* 1978; 41: 84-8.
14. Proud D, Bailey GS, Naclerio RM, et al. Tryptase and histamine as markers to evaluate mast cell activation during the responses to nasal challenge with allergen, cold, dry air and hyperosmolar solutions. *J Allergy Immunol* 1992; 89: 1098-110.
15. Cruz AA, Togias AG, Lichtenstein LM, et al. Local application of atropine attenuates the upper airway reaction to cold, dry air. *Am Rev Respir Dis* (in press).
16. Togias A, Proud D, Lichtenstein LM, et al. The osmolality of nasal secretions increases when inflammatory mediators are released in response to inhalation of cold dry air. *Am Rev Respir Dis* 1988; 137: 625-9.

17 Togias A, Lykens K, Kagey-Sobotka A, et al. Studies on the relationships between sensitivity to cold, dry air, hyperosmolar solutions and histamine in the adult nose. *Am Rev Respir Dis* 1990; *141:* 1428-33.
18 Cruz AA, Naclerio RM, Proud D, et al. Epithelial cell detachment is observed during the nasal reaction to cold, dry air (CDA). *J Allergy Immunol* 1991; *87:* 147.
19 Østberg B, Winther B, Mygind N. Cold air-induced rhinorrhea and high-dose ipratropium. *Arch Otolaryngol Head Neck Surg* 1987; *113:* 160-2.
20 Ferrer NR, Howland WC, Stevenson DD, et al. Release of leukotrienes, prostaglandins, and histamine into nasal secretions of aspirin-sensitive asthmatics during reaction to aspirin. *Am Rev Respir Dis* 1988; *137:* 847-54.
21 Christie PE, Tagari P, Ford-Hutchinson AW, et al. Urinary leukotriene E_4 concentrations increase after aspirin challenge in aspirin-sensitive asthmatic subjects. *Am Rev Respir Dis* 1991; *143:* 1025-9.
22 Borum P. Nasal methacholine challenge. *J Allergy Clin Immunol* 1979; *63:* 253-7.
23 Stjärne P, Lundblad L, Änggård A, et al. Local capsaicin treatment of the nasal mucosa reduces symptoms in patients with non-allergic nasal hyperreactivity. *Am J Rhinology* 1991; *5:* 145-51.
24 Stjärne P, Lundblad L, Lundberg JM, et al. Capsaicin and nicotine-sensitive afferent neurones and nasal secretion in healthy human volunteers and in patients with vasomotor rhinitis. *Br J Pharmacol* 1989; *96:* 693-701.
25 Togias A, Proud D, Kagey-Sobotka A, et al. Cold dry air (CDA) and histamine (HIST) induce more potent responses in perennial rhinitics compared to normal individuals. *J Allergy Clin Immunol* 1991; *87:* 148.
26 Mygind N. Perennial rhinitis. In: *Nasal allergy*, 2nd edn. Oxford: Blackwell Scientific Publications, 1979: 224-32.
27 Wihl JÅ, Petersen BN, Mygind N. The role of histamine in non-allergic perennial rhinitis. *Acta Otolaryngol (Stockh)* 1984; *214:* 99-102.
28 Sjøgren I, Juhasz J. Ipratropium in the treatment of patients with perennial rhinitis. *Allergy* 1984; *39:* 457-61.
29 Knight A, Kazim F, Salvatori VA. A trial of intranasal Atrovent versus placebo in the treatment of vasomotor rhinitis. *Ann Allergy* 1986; *57:* 348-54.
30 Dolovich J, Mukherjee J, Salvatori VA. Intranasal ipratropium bromide to control the hypersecretion of vasomotor rhinitis: A dose response study. *Am J Rhinology* 1989; *3:* 221-4.
31 Malmberg H, Grahne B, Holopainen E, et al. Ipratropium (Atrovent®) in the treatment of vasomotor rhinitis of elderly patients. *Clin Otolaryngol* 1983; *8:* 273-6.
32 Golding-Wood PH. Petrosal and vidian neurectomy in chronic vasomotor rhinitis. *J Laryngol* 1961; *75:* 232-47.
33 McAllen MK, Langman MJS. A controlled trial of dexamethasone snuff in chronic perennial rhinitis. *Lancet* 1969; *1:* 968-71.
34 Malm L, Wihl J. Intra-nasal beclomethasone dipropionate in vasomotor rhinitis. *Acta Allergol* 1976; *31:* 245-53.
35 Incaudo G, Schatz M, Yamamoto F, et al. Intranasal flunisolide in the treatment of perennial rhinitis: Correlation with immunologic parameters. *J Allergy Clin Immunol* 1980; *65:* 41-9.
36 Small P, Black M, Frenkiel S. Effects of treatment with beclomethasone dipropionate in subpopulations of perennial rhinitis patients. *J Allergy Clin Immunol* 1982; *70:* 178-82.
37 Balle VH, Pedersen U, Engby B. Allergic perennial and non-allergic, vasomotor rhinitis treated with budesonide nasal spray. *Rhinology* 1980; *18:* 135-42.
38 Marabini S, Ciabatti G, Polli G, et al. Effect of topical nasal treatment with capsaicin in vasomotor rhinitis. *Regul Pept* 1988; *22:* 121.
39 Saria A, Wolf G. Beneficial effect of topically applied capsaicin in the treatment of hyperreactive rhinopathy. *Regul Pept* 1988; *22:* 167.
40 Holzer P. Capsaicin: Cellular targets, mechanisms of action, and selectivity for thin sensory neurons. *Pharmacol Reviews* 1991; *43:* 143-201.
41 Geppetti P, Fusco BM, Marabini S, et al. Secretion, pain and sneezing induced by the application of capsaicin to the nasal mucosa in man. *Br J Pharmacol* 1988; *93:* 509-14.

CHAPTER 20

Nasal polyps

ADRIAN B DRAKE-LEE

Introduction

The word polyp was first used by Hippocrates (poly-pous means many-footed or many feet) to describe the condition that occurs in the ethmoid sinuses. Although in the past all polypoidal nasal conditions were lumped together, the term is usually employed to describe the simple, mucous polyp and it will be used in this way here. During the nineteenth century, histological examination showed that simple nasal polyps were inflammatory in nature.

Polyps have a uniform histological character and they are usually considered as a single entity. However, the nasal mucosa is only capable of acting in a limited number of ways, and the same histological picture may be produced by a number of different etiologies.

Polyps are virtually confined to humans and occur very rarely in other primates such as chimpanzees where there have been 2 case reports, separated by almost half a century, which would hardly support the conclusion of the second report that chimpanzees might be a suitable animal in which to study nasal polyps.[1,2] The difference in incidence between species is probably due to the anatomical variations of the ethmoturbinal system in animals. Therefore, there are no animal model in which to study the disease processes.

Symptoms and signs

Symptoms

All patients have nasal obstruction which is usually bilateral although it is not always equal in severity. Sneezing and rhinorrhea are present in about half the patients and may occur together. Loss of sense of smell and 'taste' occurs in three-quarters of the cases. This is usually the most difficult symptom to treat. Excess mucus results in a postnasal 'drip' which may become green if infected. Patients complain more frequently about pressure in the nose and face rather than pain. Epistaxis is uncommon and suggests malignancy in unilateral polyps.

Signs

Patients speak with a nasal twang. When the polyps are severe, they can prolapse out of the nose but they are usually seen inside the nares where they appear as semitranslucent masses in the nasal cavity. If the blood vessels are injected and the examiner cannot determine whether the structure is a polyp then it can be probed lightly. A polyp is more motile than a swollen turbinate. Polyps are relatively insensitive because they have a poor nerve supply. Examination of the nasal cavity is improved by the use of a decongestant spray.

Severe polyps occurring in children before the facial bone fuses will force the sutures apart in the growing skull and produce hypertelorism. Polyps rarely produce bone erosion, but will if a patient develops a mucocele; the latter is very rare in polyp patients and usually arises after surgery.

Investigation

Plain radiograms of the sinuses demonstrate mucosal disease in the sinuses to some degree in virtually every patient. Surgeons who use the endoscope for resecting polyps advocate computerized scanning prior to surgery to define the anatomy and the extent of the disease.

If any unusual cause for the nasal polyps is

suspected, such as cystic fibrosis, primary ciliary dyskinesia or immune deficiency, then the relevant investigations should be undertaken. No allergy work-up is required unless a coexisting allergic condition is suspected.

Histology

Patients dying in status asthmaticus have similar histological features in bronchi, sinus mucosa and polyp tissue. Respiratory epithelium lies on a thickened basement membrane which covers a grossly edematous submucosa. The edematous nature of the stroma has been well-demonstrated histologically by Taylor.[3] If there has been repeated trauma to the polyp then the ciliated epithelium may undergo squamous metaplasia.

The submucosa contains few vessels, which are mainly capillaries; the cellular infiltrate is mainly composed of plasma cells, small lymphocytes and macrophages, and the most striking feature, which is present in over 90% of polyps, is eosinophilia. The cellular infiltrate varies within and between polyps. The role of the eosinophils in the pathogenesis of polyps remains unclear. Activated eosinophils release cytotoxic proteins, and they are believed to be important in the initiation of tissue changes in patients with intolerance to acetylsalicylic acid.[4] There is little nervous tissue in polyps.[5]

Etiology

If 'polyps' are encounted before 2 years of age then a defect of the anterior cranial fossa or a dermoid cyst should be suspected and a CT (computer tomography) scan of the cranium, sinuses and nose performed. Children with cystic fibrosis may have nasal polyps after 2 years of age.[6] As benign simple polyps rarely present before age 20, every child with nasal polyps should have a sweat test performed.

There are no comparable studies between the different racial groups. The incidence of polyps is difficult to determine but between 0.2% and 1% of the UK adult population have nasal polyps at some time in their lives.

A strong male predominance is found in all studies of nasal polyps. Figures vary from series to series but the ratio is between 2 and 4 to 1. Patients who have asthma in addition to polyps have a lower ratio,[7] suggesting that this may be a different group of patients.

Despite popular misconceptions, several authors have shown that allergic diseases are no more common in polyp patients than in the normal population.[7, 8]

The ASA triad

HL-A typing has been carried out on 29 patients with nasal polyps and compared with 106 controls.[9] The only increased incidence was in the phenotype A_1B_8 which was present in 3 out of the 4 patients who had intolerance to acetylsalicylic acid (aspirin), asthma and nasal polyps (the 'ASA triad': aspirin, sinusitis, asthma). The significance of this findings is uncertain.

Metabolic abnormalities may possibly account for the development of nasal polyps, especially those involving prostaglandins where shunting occurs from the cyclo-oxygenase to the lipoxygenase pathways. These are probably related to the ASA triad alone.[10] Work with platelets looking at H_2O_2 activity showed lower activity in the ASA triad but the study concluded that ASA was a heterogenous group of patients.[11]

Cystic fibrosis and other airway diseases

Polyps occur in at least 10% of patients with cystic fibrosis (CF)[12] and they seem to be associated with the respiratory rather than the gastrointestinal manifestations of the disease.[13] Polyps usually arise in established cases of CF. The sinuses do not appear to act as a reservoir of infection for the chest disease.[14]

CF polyps have been used to study the ionic transport over the surface epithelium and compare it with that of normal tissue taken from inferior turbinates.[15] The changes in potential difference across the epithelial membrane can be measured, and a defective ion transport, caused by abnormal Cl^- secretion, can be identified and studied.

The CFTR gene on the 7th chromosome has several mutations which produce diverse phenotypes. A study of nasal polyps in 7 non-CF patients only found a positive result with 1 of 9 gene probes

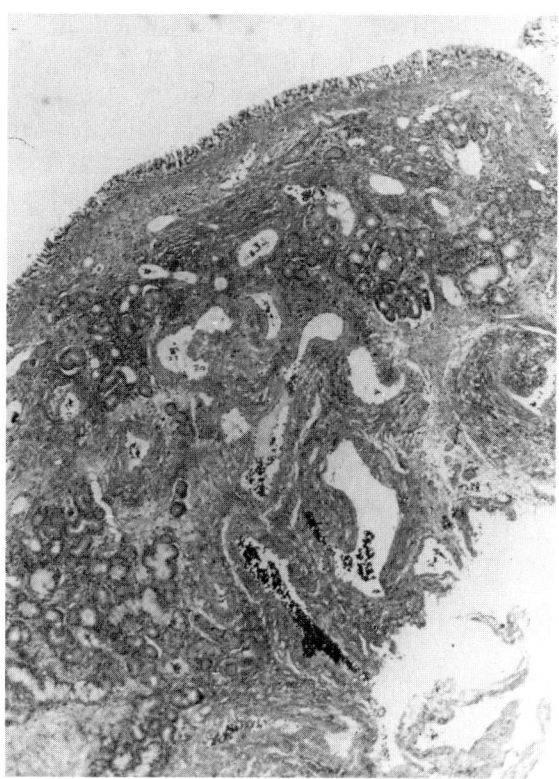

Fig. 20.1. This section through the mucosa of the normal inferior turbinate shows the large number of blood vessels. The venous sinusoids are the most easy to identify.

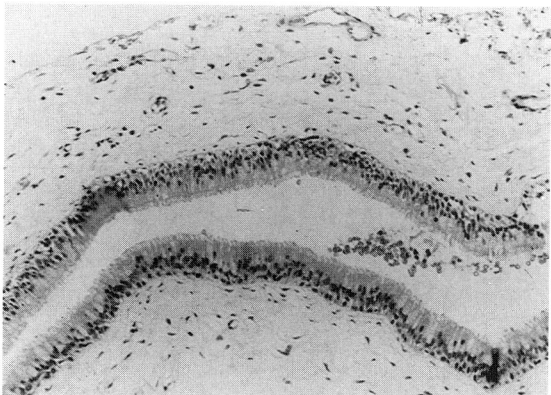

Fig. 20.2. The lining of the ethmoid sinus shows how relatively less complex the mucosa is. There are far fewer blood vessels, even allowing for the differences in magnification.

in 4 out of 112 chromosomes, suggesting no relationship between them.[16]

The abnormalities in the respiratory mucosa such as primary ciliary dyskinesia (Kartagener's syndrome), Young's syndrome and immune deficiencies may result in the formation of nasal polyps.

The association between nasal polyps and late-onset asthma, which occurs in 20-40% of patients with nasal polyps, has been well-documented by Malony & Collins.[17] The ASA triad occurs in about 8% of patients who present with nasal polyps.[18]

Blood vessels

There has been little work done on the blood supply of the nasal mucosa in patients with nasal polyps but Figs. 20.1 and 20.2 show that there are differences in the blood supply between mucous membranes in the nose and in the paranasal sinuses. This can be directly visualized when the nose and the sinuses are inspected with a Hopkin's endoscope. The linings of the sinuses are pale and transparent and the blood vessels may be seen lying deeper, whereas the whole of the nasal mucosa is pink and it is not possible to make out the deeper vessels.

Anatomical abnormalities

Whole sections of skulls can identify the anatomical variations and abnormalities but numbers limit post-mortem studies. The same information can be obtained from computerized scans of the head. Lloyd[19] studied 100 CT-scans for non-invasive orbital problems and found that anatomical variations were common (Table 20.1). The results of this study have been confirmed in a similar study of 380 persons (personal communication) using MRI (magnetic resonance imaging), which gives a more detailed presentation of the mucous membranes of the nose and paranasal sinuses. Of these persons,

Table 20.1. *Anatomical abnormalities and variations found at CT-scan examination of 100 persons examined for non-invasive orbital problems. From Lloyd G. CT of the paranasal sinuses: study of a control series in relation to endoscopic sinus surgery.* J Laryngol Otol *1990; 104: 477-81.*

Abnormality	Per cent
Concha bullosa	14
Bent uncinate process	16
Reversed middle turbinate	17
Others	5

133 had full nasal histories. There was no correlation between MRI findings and nasal symptoms, casting doubt on the clinical relevance of these anatomical variations.

Possible role of bacteria

Nasal polyp homogenates have been cultured for organisms and 24 out of 40 grew aerobic bacteria. There was a highly significant positive correlation between bacterial count and tissue neutrophilia. All cultures for mycoplasma and viruses were negative.[20]

The presence of bacterial-specific IgE in nasal polyp edema fluid has been investigated by Calenoff et al[21] but the results appear to be inconclusive. Nasal polyp tissue has been challenged with bacteria to release histamine, and a wide and variable release of histamine was seen with anti-IgE.[22] The authors concluded that bacterial allergy was only a theoretical possibility. A further indirect argument against a direct bacterial role is the dramatic response to glucocorticosteroids in most polyp patients.

Virtually every patient with nasal polyps has some degree of radiological change in the sinuses, which is not confined to the ethmoids alone. The coexisting presence of neutrophils and a positive culture from the maxillary antrum was found in 15%, which suggests a secondary role for bacteria in the mucosal changes.[23]

Pathogenesis

Histologically, polyps are characterized by massive edema and accumulation of eosinophils and mast cells. Although there is debate on the subgrouping of human mast cells, there appears to be a spectrum of cells which have metachromatic granules at light microscopy and electron-dense granules ultrastructurally. The variation in mast cell morphology in the nasal mucosa, including nasal polyps, has been well-described by Pipkorn and coworkers.[24] Metachromatic cell progenitors have also been identified in human nasal mucosa and polyps.[25] It is an important item of information that ultrastructural

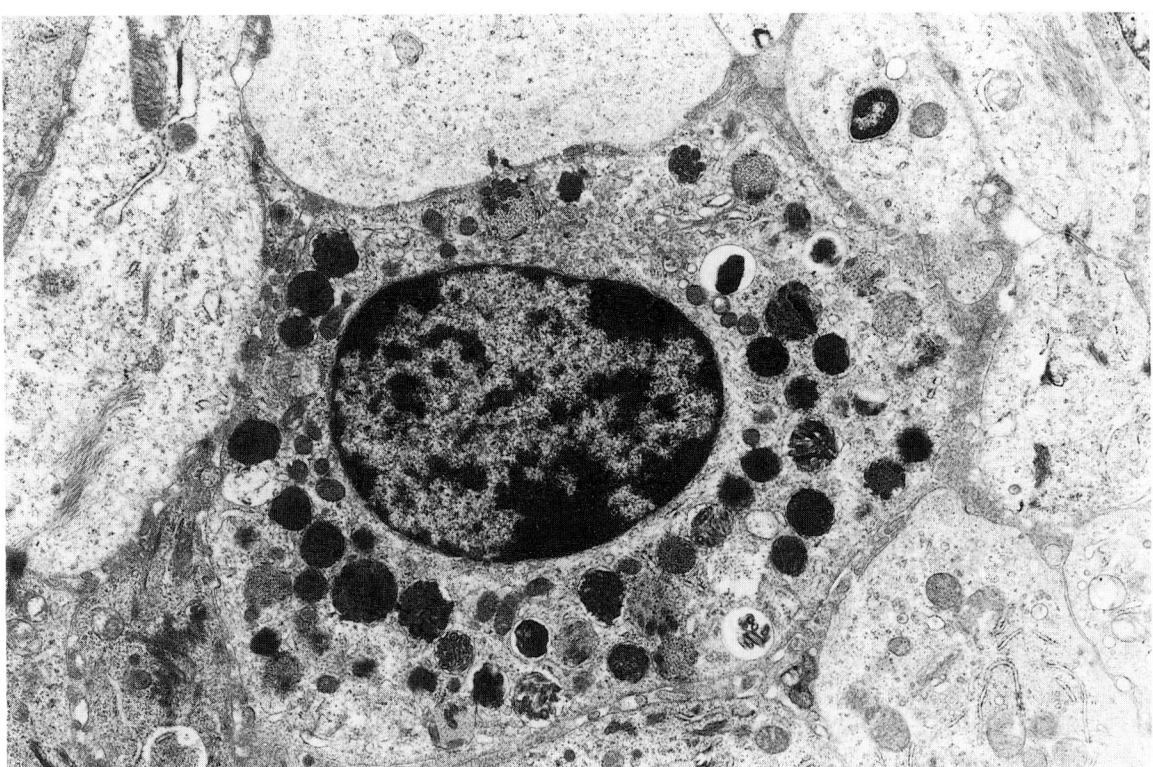

Fig. 20.3. A normal mast cell from the inferior turbinate of a normal nose. The electron-dense granules are easily identified and may be compared with the morphology of Fig. 20.4 (original magnification ×3,000).

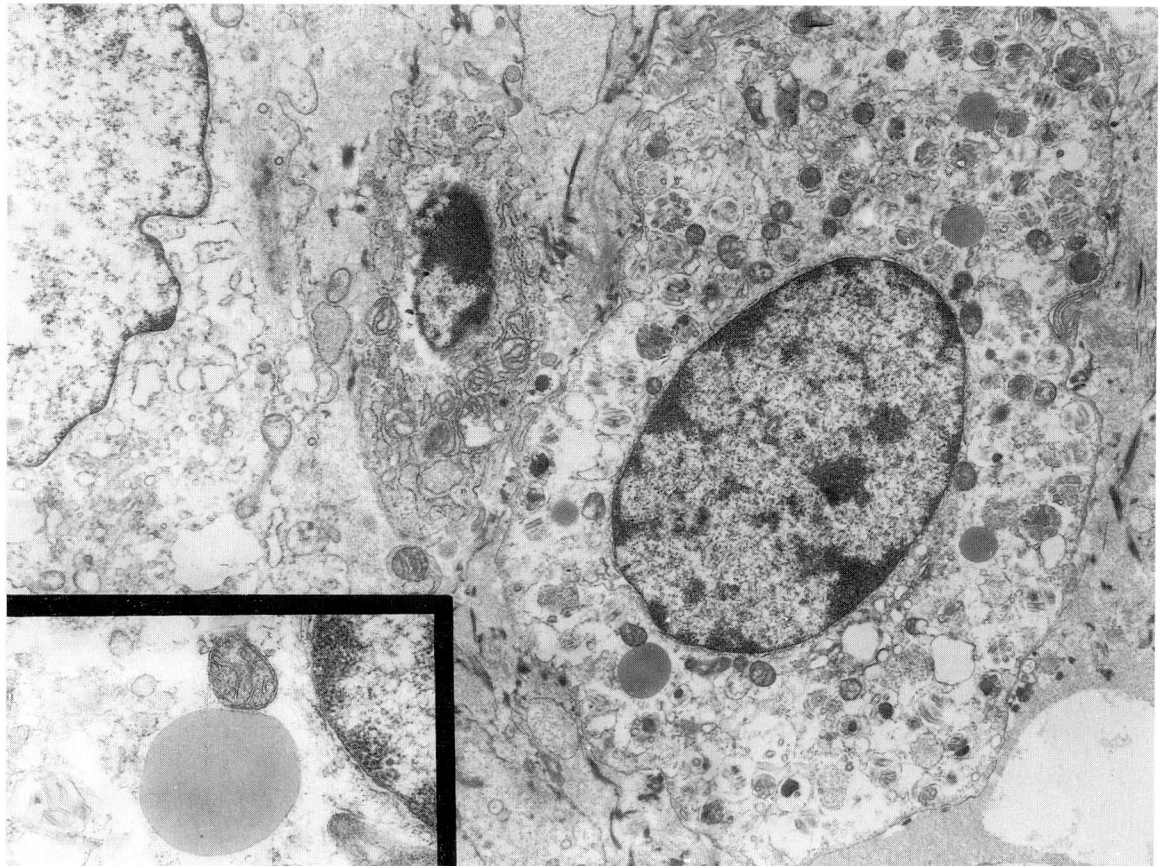

Fig. 20.4. The granules are much less obvious and this is due to the loss of architecture due to degranulation. The inclusion is a lipid body which may be found from time to time in human mast cells (original magnification × 4,000).

studies have shown that mast cells in polyps are degranulated[26, 27] (Fig. 20.3 and Fig. 20.4).

We have found a few IgE-producing plasma cells in all nasal polyps. About half of the mast cells have an intense staining for IgE, whereas the other cells appear to have very little IgE on their surface.[28]

Berdal[29] was the first to collect matched sera and centrifugated polyp fluid. Plasma proteins, including immunoglobulins, were present usually in lower concentrations than in serum. As an exception, levels of IgE and IgA in polyp edema have in other studies been found to be higher than the corresponding serum values.[30, 31, 32] High levels of IgE may be found also in nasal secretions from non-atopic patients.[33] Two studies have identified allergen-specific IgE to house dust mite and grass pollens in polyp edema fluid,[34, 35] which supports the notion of local production of antibody.

Histamine, prostaglandins and leukotrienes mediate inflammation and they can be derived from mast cells. A variable amount of histamine is found in nasal secretions,[36] but levels are far higher in polyp fluid.[32]

Kaliner and coworkers[37] used a heterogenous collection of tissue, including polyps taken from children with cystic fibrosis, and either challenged allergic tissue or passively sensitized non-allergic tissue with pollen extract, and they were able to demonstrate release of histamine.[37]

Arachidonic acid metabolites are not easy to study and quantify since they are relatively unstable and they may be generated by trauma. The results from four studies which have looked at these compounds are difficult to interpret,[38, 39, 40, 41] and there is little work on normal values in nasal tissue. Two of the studies induced the generation of metabolites by allergen challenge. It appears that the levels of thromboxanes are elevated and that allergen challenge will produce 5-, 12- and 15-hydroxyeicosatetraenoic acid (HETE), the most elevated being 15-HETE. There is some suggestion that levels are higher in patients with aspirin sensitivity but whether this is due to a more severe inflammation is not clear. Leukotriene C_4 and D_4, and prostaglandin E_2 and $F_{2\alpha}$ can also be demonstrated in polyp edema fluid. No role for any of these mediators has yet been established.

Treatment

Initial medical treatment

Most cases respond to corticosteroids. Although polyps regress when the treatment is given orally, the intranasal route is preferred because of fewer side-effects. Betamethasone drops (only avilable in UK), two each side with retention twice a day, should be tried; or an aqueous spray such as beclomethasone, budesonide or flunisolide, two puffs each side twice a day, may also be given for a month.[42, 43] If the polyps do not respond then they may be removed surgically.

Surgical treatment

There are different views on the best surgical treatment for nasal polyps. The majority of patients who have occasional recurrences may be treated effectively by simple polypectomy.

Unfortunately, no trials have ever been performed on patients who have radical surgery, despite the enthusiasms of some authors.[44] As yet, no trials have demonstrated that endoscopic nasal surgery is better at controlling recurrence but it does imply a risk of complications, particulary those of involving the orbit.[45]

Post-operative therapy

Evidence suggests that long-term post-operative treatment reduces the severity of recurrence.[46, 47] Both beclomethasone, budesonide and flunisolide may be used. Oral corticosteroids, such as prednisolone, may be required to control nasal symptoms in those patients where neither surgery nor inhaled corticosteroids prevent severe exacerbations of symptoms. Prenisolone therapy should be confined to short, 1- to 2-week periods in order to avoid side-effects.

Conclusion

Polyps are a multifactorial disease which affects the nasal lining and sinus mucosa and, in about a third of the patients, they are associated with asthma. Polyps are prone to recurrence. They may occur in other respiratory diseases such as cystic fibrosis, primary ciliary dyskinesia, Young's syndrome and immune deficiencies. Allergy does not appear to predispose to polyp formation but mast cell reactions and eosinophil activation with subsequent inflammation seem to be important and may explain why corticosteroids are effective in controlling most cases and in helping to prevent recurrence. Some cases regress on intranasal corticosteroids and do not require surgery primarily. Simple polypectomy is the treatment of choice in those cases requiring surgery and this can be followed by a corticosteroid spray in more severe cases and in those with symptoms of rhinitis. Short-term systemic corticosteroids as well as ethmoidectomy may be required in recalcitrant cases.

References

1. Nichols R. Nasal polypus in a chimpanzee. *J Am Vet Med Assoc* 1939; *47:* 56.
2. Jacobs R, Lux G, Spielvogel R, Eichberg J, Gleiser C. Nasal polyposis in a chimpanzee. *J Allergy Clin Immunol* 1984; *74:* 61-3.
3. Taylor M. Histochemical studies on nasal polyps. *J Laryngol Otol* 1963; *77:* 326-41.
4. Sasaki Y, Nakahara H. Granule core loss in eosinophils from a patient with aspirin-induced asthma: an electron microscope study. *Ann Allergy* 1989; *63:* 306-8.
5. Freedman I, Osbourne D. Miscellaneous granulomas and nasal polyps. In: Freedman I, Osbourne D, eds. *Pathology of granulomas and neoplasms of the nose and paranasal sinuses.* Edinburgh: Churchill Livingstone, 1982: 28-35.
6. Lurie H. Cystic fibrosis of the pancreas and the nasal mucosa. *Ann Otol Rhinol Laryngol* 1959; *68:* 478.
7. Drake-Lee A, Lowe D, Swanston A, Grace A. Clinical profile and recurrence of nasal polyps. *J Laryngol Otol* 1984; *98:* 783-93.
8. Settipane G, Chafee F. Nasal polyps in asthma and rhinitis. *J Allergy Clin Immunol* 1977; *58:* 17-21.
9. Moloney J, Oliver R. HLA antigens, nasal polyps and asthma. *Clin Otolaryngol* 1980; *5:* 183-9.

10 Sczeklik A, Gryglewski R, Czerniawske-Mysik G. Relationship of inhibition of prostaglandin biosynthesis by analgesics to asthma attacks in aspirin-sensitive patients. *Br Med J* 1975; *1:* 67-9.
11 Pearson D, Suarez-Mendez V. Abnormal platelet hydrogen peroxidase metabolism in aspirin sensitivity. *Clin Exp Allergy* 1990; *20:* 157-63.
12 Schwachman H, Kulcyzchi I, Mueller H, Flake C. Nasal polyposis in patients with cystic fibrosis. *Paediatrics* 1962; *30:* 389-401.
13 Drake-Lee A, Pitcher Wilmott R. The clinical and laboratory correlates of nasal polyps in cystic fibrosis. *Int J Paediat Otolaryngol* 1982; *4:* 209-14.
14 Drake-Lee A, Morgan D. Nasal polyps and sinusitis in children with cystic fibrosis. *J Laryngol Otol* 1989; *103:* 753-5.
15 Knowles M, Stutt M, Spock A, Fischer N, Gatzy J, Boucher R. Abnormal ion permeation through cystic fibrosis respiratory epithelium. *Science* 1983; *221:* 1067-9.
16 Burger J, Macek M, Stuhrmann M, Reis A, Krawczak M, Schmidtke J. Genetic influences in the formation of nasal polyps (letter). *Lancet* 1991; *337:* 974.
17 Maloney J, Collins J. Nasal polyps and bronchial asthma. *Br J Dis Chest* 1977b; *71:* 1-6.
18 Samter M, Lederer F. Nasal polyps: their relationship to allergy, particularly bronchial asthma. *Med Clin North Am* 1958; *42:* 175-97.
19 Lloyd G. CT of the paranasal sinuses: study of a control series in relation to endoscopic sinus surgery. *J Laryngol Otol* 1990; *104:* 477-81.
20 Dunnette S, Hall M, Washington J, et al. Microbiologic analyses of nasal polyp tissue. *J Allergy Clin Immunol* 1986; *78:* 102-8.
21 Calenoff E, Guilford T, Green J, Engelhard C. Bacterial specific IgE in patients with nasal polyps. *Arch Otolaryngol* 1983; *109:* 372-5.
22 Baenkler H, Schaubschlager W, Behnsen H. Antigen induced histamine release from the mucosa in nasal polyposis. *Clin Otolaryngol* 1983; *8:* 227-30.
23 Dawes P, Bates B, Watson D, Lewis D, Lowe D, Drake-Lee A. The role of bacterial infection of the maxillary sinus in nasal polyps. *Clin Otolaryngol* 1988; *14:* 447-50.
24 Pipkorn U, Karlsson G, Enerbäck L. Phenotypic expression of proteoglycan in mast cells of the human nasal mucosa. *Histochem J* 1988; *20:* 519-25.
25 Otsuka H, Dolovitch J, Richardson M, Bienenstock J, Denburg J. Metchromatic cell progenitors and specific growth and differentiation factors in human nasal mucosa and polyps. *Am Rev Respir Dis* 1987; *136:* 710-7.
26 Cauna N, Hinderer K, Manzethi G, Swanson E. Fine structure of nasal polyps. *Ann Otol Rhinol Laryngol* 1972; *81:* 41-58.
27 Drake-Lee A, Barker T, Thurley K. Nasal polyps. II. Fine structure of mast cells. *J Laryngol Otol* 1984; *98:* 783-93.
28 Drake-Lee A, Barker T. Free and cell bound IgE in nasal polyps. *J Laryngol Otol* 1984; *98:* 795-801.
29 Berdal P. Serological examination of nasal polyp fluid. *Acta Otolaryngol (Stockh)* 1954: suppl. 115.
30 Donovan R, Johansson SGO, Bannich H, Soothill J. Immunoglobulins in nasal polyp fluid. *Int Arch Allergy Appl Immunol* 1970; *37:* 154-66.
31 Chandra R, Abrol B. Immunopathology of nasal polypi. *J Laryngol Otol* 1974; *88:* 1019-24.
32 Drake-Lee A, McLaughlin P. Clinical symptoms, free histamine and IgE in patients with nasal polyps. *Int Arch Allergy Appl Immunol* 1982; *69:* 268-71.
33 Mygind N, Weeke B, Ullman S. Quantitative determination of immunoglobulins in nasal secretions. *Int Arch Allergy Appl Immunol* 1975; *49:* 99-107.
34 John A, Merret T. The radioallergosorbent test in nasal polyps. *J Laryngol Otol* 1979; *93:* 889-98.
35 Drake-Lee A. Nasal Polyps. University of Bth: Ph D thesis, 1988: 85-123.
36 Eggleston P, Owen Hendley J, Gwaltney J. Histamine in nasal secretions. *Int Arch Allergy Appl Immunol* 1978; *57:* 193-200.
37 Kaliner M, Wasserman S, Austen K. Immunologic release of chemical mediators from human nasal polyps. *N Engl J Med* 1973; *289:* 277-81.
38 Salari H, Borgeat P, Steffenrud S, et al. Immunological and non-immunological release of leukotrienes and histamine from human nasal polyps. *Clin Exp Immunol* 1986; *63:* 711-7.
39 Nigam S, Kunkel G, Herold D, Baumer F, Jusuf L. Nasal polyps and their content of arachidonic acid metabolits. *N Engl Reg Allergy Proc* 1986; *7:* 109-12.
40 Smith D, Gerrard J, White J. Comparison of arachidonic acid metabolites in nasal polyps and eosinophils. *Int Arch Allergy Appl Immunol* 1987; *82:* 83-8.
41 Jung T, Juhn S, Hwang D, Stewart R. Prostaglandins, leukotrienes and other arachidonic acid metabolites in nasal polyps and nasal mucosa. *Laryngoscope* 1987; *97:* 184-9.
42 Charlton R, MacKay I, Wilson R, Cole P. Double blind placebo controlled trial of beclomethasone nose drops for nasal polyps. *Br Med J* 1985; *2:* 788-9.
43 Dingsor G, Kramer J, Olshot R, Sonderstrom J. Flunisolide nasal spray 0.025% in the prophylactic treatment of nasal polyposis after polypectomy. *Rhinology* 1985; *23:* 49-53.
44 Hughes R. The role of radical surgery in the treatment of nasal polyps. *J Laryngol Otol* 1973; *87:* 117-22.
45 Levine H. Functional endoscopic sinus surgery: evaluation, surgery and follow-up of 250 patients. *Laryngoscope* 1990; *100:* 79-84.
46 Mygind N, Pedersen C, Prytz S, Sørensen H. Treatment of nasal polyps with intranasal beclomethasone diproprionate aerosol. *Clin Allergy* 1975; *5:* 159-64.
47 Deuschl L, Dretner B. Nasal polyps treated by beclomethasone nasal aerosol. *Rhinology* 1977; *15:* 17-23.

CHAPTER 21

Rhinitis in children

SHELDON C SIEGEL

The basic underlying pathophysiologic mechanisms, clinical features, the diagnosis and treatment of rhinitis in childhood are virtually the same as those in adults. Nevertheless, there are a few differences in rhinitis observed in children versus adults. Some of these dissimilarities relate to growth and development, prognosis, differential diagnosis, children's increased susceptibility to respiratory infections, diagnostic techniques, drug dosages, and a greater potential for prophylactic measures in children. This presentation will highlight those aspects of these disorders which primarily relate to children. Rhinitis ranks high as a common disorder that occurs in the child and often persists into adulthood. Although precise prevalence figures for all types of rhinitis are unknown, various investigations suggest that one well-defined cause of rhinitis, allergic rhinitis, affects about 10% of children, and up to 20% of adolescents and adults. While rhinitis is not life-threatening, its symptoms reduce the quality of life and cost a great deal. A U.S. National Health Survey in 1975 estimated that Americans suffer 28 million restricted days and 2 million lost school days each year from allergic rhinitis alone.[1] Physicians' bills and drug costs in the U.S. for treating this illness have been estimated to exceed 500 million dollars per year.

Allergic rhinitis

Allergic rhinitis is usually subclassified into seasonal and perennial; both types occurring frequently in children. It has been estimated that allergic mechanisms are involved in about 30% of adult patients with perennial rhinitis and about 80% of children. Allergic rhinitis has been described in the newborn period, and may have its onset during the 1st year of life.[2] Orgel et al[3] reported rhinorrhea, rather than atopic dermatitis, to be the earliest manifestation of atopy in infancy. In a prospective study of the clinical manifestations of atopic disease in infancy, Van Asperen et al[4] also observed that non-infective rhinitis occurred before 1 year of age in more than half of the 79 children they studied. However, their findings suggested that factors other than IgE-mediated allergic reactions are important in the development of rhinitis in infancy.

Usually the onset is between 5-10 years of age, with a peak occurring between 10 and 20 years. Viner & Jackman,[5] in a retrospective survey of 1,271 patients diagnosed as having perennial rhinitis found that 32% developed symptoms prior to age 10 with an established allergic cause in 64%.

As is the case with asthma, most surveys investigating the prevalence of allergic rhinitis in children and young adults have reported significant sex differences – males being more commonly affected than females. In one recent study from Denmark the preponderance of males over females was found to persist up to the age of 30.[6]

During infancy and early childhood, foods may be the offending allergenic agent. With increasing age, inhalants more commonly are the cause of the hypersensitivity reaction. However, older children and adults with pollen allergy often report hypersensitivity symptoms after the ingestion or handling of various nuts, fruits and roots.[7]

Non-allergic rhinitis

Eosinophilic subgroup

Eosinophilic non-allergic rhinitis has recently been recognized as an infrequent cause of chronic nonallergic rhinitis in children.[8] The diagnosis is established by the finding of nasal eosinophilia and the exclusion of an allergic etiology by history, negative skin tests and normal IgE blood concentrations. Patients with this nasal disorder respond exceptionally well to topical corticosteroids.

The syndrome of aspirin intolerance, hyperplastic rhinitis with or without polyps, and intrinsic asthma (the "aspirin triad") has long been recognized in adults. Recent studies have suggested that the incidence of aspirin intolerance in children with asthma is higher than previously suspected.[9, 10] The etiology of this syndrome remains unknown. There is no convincing evidence that aspirin induces the "triad" via an immunologic mechanism. The most plausible theory of its pathogenesis is that aspirin, by blocking the cyclooxygenase pathway of arachidonic acid metabolism, causes a preferential release of leukotrienes via the lipoxygenase pathway. The non-steroidal, antiinflammatory agents cross-react with aspirin in intolerant persons. Treatment of patients with this syndrome requires the strict avoidance of aspirin and cross-reacting agents. Aspirin desensitization has been reported to be beneficial in adults with rhinosinusitis; however, the procedure is dangerous and has not been studied in children.[11]

Non-eosinophilic subgroup

This diagnosis is usually reserved for those patients with chronic turbinate swelling associated with hypersecretion (non-purulent). Symptoms are frequently triggered by nonspecific factors such as temperature changes, irritants, odors and the ingestion of alcohol. A local imbalance of the autonomic nervous system with parasympathetic dominance has been postulated as the etiology. Non-allergic rhinitis of this type is infrequently diagnosed in children. Profuse rhinorrhea and marked nasal congestion in the absence of atopy or nasal eosinophilia should suggest the diagnosis.

Other causes of nasal symptoms

Atrophic rhinitis

Atrophic rhinitis is exceedingly rare in children. It is characterized by a dry crusted mucous membrane and a foul odor emanating from the nose. The etiology is often unknown and the treatment unsatisfactory. In children it is most likely secondary to removal of nasal mucosa and, rarely, Wegener's granulomatosis.

Rhinitis medicamentosa

Rhinitis medicamentosa, produced by prolonged use of topical alpha adrenergic vasoconstrictor agents, is not uncommon in children, especially in adolescent patients. Rebound congestion of the nasal mucous membranes occurs after several days use of local treatment with vasoconstrictor nose drops or sprays. Patients presenting with chronic rhinitis, no matter what the etiology, should always be carefully questioned as to the use of nose drops or sprays since the patients frequently forget to mention their use, and since other causes of rhinitis may often have led to their introduction. Discontinuation of the topical decongestants may be facilitated by stopping their use in one nostril at a time. Topical intranasal corticosteroids may also be helpful.

Rhinitis associated with systemic disorders and medications

Nasal congestion is not uncommon in infants with congenital hypothyroidism. In addition to the characteristic facial features, feeding difficulties, largely due to the enlarged tongue and nasal congestion, should help to make the diagnosis which can be confirmed by the finding of low serum levels of T_4 and T_3 and elevated levels of thyroid-stimulating hormone.

Pregnancy is obviously not a cause of rhinitis in children, but a teenager who becomes pregnant is just as susceptible as an adult to this complication. When it does occur, the type of nasal congestion can be refractory to treatment.

In adults, oral contraceptives, and antihypertensive drugs interfering with alpha adrenergic activity are also causes of nasal congestion. In children, medications are unlikely etiologic factors in causing rhinitis. An exacerbation of allergic rhinitis also commonly occurs after substituting topical corticosteroids for systemic corticosteroids in the treatment of asthma.

Recently, abnormalities in ciliary function have been recognized as causes of rhinitis in children. Both primary and secondary defects have been observed.[12] The primary ciliary disorder has been named "the immotile cilia syndrome" and more correctly "primary ciliary dyskinesia." About half of the primary congenital cases have the classical Kartagener's triad syndrome characterized by chronic rhinosinusitis, bronchiectasis and situs inversus. The diagnosis in cases not associated with situs inversus may be difficult to establish. Symptoms and signs that should alert the clinician to suspect this syndrome are: (1) a history of daily nasal discharge from early childhood; (2) chronic recurrent sinusitis; (3) chronic secretory otitis media; (4) presence of bronchitis with a productive cough; (5) bronchiectasis; (6) nasal polyps; and (7) infertility in adult male patients.

The diagnosis is established by ultrastructural examination of the respiratory cilia from the nasal mucosa or bronchi or by studying motility patterns in a phase contrast microscope. Three major types of axonemal structural defects have been described: (1) deficiency of dynein arms, (2) defective ciliary spokes, and (3) microtubular abnormalities. Lowered mucociliary clearance activity, reduced number of cells with motile cilia, asynchronous beating, and hyperfrequent beating of cilia have also been observed in patients with this syndrome.[12, 13]

It is important to keep in mind that secondary ciliary dyskinesia might result from a number of respiratory diseases. It has been observed following both bacterial and viral respiratory infections.[13]

Mucociliary dysfunction is characteristic of patients with cystic fibrosis. Recently, the identification and cloning of the cystic fibrosis gene which codes for the membrane protein that regulates transmembrane ion transport may lead to an understanding of the basic defect in this disease and to more effective treatment.[14] Abnormal ciliary function has also been observed in allergic rhinitis and in bronchial asthma.[15] Wanner and coworkers have demonstrated that inhalation challenge with specific antigen causes a further impairment of mucociliary transport rates that appears to be related to liberation of the leukotrienes.[16] Mucociliary function has also been shown to be influenced by a wide variety of physicochemical factors and pharmacologic agents.[17]

Adenoid hypertrophy

In contrast to adults a common cause of nasal stuffiness in children is obstruction of the posterior nasal choana by adenoid hypertrophy. Mouth breathing, noisy respirations, loud snoring and sleep apnea are characteristic symptoms in these children. With prolonged nasal obstruction, an open-mouthed adenoid facies becomes a common finding; in rare instances it may result in alveolar hypoventilation and cor pulmonale.[18] The diagnosis of adenoid hypertrophy is confirmed by either indirect or direct visualization (posterior rhinoscopy) of the adenoids or, better, by a lateral radiograph of the nasopharynx.

Nasal polyps

A history of progressive nasal obstruction, especially associated with a chronic viscid nasal discharge, should suggest the diagnosis of nasal polyps. These rarely occur in children; when they do, cystic fibrosis or primary ciliary dyskinesia should be strongly suspected, whereas in adolescents and adults aspirin intolerance must always be considered. The etiology of nasal polyps remains unknown. Most frequently they arise from the ethmoid sinuses and project into the nasal cavity.

The diagnosis is usually easily made on nasal examination, though the edematous nasal mucosa may have to be treated with a topical adrenergic decongestant in order to visualize the polyp adequately. Use of fiberoptic rhinopharyngoscopy in our hands has also proved to be a valuable adjunct in evaluating the presence and extent of nasal polyposis.[19] Treatment of nasal polyps usually requires surgical removal, but it is usually only of temporary benefit since they tend to recur. Topical corticosteroid aerosols have been reported to reduce the size of polyps and may obviate or delay the necessity for polypectomy.[20, 21]

Infectious rhinitis

Acute viral infections. Infectious rhinitis of viral origin is by far the most common type of rhinitis observed in children and is responsible for 50% of all acute illnesses in this age group. An average normal child gets 3-6 common colds per year. The frequency of these infections is greater in children under 5 years of age. Owing to increased exposure to a greater range of viruses and to an increased age-related susceptibility to viral respiratory infections, the frequency of these infections rises sharply when children enter pre-school or kindergarten. In general, the greater the exposure to other young children, the greater the individual attack rate for upper respiratory illnesses. When they occur in rapid succession and/or are complicated by bacterial infections it frequently becomes difficult to differentiate infectious rhinitis from allergic and non-allergic rhinitis.

Rhinosinusitis. Bacterial rhinosinusitis occurs more commonly in children than previously recognized. It may be subclassified as either acute, subacute or chronic and occurs either as a primary disorder or as a complication of some pathological process. Any type of mechanical obstruction of either the nasal passages or sinus ostia, e.g. foreign body or polyps, will usually result in this condition. We have also found sinusitis to be extremely common in allergic children (53% of 70 children) and that it often contributes to the chronicity of symptoms.[22] Numerous other factors such as immunodeficiency disorders, ciliary dyskinesia, etc., also contribute to the number and severity of rhinosinusitis. For a more detailed discussion of these factors the reader is referred to a previous publication by the author.[23]

Diagnosis

History

As in the adult patient, the history should include information pertaining to the onset of symptoms, seasonal variations, nature, duration and severity of symptoms, precipitating factors, response to medication, and complications. A history of other atopic manifestations (atopic dermatitis and/or asthma) makes it likely that the rhinitis is allergic in origin. Since a positive family history is present in only 50% of allergic children, this information by itself is of limited value in establishing the diagnosis of allergic rhinitis. In the very young child a detailed dietary history may uncover a relationship to nasal symptoms. The toddler crawling on carpets has an intimate contact with house dust mites and animal allergens. Inquiry about carpets, stuffed toys and vaporizers in the child's bedroom may provide further clues to etiologic factors. Nasal itching is a particularly bothersome symptom in children, causing nasal twitching, rubbing ('allergic salute') (Fig. 21.1), and grimacing.

Physical examination

The child with chronic allergic rhinitis can also frequently be recognized by his/her facial characteristics (Fig. 21.2) and mannerisms. Often there are infraorbital dark circles ('allergic shiners') probably related to venous plexus engorgement. An adenoid facies with open mouth is quite characteristic in patients with long-standing disease and may give rise to a high arched palate and malocclusion.[24,25] The frequent upward rubbing of the nose will often result in a transverse crease ('allergic crease') (Fig. 21.3). The lower eyelid also may have an accentuated line or atopic pleat ('Dennie's line'). The gingivae can be hypertrophic from persistent

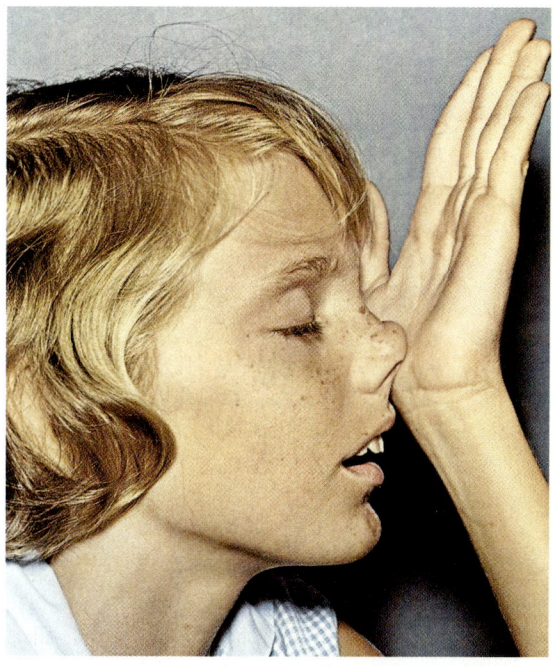

Fig. 21.1. The 'allergic salute'. From Marks MB. *Stigmata of respiratory tract allergens.* Kalamazoo: The Upjohn Company, 1972.

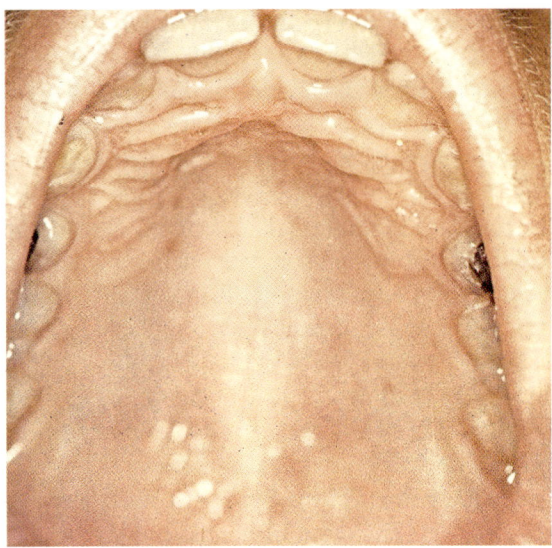
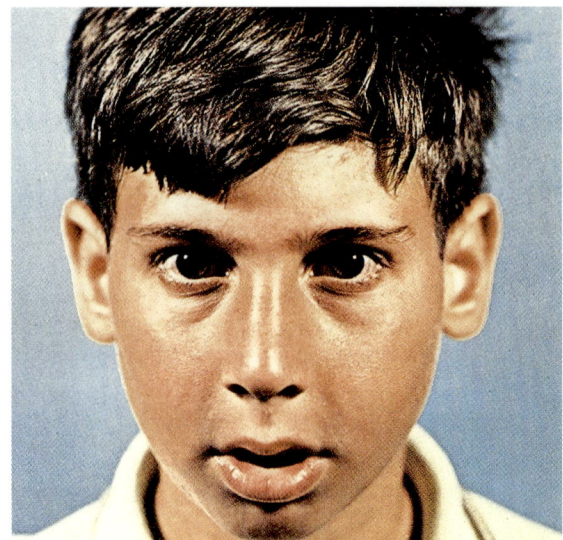

Fig. 21.2. 'Allergic shiners' and 'edema bags' in a boy with perennial allergic rhinitis since infancy (left). Chronic mouth breathing has resulted in an 'adenoid face' and a high arched palate (right). From Marks MB. *Stigmata of respiratory tract allergens*. Kalamazoo: The Upjohn Company, 1972.

mouth breathing. Nasal polyps are rarely observed in children, and contrary to previous teachings are almost never secondary to allergic rhinitis when observed in this age group. As previously stated, when they are found, a sweat chloride test must be performed to rule out cystic fibrosis.

The appearance of the nasal mucous membrane can be deceptive; a pale violaceous colored membrane is considered to be characteristic of allergic rhinitis but is not a constant finding, and some children will have a reddened inflamed mucosa usually considered the typical finding in infectious rhinitis. Because otitis media and middle ear effusions may occur with increased frequency in children with allergic rhinitis, it is essential that the physical examination include the ears. When secretory otitis media is suspected, examination with a pneumatic otoscope or obtaining a tympanogram should provide additional information on the compliance of the tympanic membrane and ossicular chain.

Laboratory tests

Nasal smear. The routine laboratory work-up for any child with rhinitis should include a cytologic examination of the nasal secretions. Usually, a smear which contains more than 10% eosinophils is indicative of allergic rhinitis.[26, 27] How-ever, it should be kept in mind that a nasal secretion eosinophilia is also seen in many patients with non-allergic rhinitis; it may be absent during periods of remission, infection, and systemic or intranasal topical corticosteroid therapy.[28] On the other hand, administration of antihistamines does not affect the presence of nasal eosinophils.[29] Studies have emphasized the importance of re-

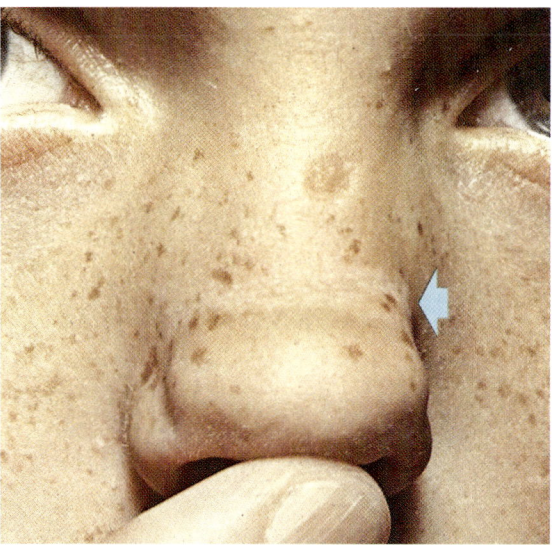

Fig. 21.3. 'Allergic crease' resulting from repeated 'allergic salutes'. From Marks MB. *Stigmata of respiratory tract allergens*. Kalamazoo: The Upjohn Company, 1972.

peating the examination of nasal secretions for eosinophils at a time when the patient is being exposed to specific allergens.[30]

The presence of basophil leukocytes and mast cells in nasal secretions and scrapings have also been reported as being indicative of allergic rhinitis.[31] However, others have shown that these cells are not uniformly found in patients with this disorder.[32]

The presence of neutrophils, especially in association with intracellular bacteria, usually connotes the presence of rhinosinusitis. Ciliocytophthoria changes in epithelial cells (margination of nuclear chromatin, nuclear pyknosis, and breakage of cilia tufts) is suggestive of virus rhinitis. Various methods for obtaining nasal secretions in children have been described. In older children, secretions can be satisfactorily obtained by having the child blow his nose into a plastic wrap or by using a cotton-tipped applicator. In small children the use of a rubber bulb syringe may facilitate obtaining the secretions. By use of either a wire applicator with a calcium alginate tip or a flexible plastic nasal probe (Rhino-Probe, Apotex Scientific, Arlington, TX), mucosal tissue scrapings as well as nasal secretions can be obtained for cytologic examination.

Peripheral eosinophilia. In contrast to allergic asthma and atopic dermatitis, peripheral blood eosinophilia is not frequently found in patients with rhinitis alone.

Skin tests. No child is too young to skin test if the history and physical examination suggest atopy. However, testing should be limited to those allergens to which the child is exposed and which will provide useful information for determining therapeutic interventions. Prick testing will usually suffice; intradermal skin testing is rarely indicated.

RAST and ELISA. *In vitro* tests to determine specific circulatory IgE antibodies – radioallergosorbent test (RAST) and enzyme-linked immunosorbent assay (ELISA) for some allergens – have been shown to be as reliable as skin testing in identifying specific offending allergens. However, it is seldom necessary to perform them since skin testing is less expensive, more sensitive, technically easier to perform, and the results can be interpreted immediately. A wider range of antigens are also available for skin testing. RAST or ELISA are advantageous in children who have concomitant dermographic or widespread atopic dermatitis.

Serum IgE. Serum IgE levels are elevated in about 50-60% of children with allergic rhinitis. In a study of 53 children with allergic rhinitis being evaluated for the efficacy of flunisolide, we found that only 56% had elevated levels.[33] Thus, a normal level does not rule out the possibility of this diagnosis. Measurement of IgE serum levels in children is rarely indicated and seldom necessary for establishing the diagnosis of allergic rhinitis. Nevertheless, serum IgE levels over 5 IU/ml in cord blood, 20 IU/ml in infants at 1 year of age and 60 IU/ml at 3 years of age are predictive that the patient will probably develop, or already has, an allergic disorder.[34]

Nasal provocation tests. Nasal provocation testing with specific allergens is rarely used in the United States to establish the diagnosis of allergic rhinitis. When performed, they are largely done for experimental purposes. Possible reasons why this procedure has not been more widely used are: (1) the cost; (2) it is a time-consuming procedure; (3) the technique is poorly standardized and results are difficult to objectively quantitate; (4) problems relating to rhinomanometric measurements. Until these problems have been resolved, it would seem unlikely that these tests will be used routinely except for experimental purposes.

Controversial techniques. It is important to mention briefly a number of controversial techniques which have been recommended for the diagnosis (and treatment) of allergic disorders. These procedures have gained some popularity in the United States and are making some inroads in Europe. These include sublingual provocation testing and desensitization treatment, serial intracutaneous titration and provocation testing, leukocytotoxic testing, the leukopenic index and pulse test, and autogenous urine injections. There is insufficient valid scientific evidence to support the use of any of these procedures in the care of patients.

Treatment

The treatment of allergic rhinitis in children is essentially the same as in adults, with only a few differences. The successful management in both age groups depends upon three therapeutic approaches: (1) avoidance of the offending allergens; (2) pharmacologic therapy; and (3) immunotherapy.

Other chapters in this book are devoted to the details of the management of allergic rhinitis. Only those aspects pertaining to the pediatric patients will be mentioned.

Environmental control

Avoidance of respiratory allergens and irritants can be readily ensured in small children since their symptoms are determined largely by the indoor environment in which they spend most of their time. Furthermore, elimination of an offending food is also easier during infancy than in older children. Because of the strong emotional attachment children have to their pets, it is often difficult to remove them from the home. More often than not, families disregard advice to remove the offending pet. When symptoms persist as a direct result of the animal remaining in the home, additional steps may have to be taken to convince the family that their child's allergy is more important than the pet.

When a family refuses to remove a pet cat, a potent allergen affecting 2% of the population in the United States, De Blay et al[35] have shown recently that vacuum cleaning with a high-efficiency filter, using little carpeting, minimizing upholstered furniture and washing the cat weekly will reduce airborne cat allergen levels. Air-cleaning devices, particularly the HEPA (High-Effeciency Particulate Air) filters also may be helpful in removing airborne allergens.

Pharmacologic management

Antihistamines. The antihistamines continue to be the primary agents used in the management of allergic rhinitis. They act as competitive inhibitors for histamine at the H_1 receptors and are most effective for controlling symptoms of nasal pruritis, sneezing and rhinorrhea. To be effective they must be given prior to histamine release and its attachment to the receptor sites. Thus, when taken on a routine basis rather than sporadically they generally give better results. In the past, because of their potential drying effects, pediatricians have been reluctant to prescribe antihistamines in patients with accompanying asthma. Evidence has been presented that these agents can be used in most children with asthma without having any adverse effects on the course of their disease.[36-38] First generation antihistamines, due to their sedative effect, should be avoided in status asthmaticus.

Despite being widely used for the treatment of allergic rhinitis since the 1940's, there have been few studies of the pharmacokinetics of H_1 antihistamines, especially in children.[39] Accordingly, the recommended therapeutic doses of these agents administered to both adults and children have largely been based on empirical guidelines. Fortunately there appears to be a wide range of dosage safety and severe toxic reactions are uncommon. However, fatal or near fatal intoxication has been reported following ingestion of large doses of antihistamines.

Children also seem to be more suceptible to idiosyncratic reactions such as facial dyskinesia and excitation. Other adverse effects (drowsiness, poor coordination, dizziness, tinnitus, blurred vision, tremor and dry mouth) are as common in children as in adults. Parents and older children should be warned about potential side-effects before allowing a child or adolescent to participate in activities that require alertness and fine motor coordination, e.g. riding a bicycle or driving a car.

Fortunately, the newly introduced nonsedating antihistamines (terfenadine, astemizole, loratadine, cetirizine) are relatively free of the sedative side-effects associated with the first-generation antihistamines and have little to no effect on psychomotor performance.

Oral decongestants. Psudoephedrine and phenylpropanolamine are the two most commonly prescribed oral decongestant alpha adrenergic agents used in the therapy of allergic rhinitis. In adults, phenylpropanolamine and pseudoephedrine tablets of 50 and 60 mg respectively are given 2-3 times daily. Exact pediatric doses of these oral and topical decongestants have not been clearly defined, and oral alpha adrenergic agents should be prescribed with care in children. In addition to occasionally causing central nervous system stimulation, insomnia, personality changes, agitation and jitteriness, they have recently been reported to cause hallucinations.[40] Employed in combination with antihistamines their effectiveness may be increased and central nervous system activity may be counterbalanced.

Topical decongestants provide quick relief of nasal congestion, but usage beyond a few days (> 3-5 days) causes rebound congestion (rhinitis medicamentosa) limiting their usefulness for the treatment of any chronic rhinitis. However, they are useful in facilitating examination of the nasal mucosa and increasing nasal patency; thus, they can be especially useful before instillation of intranasal topical corticosteroids, for decreasing obstruction of the sinus ostia during air travel and during acute sinusitis. In infants and young children, absorption of topically applied decongestants, especially with excessive use, is more likely to lead to adverse reactions.

Cromolyn sodium. Cromolyn sodium (sodium cromoglycate) (available in the U.S. in a 4% and in Europe in a 2% solution) applied topically has been shown to be effective in the treatment of allergic rhinitis in children and adolescents.[41] It has the major advantage of being free of any significant side-effects. Disadvantages relate to the necessity for its frequent administration (4-6 times per day) and that it is less effective than topical corticosteroids (see Chapter 11).

Topical corticosteroids. When the above pharmacologic agents have failed to provide adequate relief of symptoms, one can resort to the use of the newer, highly potent, topical corticosteroids. Beclomethasone dipropionate, flunisolide, and triamcinolone acetonide have been approved for use in the United States. (Triamcinolone acetonide has not been approved for use in children under 12 years of age). In other parts of the world budesonide has been extensively studied and found to be highly efficacious and safe for the treatment of rhinitis in both children and adults.[42, 43] Intranasal dexamethasone sodium phosphate is also approved in the U.S. for children over 6 years of age. However, because the absorbed part is not first-pass deactivated in the liver and produces systemic side-effects, it should not be used in either children or adults.

We have studied intranasal flunisolide in 53 children and found that 2 sprays in each nostril twice daily (200 μg/day) was highly effective in 80% of the patients.[44] We have also found that intranasal beclomethasone dipropionate administered 3 times a day in each nostril provides optimal relief in adults and that larger doses or more frequent dosing is unnecessary.[45] Once the desired effect had been obtained, the dosage should be reduced to the minimal amount that will keep the symptoms under control. Both preparations seem equally effective and no serious systemic or local side-effects have been reported (see Chapter 14).

Systemic corticosteroids. Because of their undesirable side-effects, systemic corticosteroids have limited usage for the treatment of allergic rhinitis in children. However, they may be useful in short bursts to alleviate complete obstruction of the nose, to facilitate the administration of topical corticosteroids, and to temporarily decrease the size of polyps. Short-acting preparations (prednisone, prednisolone, or methylprednisolone) should be used. The dose prescribed for children can be 2 mg/kg/day of prednisone (maximum of 30 mg/day) in 2 divided doses; after 3 days the dose is then tapered off over the next 7 to 10 days. Palatable liquid preparations containing 5 mg or 15 mg prednisone or prednisolone per 5 ml (Liquid Pred, Prelone, Muro) (Pediapred, Fisons) are now available in the U.S. for younger children who are unable to swallow pills.

Immunotherapy. Immunotherapy should be reserved for those patients who have severe symptoms unresponsive to appropriate environmental control and pharmacologic measures or if complications have arisen (see Chapter 16). Controlled studies have demonstrated that immunotherapy is beneficial in children who have a proven IgE response to specific allergens and who are able to tolerate high doses of injected allergens for several months.[46] Since clinical benefit from immunotherapy usually results in only a partial amelioration of symptoms and not a "complete cure", and is an expensive and time-consuming modality of therapy, it must not be used indiscriminately and should be prescribed only when clearly indicated. It is rarely necessary in the young child.

Conclusion

Rhinitis is a very common disorder in children and often persists into adulthood. To be successfully treated, the various causes of rhinitis must be recognized. Allergy and infection are the most frequent causes of rhinitis in children. Other recognized causes include eosinophilic non-allergic rhinitis, non-eosinophilic non-allergic rhinitis, atrophic rhinitis, rhinitis medicamentosa, and rhinitis associated with systemic disorders, medications, mechanical obstruction and abnormalities of ciliary function. The diagnosis of allergic rhinitis can usually be established by history and physical examination alone. Allergy skin tests or *in vitro* tests may be useful in identifying specific IgE offending allergens.

Treatment of allergic rhinitis in children is essentially the same as in adults: namely, 1) environmental control, 2) pharmacologic therapy and 3) immunotherapy. Avoidance of allergens remains the cornerstone of therapy. Recent advances in pharmacologic therapy, including the new nonsedating antihistamines and topical corticosteroids, have greatly improved our ability to provide symptomatic relief. In recalcitrant cases unresponsive to environmental control and pharmacologic measures, immunotherapy should be considered.

References

1. U.S. National Health Survey, Series 10, No. 100, September 1975.
2. Ingall M, Glaser J, Meltzer RS, Dreyfuss EM. Allergic rhinitis in early infancy. *Pediatrics* 1965; *35:* 108.
3. Orgel H, Kemp J, Meltzer E. Atopy and IgE in a pediatric practice. *Ann Allergy* 1977; *39:* 161.
4. Van Asperen PP, Andrew SK, Mellis GM. A prospective study of the clinical manifestations of atopic disease in infancy. *Acta Paediatr Scand* 1984; *73:* 80.
5. Viner AS, Jackman N. Retrospective survey of 1271 patients diagnosed as perennial rhinitis. *Clin Allergy* 1976; *6:* 251.
6. Pedersen PA, Weeke ER. Allergic rhinitis in Danish general practice: Prevalence and consultation rates. *Allergy* 1981; *36:* 375.
7. Løwenstein H, Eriksson NE. Hypersensitivity to foods among birch pollen-allergic patients. *Allergy* 1983; *38:* 577.
8. Rupp GH, Freidman AA. Eosinophilic nonallergic rhinitis in children. *Pediatrics* 1982; *70:* 437.
9. Rachelefsky GS, Coulson A, Siegel SC, Stiehm ER. Aspirin intolerance in chronic childhood asthma: detected by oral challenge. *Pediatrics* 1975; *56:* 443.
10. Weinberger M. Analgesic sensitivity in children with asthma. *Pediatrics* 1978; *62 (suppl):* 910.
11. Stevenson DD, Pleskow WW, Simon RA, et al. Aspirin-sensitive rhinosinusitis asthma: A double-blind cross-over study of treatment with aspirin. *J Allergy Clin Immunol* 1981; *73:* 500.
12. Mygind N, Pedersen M, Nielsen MH. Primary and secondary ciliary dyskinesia. *Acta Otolaryngol (Stockh)* 1983; *95:* 688.
13. Karja J, Nuutinen J. Immotile cilia syndrome in children. *Int J Ped Otorhinolaryngol* 1983; *5:* 72.
14. Rich DP, Anderson MP, Gregory RJ. Expression of cystic fibrosis-transmembrane conductance regulator corrects defective chloride channel regulation in cystic fibrosis airway epithelial cells. *Nature* 1990; *347:* 382.
15. Mygind N, Bretlau P. Scanning electron microscopic studies of the human nasal mucosa in normal persons and in patients with perennial rhinitis. *Acta Allergol* 1973; *28:* 9.
16. Wanner A. Allergic mucociliary dysfunction. *Laryngoscope* 1983; *93:* 68.
17. Irvani J, Melville GN. Mucociliary function in the respiratory tracts as influenced by physiochemical factors. In: Widdicombe JG, ed. *Respiratory pharmacology.* New York: Permagon Press, 1981: 477.
18. Myer C 111, Cotton RT. Nasal obstruction in the pediatric patient. *Pediatrics* 1983; *72:* 766.
19. Rohr A, Hassner A, Saxon A. Rhinopharyngoscopy for the elevation of allergic immunologic disorders. *Ann Allergy* 1983; *50:* 380.
20. Mygind N, Petersen CG, Prytz S, Sørensen H. Treatment of nasal polyps with intranasal beclomethasone dipropionate aerosol. *Clin Allergy* 1975; *5:* 159.
21. Mygind N. Nasal Polyposis. *J Allergy Clin Immunol* 1990; *86:* 877.
22. Rachelefsky GS, Goldberg M, Katz RM, et al. Sinus disease in children with respiratory allergy. *J Allergy Clin Immunol* 1978; *61:* 310.
23. Seigel SC. Recurrent and chronic upper respiratory infections and chronic otitis media. In: Bierman CW, Pearlman DS, eds. *Allergic disease of infancy, childhood and adolescence.* Philadelphia: WB Saunders, 1980: 715.
24. Marks AB. The gaping allergic child. *Ann Allergy* 1965; *23:* 616.
25. Trask GM, Shapiro PA. Nasal obstruction and facial development. In: Naspitz CK, Tinkelman DG, eds. *Childhood rhinitis and sinusitis,* New York: Marcel Dekker, 1990: 217.
26. Miller RE, Paradise JL, Friday GA, Fireman P, Voith D. The nasal smear for eosinophils. Its value in children with seasonal allergic rhinitis. *Am J Dis Child* 1982; *34:* 1009.
27. Malmberg H, Holopainen E. Nasal smear as a screening test for immediate type nasal allergy. *Allergy* 1979; *34:* 331.
28. Goldenhersh MJ, Rachelefsky GS, Dudley J, et al. The microbiology of chronic sinus disease in children with respiratory allergy. *J Allergy Clin Immunol* 1990: *85:* 1030.
29. Smith RE, Casanova-Roig R, Wells DE. Effect of antihistamines on nasal smear eosinophils in patients with allergic rhinitis. *Ann Allergy* 1968; *26:* 80.
30. Pelikan Z. The changes in the nasal secretions of eosinophils during the immediate nasal response to allergen challenge. *J Allergy Clin Immunol* 1983; *72:* 657.
31. Okuda M, Kawabori S, Ohtsuka H. Basophil leukocytes and mast cells in the nose. *Eur J Resp Dis* 1983; *64 (suppl 128):* 65.

32 Wihl JÅ, Brofeldt S, Grønborg H, Borum P, Mygind N. Blind study of basophilic cells in nasal smears from patients with grass pollen hayfever. *Eur J Respir Dis* 1983; *64 (suppl 128):* 383.
33 Siegel SC. Unpublished data.
34 Hamburger RN. The immunogenetics of IgE provides predictive value for the development of allergy. *Ann Allergy* 1982; *49:* 9.
35 De Blay F, Chapman MD, Platts-Mills TAE. Airborne cat allergen (Fel d1), environmental control with the cat in situ. *Am Rev Respir Dis* 1991; *143:* 1334.
36 Karlin JM. The use of antihistamines in asthma. *Ann Allergy* 1972; *30:* 342.
37 Schuller DE. Adverse effects of brompheniramine on pulmonary function in a subset of asthmatic children. *J Allergy Clin Immunol* 1983; *72:* 175.
38 Clark TJH. Histamine antagonists and asthma. *Pharmac Ther* 1982; *17:* 239.
39 Simons EER, Simons KJ. H1 receptor antagonists clinical pharmacology and use in allergic disease. *Pediatr Clin N Am* 1983; *30:* 899.
40 Editorial comment. More on hallucinations in children receiving decongestants. *Pediatric Alert* 1984; *9:* 49.
41 Backman A, Holopainen E, Salo OP. Sodium cromoglycate in chronic allergic rhinitis. *Acta Allergol* 1977; *13 (suppl):* 55.
42 Day JH, Andersson B, Briscoe MP. Efficacy and safety of intranasal budesonide in the treatment of perennial rhinitis in adults and children. *Ann Allergy* 1990; *64:* 445.
43 Clissold SP. Rhinitis. In: Barnes P, Mygind N, eds. *Budesonide. Clinical experience in asthma and rhinitis.* Mancheste: Adis Press, 1988: 51.
44 Siegel SC. Clinical results with flunisolide. In: Norman PS, ed. *Allergic Rhinitis: The state of the art.* New Jersey, Princeton Junction: Communication Media for Education, 1982: 33.
45 Siegel SC, Katz RM, Rachelefsky GS, et al. Multicentric study of beclomethasone dipropionate nasal aerosol in adults with seasonal allergic rhinitis. *J Allergy, Clin Immunol* 1982; *69:* 345.
46 Zeiger RS, Schatz M. Immunotherapy of atopic disorders. Present state of the art and future perspectives. *Med Clin N Am* 1986; *65:* 987.

CHAPTER 22

Rhinitis and asthma

RONALD DAHL

Introduction

Bronchial asthma and rhinitis belong to the group of diseases that, several years ago, were named atopic disorders, which means strange and unexplainable diseases. The atopic disorders frequently occur in the same individual. The reason for the co-existence of disorders from different organ systems can still only be partly explained. Allergy frequently occurs in atopic diseases, but not invariably. In a way it has been unfortunate that, during recent years, atopy and allergy have become synonyms, which has not helped in the understanding of the disease or the attitude towards diagnoses and treatment. In the following chapter, similarities and differences between rhinitis and asthma will be considered.

Epidemiology

Asthma and rhinitis are diseases found all over the world, but the frequency varies widely. Asthma is the most frequent chronic disease in childhood in the western world. The true prevalences of asthma in adults are difficult to establish precisely because internationally accepted criteria for definition and classification of asthma, in contrast to other obstructive lung diseases and lung symptoms, do not exist. It may be difficult to compare epidemiological data from different parts of the world because studies have been performed with different protocols with different questions and tests performed. In children, published data on asthma prevalence as a history of asthma at any time varies from almost 0 in Gambia, Africa[1] to 17% in New Zealand, in 12-year-old schoolchildren.[2] In Europe the asthma prevalence has been reported also to vary widely, between 1.4% in Switzerland[3] and 9.3% in England.[4] The prevalence of asthma in children and young adults seems to have risen during the last 20-30 years. In Sweden, asthma increased from 1.9 to 2.8% during the years 1971 to 1981,[5] in Finnish young men, asthma prevalence seemed to increase from 0.3% to 1.8% between 1966 and 1989[6], and in Melbourne schoolchildren the prevalence of a history of asthma among 7-year-olds had increased from 19.1% in 1964 to 46% in 1986.[7]

These studies are supported by a very strong increase in the hospitalization rate for acute asthma since the 1970s.[8]

Rhinitis is even more common than bronchial asthma and geographical variation in the prevalence of rhinitis also occurs. Seasonal allergic rhinitis is especially frequent in children from puberty and in young adults, and the prevalence in Danish students was 15%,[9] but even higher prevalence figures have been reported from the USA.[10]

Similar to asthma, increased prevalence of rhinitis seems to have occurred during the last 2 or 3 decades. The prevalence of allergic rhinitis increased from 4.4% to 8.4% in Swedish conscripts during the years 1971 to 1981[5] and a similar increased prevalence seems to have occurred throughout the western world. It is very strange that allergic rhinitis was practically unknown 200 years ago and has only become a common disease since the industrial revolution, and especially so in our century.[11]

The reason behind the increased prevalence of asthma and rhinitis is not known, but epidemiological data point towards urbanization and environmental pollution playing a role. This is not only a question of outdoor pollution but also of indoor pollutants, especially tobacco smoke. Several other theories have been put forward, such as eradication of infectious diseases. Especially the conquest of parasitic infestations may have increased a susceptibility to allergic manifestations because a regulation of immunoglobulin production might be disturbed. Especially immunoglobulin E production it would no longer be naturally stimulated and the human organism, instead of reacting towards infections and parasites, now reacts with allergic manifestations towards environmental allergens and irritants.[12]

Dietary changes have also been suggested as important, not only the role of breastfeeding[13] but also the composition of food intake. Environmental factors seem of greater importance than genetic determinants and in recent years specific attention has been focussed upon the role of active and passive exposure to tobacco smoke.[14]

Rhinitis occurs in almost 3/4 of patients with allergic asthma. Rhinitis in these cases may be of seasonal or perennial type. Very often the treatment of rhinitis is neglected in patients with bronchial asthma, possibly because more attention and focus is given the bronchial component of the disease. This is rather unfortunate because effective treatment exists that may relieve the patient from symptoms interfering with daily life.

In the population at large, rhinitis occurs much more frequently than asthma and this is the reason for asthma prevalence in patients with rhinitis being much lower and found in less than 20%.[15] In patients with concomitant asthma and rhinitis the diseases start at about the same time in 25% and, in the remainder, half develop asthma first and half rhinitis first.[16]

Respiratory tract hyperreactivity

Bronchial hyperreactivity is so closely connected with bronchial asthma that this feature is part of the current asthma definition.[17] The clinical expression of hyperreactivity is bronchoconstriction after great variety of stimuli such as cold air, strong smells, dust, smoke, or fog in the air. In the laboratory, bronchial hyperreactivity is quantified by inhalation challenge test with methacholine or histamine or by exercise. There is an association between the degree of hyperreactivity and clinical severity of asthma although it is not very strong.[18]

Patients with rhinitis seem to differ in their degree of respiratory tract hyperreactivity compared to bronchial asthma. Patients with allergic rhinitis do not have exercise-induced bronchoconstriction[19] and in pollen-allergic asthma an increase in exercise-induced asthma is found during the pollen season whereas no influence on exercise reactivity is found in patients with only allergic rhinitis.[19]

In groups of patients with allergic rhinitis it has repeatedly been demonstrated that they have increased bronchial reactivity towards methacholine although they have no symptoms of asthma.[20] This is not just related to the frequent occurrence of increased methacholine responsiveness in the general population.[21] Although the methacholine responsiveness in rhinitis patients usually is lower than in asthmatics, it is not known if rhinitis patients with reactivity in the asthmatic range in fact later may become asthmatics and develop respiratory symptoms. In seasonal allergic rhinitis there seems to be a slight increase in functional residual capacity and volume of trapped gas during the season[22] which may indicate a subclinical bronchospasm in small airways.

Specific features in the bronchial tissues and the nasal mucosa may determine the type of reaction encountered after allergen or irritant exposure. The degree of mediator release during exposure of allergic individuals to a relevant antigen may differ between asthma and rhinitis. It was found that patients with bronchial asthma were more sensitive in the skin towards allergen skin test titration and more sensitive, and with a larger bronchoconstrictor response, to inhaled allergen. Patients with bronchial asthma were found to develop greater increases in serum neutrophil chemotactic activity and plasma histamine after allergen inhalation challenge and they released more histamine into skin chambers after antigen incubation.[23] These results indicate that patients reacting with bronchial asthma are more sensitive to allergen and release more mediators when challenged with allergen.

It is frequent and possible to obtain bronchoconstriction in patients with allergic rhinitis when an allergen inhalation challenge is given to the bronchi. It has been shown that segmental antigen bronchoprovocation in allergic rhinitis results in an immediate release of histamine and tryptase in bronchoalveolar lavage and also increases in eosinophils and eosinophil granule proteins in lavage fluid after

48 hours.[24] These are features previously shown to occur in response to allergen challenge of patients with bronchial asthma and again points towards quantitative instead of qualitative differences in the bronchial mucosa between asthma and rhinitis.

The occurrence of late asthmatic reaction in response to bronchial allergen challenge is much more frequent in asthmatic patients compared with rhinitis patients, whereas the degree of immediate bronchial reactivity seems similar.[25] This indicates that patients with bronchial asthma are more prone to develop an inflammatory response in the bronchi and indeed it has recently been shown that the basis for this may be in the degree of bronchial inflammatory cells present in the bronchial wall. In patients with bronchial asthma a significant increase in mononuclear cells, eosinophils, and mast cells has been established when compared with normals and it has recently been found that patients with rhinitis exhibit increases in the number of inflammatory cells in the bronchial mucosa in a quantity between those of normal controls and patients with bronchial asthma (Len Poulter, personal communication).

The bronchial response to a challenge can be measured by variation in lung function and symptom scores. The nasal response to an intranasal challenge can also be measured as a change in nasal airway resistance or by symptoms. Recently, acoustic rhinomanometry has been introduced and seems promising.[26] The nasal response measured with nasal airway resistance after challenge with increasing doses of histamine or methacholine does not differ substantially between patients with rhinitis and normal controls. Patients with rhinitis, however, more frequently respond with symptoms and increased nasal secretion.[27]

Occupational asthma and rhinitis

Sensitization towards an environmental allergen at the work place can occur and the exposure may lead to occupational asthma and rhinitis. Occupational sensitization seems to be facilitated in tobacco smokers and in patients with previous atopic manifestations.[29] The diagnosis of occupational allergy is performed along the lines of usual diagnostic procedures for detection of IgE antibodies but in cases of previously unanticipated and unknown allergies the elucidation and validation demands specialist skills in diagnostic *in vivo* and *in vitro* tests. This is also the case in those instances where sensitization does not involve IgE antibodies but is caused by other pathogenetic mechanisms. It has been suggested that advice should be given to young atopic persons about the risks of employment in specific work environments. It has also been advocated that companies working with potential sensitizers should perform tests for allergy to exclude atopic individuals from employment. It has been found that about 50% of cases who develop occupational bronchial asthma towards laboratory animals could have been spared by rejection of atopic individuals with a history of inhalant allergy.[30] A very large number of persons would in this way be excluded from work because positive skin prick tests are very frequent in the population. The exclusion of atopic individuals will not eradicate the problem of occupational sensitization because non-atopic individuals also are known to develop allergies of the occupational type. More emphasis should therefore be placed on primary prevention of sensitization.

Sensitization occurs after a latent period that may vary from months to years after the first exposure. Occupational allergy is suspected when asthma or rhinitis occurs at the work place shortly after exposure and improvements are present during weekends and holidays. Persistent symptoms may, however, develop and chronic hyperreactive airways may persist. Questions relating to the possibility for an occupational origin of disease should always be asked of a patient.

Rhinitis and sinusitis

Infection of the paranasal sinuses can complicate rhinitis, which is a predisposing factor. Swelling of the nasal mucosa may obstruct the openings to the sinuses and impair removal of secretion. Sinus mucosa may also be primarily engaged in the allergic mucosal reaction which also may predispose for sinusitis because of mucosal swelling, edema, and secretions. It has been argued that persistent sinusitis is a major factor in chronic asthma but the evidence for a supposed nasal/sinus-bronchial reflex mechanism is circumstantial.[31]

Aspirin disease, rhinitis, asthma and nasal polyps

Aspirin intolerance rarely occurs in children, whereas in adults with severe asthma intolerance to aspirin occurs in 5-10%. The characteristic feature of aspirin intolerance is that a majority of patients first experience their symptoms after the age of 30. Their disease usually includes vasomotoric rhinitis with attack series of sneezing and rhinorrhea and later develops into chronic nasal obstruction and polyp formation. Chronic bronchial asthma usually accompanies the nasal disease. Severe reactions can be seen following ingestion of aspirin and other non-steroidal antiinflammatory drugs. The pathogenesis for this specific hyperreaction is not known, but an IgE-mediated reaction has not been detected. Diagnoses can be accepted only by a typical history and, if absolutely necessary, by oral challenge with aspirin or inhalation challenge with a soluble aspirin form (lysine-acetylsalicylate). Challenges should only be performed in specialist clinics with facilities for resuscitation. It is possible to desensitize patients with aspirin disease by having them ingest increasing amounts of aspirin over some days. It is possible that desensitization can result in improvement of nasal symptoms, whereas no influence on the asthmatic component of the disease has been found.[32] Aspirin desensitization can be indicated in special circumstances where treatment with non-steroidal antiinflammatory drugs is indicated, such as rheumatoid arthritis with co-existing aspirin disease.

Conclusion

Rhinitis and asthma are very common diseases throughout the world and occur in all age groups. The underlying abnormalities are associated with an increased responsiveness in the nasal and bronchial mucosa to environmental stimuli in conjunction with and partly caused by an inflammatory reaction in the mucosal membranes. A genetic factor plays a role, but environmental factors are of the greatest importance. Environmental allergic sensitizers and factors having an adjuvant effect on the development of respiratory diseases should be found and the diseases thus controlled.

References

1. Godfrey RC. Asthma and IgE levels in rural and urban communities of the Gambia. *Clin Allergy* 1975; *5:* 201-7.
2. Barry DMJ, Burr ML, Limb ES. Prevalence of asthma among 12 year old children in New Zealand and New South Wales: a comparative survey. *Thorax* 1991; *46:* 405-9.
3. Varonier HS. Prevalence of allergy among children and adolescents in Geneva, Switzerland. *Respiration* 1970; *27 (suppl):* 115-20.
4. Wollock AJ. The problems of asthma worldwide. *Eur Respir Rev* 1991; *1, 4:* 243-6.
5. Åberg N. Asthma and allergic rhinitis in Swedish conscripts. *Clin Exp Allergy* 1989; *19:* 59-63.
6. Haahtela T, Lindholm H, Björkstein F, Koskenvuo K, Laitinen LA. Prevalence of asthma in Finnish young men. *Br Med J* 1990; *301:* 266-8.
7. Robertson CF, Heycock E, Bishop J, Nolan T, Olinsky A, Phelan PD. Prevalence of asthma in Melbourne schoolchildren: changes over 26 years. *Br Med J* 1991; *302:* 1116-8.
8. Burr ML. Is asthma increasing. *J Epidemiol Commun Health* 1987; *41:* 185-9.
9. Mygind N. *Nasal allergy*, 2nd edn. Oxford: Blackwell Scientific Publications, 1979: 219.
10. Broder I, Higgins MW, Matthews KP, Keeler JB. Epidemiology of asthma and allergic rhinitis in a total community. Tecumseh, Michigan. 3: Second survey of the community. *J Allergy Clin Immunol* 1974; *53:* 127-38.
11. Emanuel MB. Hay fever, a post industrial revolution epidemic: a history of its growth during the 19th century. *Clin Allergy* 1988; *18:* 295-304.
12. Lynch NR, Medouze L, De Prisco-Fuenmayor MC, Verde O, Lopez RI, Malave C. Incidence of atopic disease in a topical environment: partial independence from intestinal helminthiasis. *J Allergy Clin Immunol* 1984; *73:* 229-33.
13. Saarinen UM, Kajossari M, Backman A, Siimes MA. Prolonged breast-feeding as prophylaxis for atopic disease. *Lancet* 1979; *ii:* 163-6.
14. Ownby DR. Environmental factors versus genetic determinants of childhood inhalant allergies. *J Allergy Clin Immunol* 1990; *86:* 279-87.
15. Smith IM. Epidemiology and natural history of asthma, allergic rhinitis and allergic dermatitis (eczema). In: Middleton Jr E, Reed CE, Ellis EF, eds. *Allergy: principles and practice*, 2nd end. St Louis: CV Mosby Company 1983: 771-804.
16. Pedersen PA, Weeke ER. Asthma and allergic rhinitis in the same patients. *Clin Allergy* 1983; *38:* 25-9.
17. American Thoracic Society: chronic bronchitis, asthma, and pulmonary emphysema. *Am Rev Respir Dis* 1987; *136:* 224-5.
18. Salome CM, Peat JK, Britton WJ, Woolcock AJ. Bronchial hyperresponsiveness in two populations of Australian schoolchildren. I. Relation to respiratory symptoms and diagnosed asthma. *Clin Allergy* 1987; *17:* 271-81.
19. Henriksen JM. Exercise induced bronchoconstriction. Seasonal variation in children with asthma and in those with rhinitis. *Allergy* 1986; *41:* 499-506.

20 Ramsdal EH, Morris MM, Roberts RS, Hargreave FE. A symptomatic bronchial hyperresponsiveness in rhinitis. *J Allergy Clin Immunol* 1985; *75:* 573-7.
21 Bakke PS, Baste V, Gulsvik A. Bronchial responsiveness in a Norwegian community. *Am Rev Respir Dis* 1991; *143:* 317-22.
22 Svenonius E, Arborelius Jr M, Kautto R, Lilja B. Lung function studies in children with allergic rhinitis. *Allergy* 1982; *37:* 87-92.
23 Atkins PC, Bedard P-M, Zwelman B, Dyer J, Kallmer MA. Increased antigen-induced local and systemic mediator release in rhinitis subjects with pulmonary symptoms in the pollen season. *J Allergy Clin Immunol* 1984; *73:* 341-7.
24 Sedgwick JB, Calhoun WJ, Gleich GJ, et al. Immediate and late airway response of allergic rhinitis patients to semental antigen challenge. *Am Rev Respir Dis* 1991; *144:* 1274-81.
25 Stevens WJ, Van Bever HP. Frequency and intensity of late asthmatic reactions after bronchial allergen challenge in asthma and rhinitis. *Allergy* 1989; *44:* 471-6.
26 Hilberg O, Jackson AC, Swift DL, Pedersen OF. Acustic rhinometry: evaluation of nasal cavity geometry by acoustic reflection. *J Appl Physiol* 1977; *43:* 523-36.
27 Davies RJ, Corrado OJ, Änggaard A, Borum P. Rhinitis and asthma. In: Mygind N, Weeke B, eds. *Allergic and vasomotor rhinitis: clinical aspects*. Copenhagen: Munksgaard, 1985: 65-79.
28 Zetterström O, Osterman K, Machado L, Johansson SGO. Another smoking hazard: raised serum IgE concentration and increased risk of occupational allergy. *Br Med J* 1981; *283:* 1215-7.
29 Cockroft A, Edwards J, McCarthy P, Andersson N. Allergy in laboratory animal workers. *Lancet* 1981; *1:* 827.
30 Platts-Mills TAE, Longbottom J, Edwards J, Cockroft A, Wilkins S. Occupational asthma and rhinitis related to laboratory rats: serum IgG and IgE antibodies to the rat urinary allergen. *J Allergy Clin Immunol* 1987; *79:* 505-15.
31 Slavin RG. Sinusitis in adults and its relation to allergic rhinitis, asthma, and nasal polyps. *J Allergy Clin Immunol* 1988; *82:* 950-6.
32 Pleskow WW, Stevenson DD, Mathison DA, Simon RA, Schatz M, Zeiger RS. Aspirin desensitization in aspirin-sensitive asthmatic patients: clinical manifestations and characterization of the refractory period. *J Allergy Clin Immunol* 1982; *69:* 11-9.

Chapter 23

Rhinitis and otitis

PAUL VAN CAUWENBERGE
K INGELS

No clinician has any doubt that there is a relationship between inflammation of the nasal cavity and the middle ear mucosa. There are, however, still many unanswered questions, and existing reports are controversial. For example, do adenoid hyperplasia and chronic adenoiditis predispose to secretory otitis media or otitis media with effusion (OME), and does adenoidectomy have a beneficial effect on the prevalence of OME and of acute otitis media (AOM)? Does a child with allergic rhinitis have a higher incidence of middle ear disease? Can OME be cured by treating the underlying nasal or sinus infection?

Something about the diseases

When discussing the relationship between rhinitis and otitis, one should distinguish the various types of nasal and middle ear inflammation. Infectious rhinitis (common cold) is probably the most common pathology in human beings. Children below the age of 7 years have 6 to 7 episodes of common cold per year;[1] adults have fewer episodes, although there is a wide range of individual data. Infectious rhinitis is usually of viral origin, rhinoviruses and coronaviruses being the most common species in adults, while in children parainfluenza, RSV and adenoviruses also play a major role.[2] Another type of inflammation, allergic rhinitis and non-allergic nasal hyperreactivity are extensively discussed in other chapters in this book.

AOM, defined as an acute episode of middle ear infection with earache and general symptoms such as fever, has the highest prevalence in the second part of the 1st year of life,[3] while OME reaches its peak prevalence between 2 and 4 years of age, varying from 10 to 25% in a normal population of schoolchildren[4-5] (Fig. 23.1).

OME, defined as fluid accumulation in the middle ear without acute symptoms, results on average in a hearing loss of about 30 dB with a range from 0 to 50 dB.[6] The spontaneous cure rate of OME is high and only a minority of children will keep their OME fluid in the middle ear for several consecutive months.[7]

Infectious rhinitis and otitis

Grote & Kuijpers[8] reported the simultaneous finding of sinusitis and OME in children, and the presence of *Haemophilus influenzae* in nasal and adenoidal infectious foci suggested that infection with this microorganism predisposes to the devel-

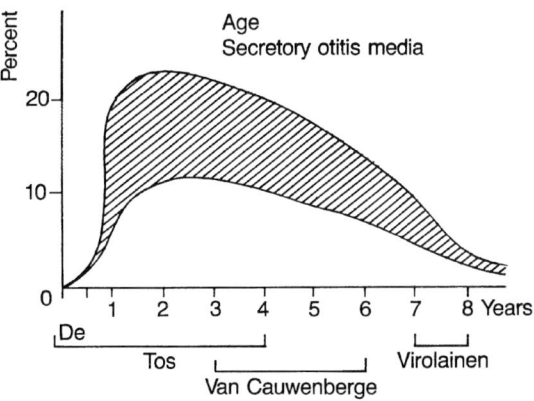

Fig. 23.1. The incidence of secretory otitis media at different ages in a general population of children according to different authors. The hatched area represents the possible range which varies with author, region and season.

opment and/or maintenance of OME. Furthermore, Otten & Grote[9] have shown in children between 3 and 10 years that persistence of chronic uppper respiratory tract infection is a negative prognostic factor with respect to the cure of OME.

In this chapter we present the results obtained from an epidemiological study performed in more than 2,000 preschool children. We investigated the relationship between rhinitis and otitis to determine the importance of nasal infections and allergy as predisposing factors to acute and secretory middle ear disease.

The Ghent epidemilogical study on infectious rhinitis and otitis[7]

There was a highly statistically significant correlation ($p < 0.001$, both with the multiple linear regression analysis and with the chi-square test) in the annual frequency between common cold and AOM (Fig. 23.2). If the child, e.g., never had a common cold, he had a 90% change of being free of AOM; on the other hand, it dropped to 55% if the child had 4 or more episodes of common cold per year. This strong correlation supports a relationship between the nasal and middle ear cavity. The eustachian tube is probably an important link between nasal and middle ear pathology: normal function of the middle ear depends on normal function of the eustachian tube. Up to the age of 7 years, the functioning of the eustachian tube is not yet optimal,[10] but marginally able to provide a middle ear pressure ventilation in normal conditions. However, in the presence of a concomitant pathology interfering with eustachian tube function, e.g. edema of the nasal and eustachian tube mucosal lining, the pressure equilibrating function of the eustachian tube will be lost, resulting in middle ear hypoventilation and a negative middle ear pressure. A cascade of tissue processes follows in the middle ear mucosa, which may lead to AOM, OME and chronic suppurative otitis media.[6]

Some children with a normal functioning eustachian tube do not develop middle ear pathology, even in the presence of nasal pathology, while others have a poor eustachian tube function which can be the cause of a middle ear pathology even in the absence of nasal disease.

The relationship between nasal and middle ear inflammation was also demonstrated by evaluating the tympanometric results against several nasal parameters: annual frequency of common cold, the time between the last episode of common cold and the rhinoscopic findings. The number of flat tympanograms, indicating OME, increased with the number of annual common colds ($p < 0.01$), while the number of normal middle ears decreased, and the number of negative middle ear pressures only slightly increased. The correlation between tympanometric findings and annual frequency of

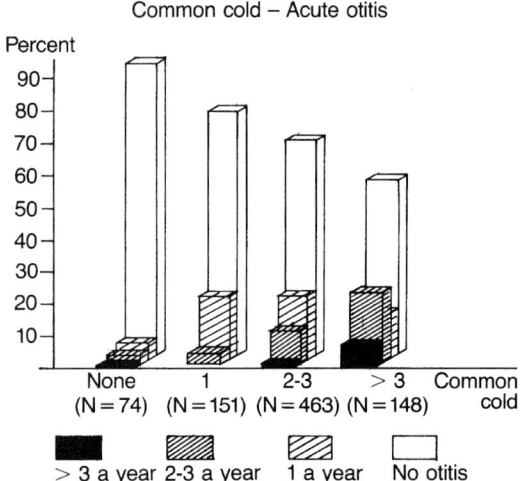

Fig. 23.2. Relationship between the annual incidence of common cold and that of acute otitis media.

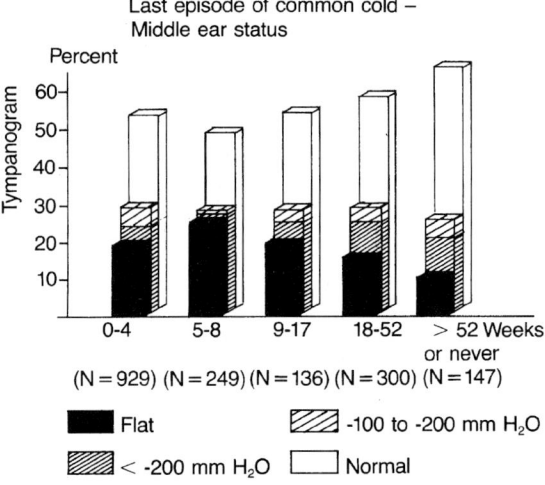

Fig. 23.3. The influence of the time to the last episode of common cold on the tympanometric finding. Note that the highest per cent of flat curves (=OME) is noted 5 to 8 weeks after the last cold.

common cold is not as strong as that between the annual episodes of AOM and of common cold, indicating that OME probably involves more factors in its pathophysiology than AOM and that the influence of the annual frequency of common cold on OME is indirect. The highest prevalence of OME is seen 5 to 8 weeks after the last episode of common cold, after which period there is a progressive improvement of the middle ear status (Fig. 23.3).

When plotting the tympanometric results against the overall rhinoscopic findings (with special regard to the signs of nasal infection) we found that in all types of infectious rhinitis the number of normal tympanograms was reduced (Fig. 23.4). Rhinitis with viscid mucoid secretions was more frequently associated with flat curves and negative middle ear pressure than rhinitis with purulent or watery hypersecretion. The investigation of infectious rhinitis was performed on a selected group of children (n = 842), which explains the higher number of pathological typanograms compared to the whole group of children screened.

From these figures we can conclude that there is a well-defined, strong correlation between nasal infection and the middle ear status.

Allergic rhinitis and otitis

The role of allergy as an etiologic factor in the pathophysiology of OME is controversial. It is still difficult to tell whether OME is a complication of nasal allergy or whether its presence is simply coincidental.

Until 1975, there were no clinical studies available in which an unselected group of children from an otology practice was screened both for allergy and for OME. Before that period it was assumed by many otologists and allergists that allergy should be ranked high on the list of factors predisposing to OME.

In 1975, Reisman & Bernstein[11] published the first report on the relationship between allergy and OME arising in an unselected group of children from an otology practice: 23% of the children who were tested for OME had an atopic disease; this figure was only slightly higher than could be expected from a random examination of unselected children. These findings were confirmed by De[12] and Ruokonen et al,[13] while Kjellman et al[14] found the incidence of atopic disease in their material to be significantly higher ($p < 0.001$) than in an unselected control group. We can state, however, that from all the clinical studies it is obvious that the incidence of allergy in children with OME is, at most, slightly greater than might be expected in the general population.

Not only clinical studies but also the measurement of IgE levels in the middle ear effusions gave rise to controversial findings. It was suggested[15] that the presence of an elevated level of IgE in the

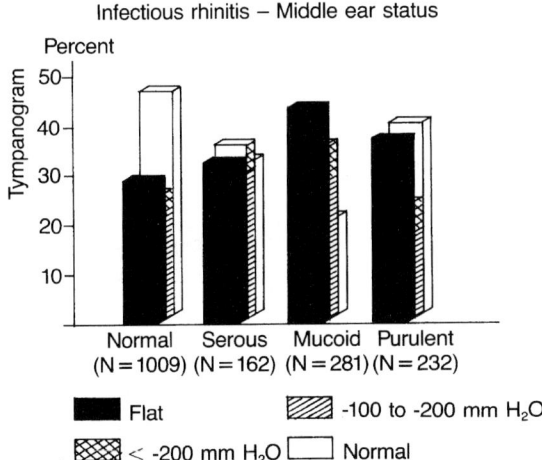

Fig. 23.4. The relationship between rhinoscopical and tympanometric findings in a selected group of children, with special regard to the character of the nasal secretions.

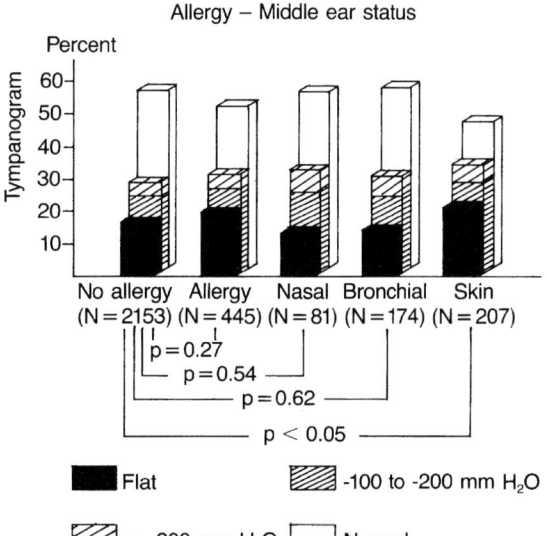

Fig. 23.5. Relationship between the presence of allergic disorders and the tympanometric findings.

middle ear effusion, found in a number of patients, should not be considered as proof of a Type I-allergic reaction, but that IgE may function as a "gatekeeper" antibody causing an increase in vascular permeability and thus permitting the translocation of specific serum antibodies of other immunoglobulin classes. Experimental studies showed that administration of the reponsible antigen into the nose of sensitized guinea pigs did not produce any changes in the eustachian tube or tympanic cavity.[16] However, Skoner et al[17] showed that intranasal challenge with pollen and with house dust mite (*Dermatophagoides pteronyssinus*) can provoke immune-mediated eustachian tube dysfunction in sensitized human subjects; no subject, however, developed fluid in the middle ear. Similar observations were made by Bellioni et al[18] in children with grass pollen allergy. In addition, Skoner et al[19] demonstrated that allergic subjects have a nasopharyngeal wall and/or tubal mucosa that is hyperresponsive to histamine, and they suggested that allergic rhinitis may predispose these patients to OME.

From these previous results we can conclude that allergy is probably not a common etiological factor in OME, although a Type I-allergic reaction may be the cause of eustachian tube obstruction in atopic children and adults and may be responsible for recurrences of some cases of OME. Indeed, if we focus only on children with OME who require several tubings (the worst cases) we can find a significantly increased number of children with an atopic disease.[20, 21]

The Ghent epidemiological study on allergic rhinitis and otitis[7]

In this epidemiological study (n = 2,360 ears) there was no statistically significant difference in middle ear findings between allergic children and those who were reported to be free of allergy (Fig. 23.5). When, however, we divided the group of allergic children into three subgroups: (1) children with allergic rhinitis; (2) children with allergic asthma; and (3) children with atopic dermatitis (alone or in combination), we found a statistically significantly higher number of OME in children with skin disease compared with non-allergic children and children with nasal or bronchial allergy.

These figures suggest that there is no direct relationship between allergy of the nasal and bronchial mucosa, and formation of effusion in the middle ear, confirming the results of other studies. The higher number of OME cases in children with atopic dermatitis, which is often not a Type I-allergic reaction, may suggest that other processes may be involved in the pathophysiology of OME.

From all the data available, including our own, we may conclude that, in a large population, allergic rhinitis is not a major predisposing factor to OME. On the other hand, when we consider the group of OME patients, atopy may be responsible for recurrences and maintenance of the middle ear disease in some patients.

Conclusion

Because of the close correlation between nasal and sinus infection on the one hand, and AOM and OME on the other, a thorough examination of nose, sinuses and nasopharynx is indicated in a child with recurrent/chronic middle ear problems. Before treating the middle ear disease, it is recommended first to treat any underlying disorder in nose or nasopharynx. Allergy seems to be a predisposing factor to relapsing, chronic OME, and an allergy examination is relevant in selected cases where allergic nasal symptomatology is present.

References

1 Van Cauwenberge P. Epidemiology of common cold. *Rhinology* 1985; *23:* 273-82.
2 Gwaltney JM, Hayden FG. The nose and infection. In: Proctor DF, Andersen I, eds. *The nose*. Amsterdam: Elsevier, 1982: 339-42.
3 Ingvarsson L. Acute otitis media in children. Lund, Thesis, 1982.
4 Van Cauwenberge P, Kluyskens P. Some predisposing factors in OME. In: Lim DJ, Bluestone CD, Klein JO, Nelson JD, eds. Proceedings of the Third International Symposium. Recent advances in otitis media with effusion. Philadelphia: Decker, 1984: 28-32.

5. Virolainen E, Puhakka H, Aanatta E, et al. Prevalence of secretory otitis media in seven- to eight-year-old school children. *Ann Otol (St Louis)* 1980: *89 (suppl 68):* 7-11.
6. Van Cauwenberge P. Otitis media with effusion. *Acta Otorhinolaryngol (Belg)* 1982; *36:* 5-240.
7. Van Cauwenberge P. Secretoire otitis media. Een epidemiologische, klinische en experimentele studie. Thesis, Ghent, 1988.
8. Grote JJ, Kuijpers W. Middle ear effusion and sinusitis. *J Laryngol* 1980; *94:* 177-83.
9. Otten FW, Grote JJ. Otitis media with effusion and chronic upper respiratory tract infection in children: a randomized, placebo-controlled clinical study. *Laryngoscope* 1990; *100:* 627-33.
10. Bylander A. Comparison of Eustachian tube function in children and adults with normal ears. *Ann Otol (St Louis)* 1980; *89 (suppl 68):* 20-4.
11. Reisman RE, Bernstein JM. Allergy and secretory otitis media. *Pediatr Clin N Am* 1975; *22:* 251-7.
12. De PR. Secretory otitis media and allergic rhinitis. *J Laryngol* 1980; *94:* 185-9.
13. Ruokonen J, Holopainen E, Palva T, Backman A. Secretory otitis media and allergy. *Allergy* 1981; *36:* 59-68.
14. Kjellman NIM, Synnerstad B, Hansson LO. Atopic allergy and immunoglobulins in children with adenoids and recurrent otitis media. *Acta Paediat Scand* 1976; *65:* 593-600.
15. Lim DJ, Liu YS, Schram J, Birck HG. Immunogloublin E in chronic middle ear effusions. *Ann Otol (St Louis)* 1976; *85 (suppl 25):* 117-23.
16. Yamashita T, Okazaki N, Kumazawa T. Relation between nasal and middle ear allergy. Experimental study. *Ann Otol (St Louis)* 1980; *89 (suppl 68):* 147-52.
17. Skoner DP, Doyle WJ, Chamovitz AH, Fireman P. Eustachian tube obstruction after intranasal challenge with house dust mist. *Arch Otolaryngol Head Neck Surg* 1986; *112:* 840-2.
18. Bellioni P, Cantani A, Salvinelli F. Allergy: a leading role in otitis media with effusion. *Allergol Immunopathol* 1987; *15:* 205-8.
19. Skoner DP, Doyle WJ, Fireman P. Eustachian tube obstruction after histamine nasal provocation: a double-blind dose-response study. *J Allergy Clin Immunol* 1987; *79:* 27-31.
20. Bernstein JM, Lee J, Conboy K, Ellis E, Li P. The role of IgE mediated hypersensitivity in recurrent otitis media with effusion. *Am J Otol* 1983; *5:* 66-9.
21. Bain D. Secretory otitis media and grommets. *Br Med J* 1981; *282:* 1316.

Index

α-adrenergic agents 96
α$_1$-agonist 97
α$_2$-agonist 98
acaricides 27
acetylcholine 97, 105, 156
acoustic rhinometry 186
acute inflammatory response 35
adenoids 13, 176
adenoviruses 189
adrenalin 49, 97, 98, 144
adrenergic agents 74, 77, 180, 181
aeroallergens 23, 29, 153
aerobiology 29
aerodynamic characteristics 23
aerosol 33, 34, 36, 38, 39, 77, 118, 176
airborne allergens 180
air pollution 12, 32, 33, 34, 35, 36, 38, 41, 42
airways 12, 24, 37, 66, 67, 101, 102, 127, 185, 186
albumin 37, 38, 40, 41, 42, 67, 105, 106, 124, 125, 131, 157
alcohol 68, 133, 134, 175
allergen avoidance 23, 144, 145
allergens 15-20, 23-31, 33, 34, 51, 52, 54, 67, 82-92, 128, 137, 138, 141-148, 153, 157, 161, 177, 178, 179, 180, 181, 185
allergic diagnosis 73
allergic rhinoconjunctivitis 111, 112, 123, 127, 128, 129, 130, 131, 133, 134
allergic salute 177, 178
almond 46
alpha-adrenergic receptors 131
alternaria 25, 144, 145
ambrosiaceae 141
analgesia 95, 98
anaphylaxis 41, 46, 49, 144, 145
angioedema 46
animal danders 17, 23, 28
anticholinergic agents 77, 164
antidepressants 133, 159
antigens 16, 32, 35, 36, 123, 145, 172, 179
antihistamines 13, 76, 90, 91, 103, 111, 117, 118, 123-136, 145, 178, 180, 181
antihypertensives 12, 13, 159
apple 46, 83, 141
ASA 168, 169
aspergillus 25
aspirin 47, 71, 162, 163, 168, 171, 172, 175, 187
aspirin intolerance 47, 111, 175, 176, 187
astemizole 117, 123, 126, 128, 129, 131, 132, 133, 134, 135, 180

asthma 15, 17, 18, 117, 120, 133, 137, 138, 142, 144, 145, 162, 168, 174, 184-188, 192
atopic dermatitis 46, 174, 177, 179, 192
atopic disorders 184
atopy 15, 16, 17, 19, 20, 87, 174, 175, 179, 184, 192
atrophic rhinitis 66, 76, 159, 175
atropine 105, 106, 108, 109, 162, 163
azelastine 123, 126, 129, 133, 134

B
β-phenylethylamine derivatives 96
baker's asthma 19, 46, 47, 49
basophilic cells 66-81
beclomethasone dipropionate 77, 132, 134, 181
benzyl benzoate 27
Bermuda grass 25, 141
birch 46, 71, 72, 83, 86, 126, 141
blood-brain barrier 105, 131
bronchial asthma 11, 176, 184-187
bronchial hyperreactivity 185
bronchial membranes 20
bronchial symptoms 144
bronchoalveolar lavage 42, 101, 185
bronchoconstriction 38, 185, 187
bronchodilatation 105
bronchodilator 101
budesonide 77, 107, 115-122, 137, 172, 181

C
capacitance vessels 97, 115, 128
capsaicin 40, 41, 42, 163
cardiac arrest 132, 133
cat allergen 28, 29, 34, 82, 83, 180
cataract 112, 120
cereals 141
cetirizine 76, 123-134, 180
C-fiber neurons 41
challenge studies 24, 37, 38, 39, 40
chemosis 111
chlorpheniramine 38, 123-136
chronic otitis media 64
ciliary function 66, 176
ciliocytophthoria 69, 70, 71, 75, 76, 179
ciliostasis 36, 37
cladosporium 25, 145
clavulanate potassium 79
CNS 96, 98, 131, 132
cocaine 95, 97, 98
cockroaches 23, 29, 33, 34, 153
common cold 13, 108, 109, 177, 189, 190, 191, 192

complement 36, 117
compositeae 141
concha bullosa 51, 54, 55, 59, 60, 61, 63, 150, 169
congenital choanal atresia 12, 13
conjunctivitis 46, 84, 111, 127, 129, 133, 137, 138, 144, 145
contact eczema 46
coronary artery disease 99
coronaviruses 189
cough 59, 111, 133, 155, 176
cromoglycate 49, 77, 101-104, 181
cromolyn 77, 117, 118, 130
cromolyn sodium 77, 102, 103, 118, 131, 181
cross reactivity 25
crusting 159
CT-scan 12, 52, 54, 55, 58-65, 169
cushingoid features 112
cypress 137
cystic fibrosis 13, 17, 111, 151, 159, 168, 171, 172, 176, 178
cytochrome 126, 127, 133
cytology 66-81, 106, 164

D

decongestant 37, 59, 76, 97, 99, 111, 112, 117, 118, 119, 129, 133, 159, 161, 164, 167, 175, 176, 180, 181
dermatitis 88, 187
dermatitis herpetiformis 46
dermatophagoides 26, 192
dexamethasone isonicotinate 115
D. farinae 26
diabetes mellitus 99, 112
diphenhydramine 123, 130, 132, 133, 134
D. microceras 26
dog allergen 28, 83
D. pteronyssinus 26
dryness 37, 38, 106
dust 15, 17, 23-31, 32-45, 60, 63, 82, 83, 86, 145, 153, 159, 161, 171, 184, 185, 187, 192
dysplasia 74, 76

E

ebastine 123
ecchymoses 112
eczema 17, 20, 187
egg 26, 29, 47, 87, 156
ELISA 24, 179
emotional factors 24
endoscopy 13, 53, 59, 64, 150, 161
environmental control 25, 26, 27, 28, 29, 180, 181
eosinophil duodenitis 46
eosinophilia 12, 13, 55, 71-81, 102, 107, 111, 112, 117, 160, 164, 168, 175, 178, 179
eosinophils 12, 37, 66-81, 101, 116, 156, 157, 168, 170, 172, 178, 179, 185, 186
ephedrine 95, 96, 97, 99, 129, 130, 180
epidemiologic studies 20, 35, 38, 39
epidemiology 15, 16, 17, 160, 184, 187, 192

epistaxis 159, 167
epithelium 35, 36, 38, 67, 68, 69, 74, 78, 99, 108, 153, 154, 168, 173
estrogen 74, 159
ethmoidal cells 60, 61, 62
euroglyphus maynei 26
eustachian tube 190, 192
eustachian tube dysfunction 118, 192
exercise 36, 37, 38, 95, 97, 185, 187
exocytosis 96
extrinsic asthma 16, 20
eye symptoms 117, 129

F

facial pain 149, 150
flunisolide 77, 115, 116, 118, 119, 172, 179, 181
fluocortin butylester 118
fluticasone propionate 78, 118
food allergy 12, 46, 47
food intolerance 46, 49
formaldehyde 33, 34, 38, 39, 74, 138
fungicides 26

G

genetic factors 18
giant ragweed 25
glaucoma 112
glucocorticosteroids 12, 114, 170
glutaraldehyde 138
glycoproteins 23, 157
goblet cells 38, 69, 70, 71
grass 23, 25, 60, 133, 137-147, 153, 171, 192
guinea pig 41, 42, 192
gustatory rhinitis 49

H

Haller cell 59, 60, 63
hay fever 11, 12, 16, 17, 18, 19, 20, 98, 118, 132, 187
hazelnut 46
headache 106, 149, 150, 162
histamine 41, 47, 72, 101, 106, 109, 115, 123-134, 156, 157, 163, 164, 170, 171, 180, 185, 186
host factors 20
house dust mites 15, 143, 177
humidifiers 26, 27, 39
hydrocortisone 114
hyperplasia 38, 189
hyperreactivity 82, 85, 86, 88, 157, 163, 185, 189
hypersecretion 105, 106, 107, 109, 163, 175
hypertension 99, 112
hyperthyroidism 99
hypnotics 133
hyposmia 149

I

IgA 105, 106, 109, 157, 171
IgE 16, 19, 20, 82-92, 102, 111, 116, 137-146, 153, 154, 157, 161, 170, 171, 174, 175, 179, 181, 186, 187, 191, 192
IgG 42, 92, 105, 106, 145, 157

IgM 157
IL-4, 153
imidazoline derivatives 95, 96
immunodeficiency 13, 177
immunotherapy 25, 49, 54, 56, 79, 86, 91, 103, 114, 117, 137-148, 153, 180, 181
infantile eczema 16, 20
infection 12, 13, 17, 19, 51, 64, 66, 69, 71, 73, 74, 105, 108, 151, 159, 168, 174, 176, 186, 189
infectious rhinitis 12, 66, 74, 176, 177, 178, 189, 190, 191
inflammation 11, 32, 38, 52, 73, 85, 116, 119, 127, 145, 156, 161, 163, 164, 171, 172, 189, 190
inflammatory cells 17, 71, 75, 77, 78, 105, 108, 109, 156, 186
inhalant allergens 30, 85, 89
inhalation challenge 162, 176, 185, 187
insomnia 111, 133, 181
interferon-gamma 153
interleukin 38, 92
ipratropium bromide 77, 105-110, 149, 163, 164
irritant rhinitis 74
irritants 34, 39, 74, 76, 105, 161, 163, 175, 180, 185

K
Kartagener's triad 176
kinins 40, 41, 115, 124, 131, 156

L
lactation 133
lactoferrin 105, 106, 109, 157
latent allergy 83, 89
leprosy 13
leukocytes 68, 69, 72, 73, 74, 75, 108, 179
levocabastine 123, 126, 129, 130, 133, 134
lipopolysaccharides 35
loratadine 123-136
lower respiratory tract infection 17, 19
lysosyme 105, 109

M
macrophages 35, 168
MAO-inhibitors 97
masks 25
mediators 36, 92, 155, 156, 157, 162, 172, 185
metaoxedrine 97
metaplasia 39, 74, 76, 78, 168
methacholine 37, 86, 105, 106, 108, 109, 126, 163, 185, 186
microabscesses 75
middle ear 59, 178, 189, 190, 191, 192
milk allergy 50
mites 12, 15, 17, 19, 23, 26, 27, 33, 34, 153
molds 12, 25, 26, 35, 88, 143, 145, 153
mononuclear cells 37, 68, 79, 186
monosensitized 141
mountain cedar 137
mouse allergen 31
MR-imaging 58
mucociliary clearance 32, 37, 39, 75, 151, 164, 176
mucociliary transport 36, 53, 99, 116, 176

mucous membrane 11, 13, 36, 39, 58, 63, 64, 74, 111, 112, 156, 169, 175, 178
mucus 36, 74, 101, 156, 167
muscarinic receptors 131
mycelial antigens 25

N
naphazoline 95, 96
NARES 13, 52, 55, 56, 74, 75, 76, 160
narrow angle glaucoma 99
nasal burning 41, 42
nasal cavity 38, 58, 64, 67, 103, 106, 108, 109, 150, 167, 176, 189
nasal congestion 12, 36, 37, 74, 112, 124, 149, 155, 156, 159, 161, 162, 163, 175, 181
nasal itching 103, 127, 177
nasal lavage 35, 37, 38, 39, 40, 44, 47, 67, 71, 72, 74, 116, 125
nasal lavage fluid 36, 38, 41, 68, 74, 76, 124, 163
nasal mastocytosis 73
nasal obstruction 12, 13, 52, 54, 55, 59, 97, 98, 99, 106, 107, 118, 149, 150, 159, 161, 167, 176, 187
nasal polyposis 55, 66, 111, 112, 159, 172, 176
nasal polyps 12, 13, 16, 17, 20, 53, 56, 61, 74, 75, 76, 102, 111, 112, 117, 120, 149, 150, 167-173, 176, 178, 187
nasal provocation 47, 79, 85, 109, 116, 163, 164, 179
nasal resistance 32, 36, 37, 38, 39, 40, 151
nasal surface fluid 36, 37
nasal symptom scores 79, 132
nasopharyngitis 71
nasopharynx 13, 164, 176, 192
natamycin 27
necrosis 38, 157
nedocromil sodium 101, 102, 103
nerves 99, 105, 128, 153, 155, 156, 163, 164
neurons 36
neuropeptide Y 96
neutrophilia 12, 170
neutrophils 37, 39, 67-81, 156, 157, 170, 179
nitrogen oxides 32
noberastine 135
non-allergic rhinitis 11, 12, 13, 55, 73, 74, 99, 106, 111, 149, 150, 159, 174, 175, 177, 178
non-atopic 73, 74, 87, 89, 171, 186
non-eosinophilic rhinitis 12
non-purulent rhinitis 12
noradrenaline 95, 97
NPY 96
NSAID 12, 159, 162

O
occupational allergy 186
occupational asthma 17, 19, 186
ocular symptoms 111, 130, 134
oleaceae 141
olfaction 150
orchard grass 25, 141, 142
osteoporosis 112
otitis media 176, 178, 189, 190, 192

oxymetazoline 96, 97, 98, 99
ozone 32-38, 41, 42

P
parainfluenza 189
paranasal sinuses 13, 51, 58, 61, 62, 63, 64, 149, 169, 172, 186
parasites 16, 185
particles 23, 24, 26, 28, 29, 32, 33, 34, 36, 40, 53
pathogenetic mechanisms 32, 186
pathophysiology 13, 51, 98, 115, 159, 162, 163, 164, 191, 192
penicillium 25
perennial rhinitis 12, 64, 74, 77, 82, 83, 102, 105, 106, 112, 129, 164, 174
pets 24, 27, 28, 29, 34, 35, 83, 161, 177, 180
phagocytes 36
pharynx 37, 38
phenylephrine 37, 95, 96, 98
phenylpropanolamine 95, 96, 97, 99, 180
plasma proteins 115, 157, 171
pollen 12, 17, 18, 20, 23, 24, 60, 63, 71, 73, 74, 77, 84, 86, 88, 102, 111, 117, 118, 119, 120, 126, 132, 133, 134, 137, 138, 141-145, 157, 171, 174, 185, 192
pollen counts 25, 72, 82, 128, 129
pollinosis 11, 12, 83, 86, 137, 145
pollution 34, 184
polyethylene-glycol 76
polyps 17, 52-61, 75, 76, 111, 112, 167-173, 175, 176, 177, 181
polysensitized 141
post nasal drip 149
prednisone 78, 112, 118, 181
pregnancy 12, 13, 66, 74, 76, 133, 142, 159, 175
prevalence of rhinitis 15, 49, 162, 184
primary ciliary dyskinesia 13, 111, 168, 169, 172, 176
processus uncinatus bullosa 59
progesterone 74
proteins 23, 34, 83, 87, 88, 92, 106, 109, 115, 143, 145, 156, 157, 168, 185
pruritus 128, 129, 156, 161
pseudoephedrine 95-100, 130, 134, 180
psychosedatives 12
purulent sinusitis 111

R
race 19, 52, 66, 69, 70, 71, 75, 76, 97, 123, 157, 159, 172, 175, 179
ragweed 25, 79, 102, 116-121, 125, 129, 137, 138, 141, 153, 155
ragweed hay fever 19, 134, 137
RAST 12, 24, 47, 60, 87, 88, 92, 179
rat allergen 28
resistance vessels 97, 115
respiratory tract 20, 36, 37, 38, 40, 41, 46, 74, 131, 153, 177, 178, 185, 190
rheumatoid arthritis 187
rhinitis medicamentosa 12, 13, 66, 76, 98, 99, 111, 159, 175, 181
rhinomanometry 54, 78, 149, 151

rhinometry 40, 54
rhinopathy 11, 73, 74, 111
rhinorrhea 40, 41, 49, 74, 102, 103, 105-110, 111, 124, 127, 128, 129, 130, 155, 161, 162, 163, 164, 167, 174, 175, 180, 187
rhinoscopy 12, 51, 52, 56, 61, 66, 106, 176
rhinosinusitis 51, 52, 53, 54, 59, 64, 74, 75, 175, 176, 177, 179
rhinoviruses 189
risk factor 24, 27
rodents 28, 33, 34
RSV 189
rye grass 25, 141

S
seasonal allergic rhinitis 11, 12, 23, 25, 37, 73, 76, 78, 102, 103, 129, 130, 134, 145, 161, 184, 185
secretory rhinitis 106
secretory rhinopathy 106
sedation 129, 130, 132, 133, 134
sedatives 133
sensitization 20, 27, 41, 42, 46, 82, 83, 85, 89, 92, 125, 133, 137-148, 149, 153, 175, 179, 186, 187
septal deviation 13, 51, 53, 59, 60, 61, 62, 63
septum 37, 53, 55, 56, 64, 67, 111, 149, 150
short ragweed 25
sick building syndrome 39
silver birch 25
sinusitis 12, 13, 58-65, 71, 73, 74, 75, 76, 79, 159, 160, 162, 168, 173, 176, 177, 181, 186, 189
skin test 12, 16, 17, 18, 19, 20, 34, 60, 72, 74, 83, 92, 111, 138, 141, 153, 160, 161, 175, 179, 185
sneezing 11, 12, 13, 36, 47, 48, 55, 72, 97, 102, 103, 106, 107, 111, 119, 124, 125, 127, 129, 130, 149, 155, 156, 161, 163, 164, 167, 180, 187
sodium laurel sulfate 34
status asthmaticus 168, 180
steroids 77, 78, 98, 103, 111-113, 114-122, 130, 134, 145, 151, 164, 172, 175, 176, 181
steroid spray 13, 172
stramonium 105
striae 112
submucosal glands 157
submucous glands 105, 108, 128
sulfur dioxide 32, 33, 34, 36, 38, 39, 42
surgery 52, 53, 54, 55, 56, 64, 98, 112, 149-152, 159, 167, 169, 172
systemic corticosteroids 137, 172, 176, 181

T
TAME-esterase 40, 41, 42, 72, 115, 124, 125, 131
tannic acid 27, 28
tartrazine 47
terfenadine 76, 123-136, 180
tetracosactrin 113
tetrahydrozoline 97
Timothy grass 25
tobacco smoke 23, 33, 34, 40, 41, 184, 185, 186
tomography 53, 55, 58, 168
topical eyedrops 117

tricyclic antidepressants 97
tripelennamine 130
triprolidine 99, 130
tumors 13, 38, 159, 163
turbinates 69, 72, 149, 150, 151, 168
twins 18, 19
tympanometric 190, 191

U
urticaria 46, 47, 111, 134, 144

V
vaporizers 26, 177
vasoconstrictor 12, 68, 95-99, 103, 150, 175
vasomotor rhinitis 12, 66, 74, 76, 98, 99, 105-110, 159
ventricular arrhythmia 132
vibrissae 36

viral infection 12, 13, 17, 19, 20, 66, 67, 71, 75, 76, 159, 176, 177, 189
viral infection-induced rhinitis 131

W
watery hypersecretion 191
watery rhinorrhea 47, 102, 106, 109, 149, 151
Wegener's granulomatosis 13, 175
weight gain 112, 133
wheeze 133
wheezing 111
wood 23, 29, 33, 34, 37, 53, 72, 151, 164

X
xenon 115
x-ray 12, 56, 58, 64, 75
xylometazoline 96, 97, 103